Food and Nutrition

for **Home Science, Food Science and Food Technology**

Other Books by the Same Author

- *Textbook of Biochemistry, 5th ed*
- *Biochemistry for BSc Nursing Students, 4th ed*
- *Food and Nutrition: Medical, Nursing and Allied Sciences, 2nd ed*
- *MCQs in Biochemistry, 2nd ed*
- *Essentials of Pharmaceutical Biochemistry, 2nd ed*
- *Essentials of Biochemistry for BSc Nursing Students*

Food and Nutrition

for Home Science, Food Science and Food Technology

Harbans Lal PhD FIAO FACBI FSOBSI

Former Senior Professor and Head
Department of Biochemistry
Maharaja Agrasen Medical College, Agroha (Hisar)

Former Senior Professor
Department of Biochemistry
Pt BD Sharma Postgraduate Institute of Medical Sciences
Rohtak (Haryana)

Ex-WHO Fellow

CBSPD

CBS Publishers & Distributors Pvt Ltd

New Delhi • Bengaluru • Chennai • Kochi • Kolkata • Lucknow • Mumbai
Hyderabad • Jharkhand • Nagpur • Patna • Pune • Uttarakhand

Disclaimer

Science and technology are constantly changing fields. New research and experience broaden the scope of information and knowledge. The author has tried his best in giving information available to him while preparing the material for this book. Although, all efforts have been made to ensure optimum accuracy of the material, yet it is quite possible some errors might have been left uncorrected. The publisher, printer and the author will not be held responsible for any inadvertent errors or inaccuracies.

Food and Nutrition

for Home Science,
Food Science and Food Technology

ISBN: 978-93-54667-98-5

First Edition: 2025

Published by **Satish Kumar Jain** and produced by **Varun Jain** for

CBS Publishers & Distributors Pvt Ltd

4819/XI Prahlad Street, 24 Ansari Road, Daryaganj, New Delhi 110 002, India
Ph: 011-23266838, 23289259 Website: www.cbspd.com
e-mail: delhi@cbspd.com

Corporate Office: 204 FIE, Industrial Area, Patparganj, Delhi 110 092, India
Ph: 011-49344934 Fax: 011-49344935 e-mail: publishing@cbspd.com; publicity@cbspd.com

Branches

- **Bengaluru:** Seema House 2975, 17th Cross, K.R. Road, Banasankari 2nd Stage, Bengaluru 560 070, Karnataka, India
Ph: +91-80-26771678/79 Fax: +91-80-26771680 e-mail: bangalore@cbspd.com
- **Chennai:** 18/8B, Subbarayan Street, Shenoy Nagar, Chennai 600 030, Tamil Nadu, India
Ph: +91-044-42032115, 26681266 e-mail: chennai@cbspd.com
- **Kochi:** 42/1325, 1326, Power House Road, Opposite KSEB, Power House, Ernakulum 682018, Kochi, Kerala, India
Ph: +91-484-4059061–65 Fax: +91-484-4059065 e-mail: kochi@cbspd.com
- **Kolkata:** 147, Hind Ceramics Compound, 1st Floor, Nilgunj Road, Belghoria, Kolkata 700056, West Bengal, India
Ph: +91-33-25633055/56 e-mail: kolkata@cbspd.com
- **Lucknow:** Basement, Khushnuma Complex, 7 Meerabai Marg (behind Jawahar Bhawan), Lucknow 226001, UP, India
Ph: +91-522-4000032 e-mail: tiwari.lucknow@cbspd.com
- **Mumbai:** PWD Shed, Gala No. 25/26, Ramchandra Bhatt Marg, Next JJ Hospital, Gate No. 2, Opp. Union Bank of India, Noorbaug Mumbai 400009, Maharashtra, India
Ph: +91-22-66661880/89 e-mail: mumbai@cbspd.com

Representatives

- **Hyderabad** 0-9885175004
- **Jharkhand** 0-9811541605
- **Nagpur** 0-8692091830
- **Patna** 0-9334159340
- **Pune** 0-9664372571
- **Uttarakhand** 0-9716462459

Printed at: SRK Graphics, Delhi, India

Preface

It gives me pleasure to present the first edition of the book *Food and Nutrition*. It has been written in a very lucid and simple language with a major goal to provide a book to the students studying basic course in nutrition, such as home science, and food science and technology, who are to study general aspects of nutrition, which forms a part of their course curriculum. All the chapters have been presented with the text keeping in mind the needs of the students. Major goal, though continues to provide the book on nutrition to the students of various disciplines, the study material in each chapter has been supplemented with suitable tables, flowcharts and figures. Some important questions have also been included at the end of each chapter. Various dietary recommendations have been revised as per ICMR-NIN (2020) Guidelines. At the end definition of various terms related to nutrition have also been given to apprise the students of various terms related to nutrition.

I express my sincere thanks to the Director, National Institute of Nutrition-Indian Council of Medical Research, Hyderabad, for allowing me to use the data of dietary recommendations as per ICMR-NIN 2020. I am also thankful to Mr Satish Kumar Jain and the entire team of CBS Publishers & Distributors, New Delhi, for bringing out the book in a responsive way with their earliest efforts. Comments from the readers are welcome to improve the book.

Harbans Lal
hl.biopgimsr@gmail.com

Preface to the First Edition

This textbook on "general nutrition" has been compiled with the aim to provide an elementary but updated knowledge of the nutrition for students of undergraduate courses in nursing, home science, nutrition and dietetics and all others who are to acquire preliminary knowledge in nutrition and nutritional biochemistry. The text has been presented in a simple and easily understandable language. It is divided into 25 chapters beginning with Introduction to the Science of Nutrition followed by digestion and absorption of nutrition and their chemistry and metabolism. In the next chapter RDAs have been mentioned. Next three chapters describe the requirements during specific period of life. Exercise and sports activities and some common disorders, nutritive values of foods, assessment of the nutritional status, nutritional support, malnutrition and eating disorders follows the above text. The last three chapters include food fads, food safety and food cost and marketing. In the end certain terms have been defined.

Data relating the dietary requirments and presented in Indian context and have been compiled from the work of Indian experts. Data regarding nutritive values of foods have been compiled from ICMR as well as those from the foreign experts. I owe my heartful thanks to all of them. I am also grateful to all my friends who have helped me directly or indirectly in the completion of this book. Special thanks are also due to Mr SK Jain and the team of CBS Publishers and Distributors, New Delhi, for bringing out this volume. Though every effort has been made to make it error free, I regret for the mistakes. Suggestions for improvement of the book are cordially invited from all quarters.

Harbans Lal
hl.biopgimsr@gmail.com

Contents

CHAPTER 1

Introduction to Nutrition

Nutrition is the study of nutrients and their relationship with the food and the living beings. It can be defined as **a science of food and its relationship to health.**

The **science of nutrition** interprets the **interaction of nutrients** and other substances in food, **in relation to the maintenance, growth, reproduction, health and disease of an organism.** It also includes **food intake** and **absorption, assimilation and catabolism of nutrients, and excretion of waste products**.

The diet refers to the **amount of food that a person,** normally, **takes every day**.

A **proper diet is essential** from the beginning of life **for proper growth, development** and to **remain active. Healthy diet** includes **preparation of food** and **its storage** in the way **that reduces the risk of diseases**.

HISTORY OF NUTRITION

Study of nutrition, probably, began during the 6th century BC, although the **first recorded dietary advice,** carved into a Babylonian stone tablet in about **2500 BC,** cautioned those with pain to avoid eating onions for three days.

Later **in 1500 BC**, it was first described that scurvy is due to **vitamin C deficiency**.

- **In 1747, James Lind,** a physician in the British navy, performed the first scientific nutrition experiment. He **discovered that lime juice can save sailors** (who had been at sea for years) **from scurvy** (a deadly and painful bleeding disorder).
- Later in **1794, Lavoisier** demonstrated that **oxidation of food is the source of body heat** and thus, described the process of metabolism.
- **In 1816, Francois Magendie** identified **protein as an essential dietary component.** He **discovered** that dogs fed on only carbohydrates (sugar), fat (olive oil) and water died evidently of starvation, but those who were also fed protein had survived.
- **In 1820, Coindet** discovered the **role of iodine in the treatment of goiter.**
- **In 1824, Shutter** invented the **role of cod liver oil in the treatment of rickets.**
- **In 1849, Regnault** explained the process of the **determination of respiratory quotient.**
- **In 1880, Carl Voil** performed studies on **protein requirement** and its **metabolism**.
- **In 1887, Takaki** reported that **beriberi can be prevented**.
- **Thereafter in 1897, Eijkman** performed more studies about beriberi and observed that one of its causes is **polished rice**, which **develops polyneuritis**.

- **In the early 20th century, Voit and Rubner,** independently, by applying the principle of physics in nutrition, **measured calorie (energy) expenditure** in different species of animals.
- **In 1906, Willcock and Hopkins** demonstrated that **amino acid tryptophan is essential for life.**
- **In 1941,** the **first Recommended Dietary Allowances** (RDAs) **were established by** the **Food and Nutrition Board** of the **National Research Council** (NRC), **USA.**
- **In 1992,** The **US Department of Agriculture** (USDA) **introduced** the **Food Guide Pyramid.**

ADVANCES IN NUTRITION RESEARCH

As mentioned above, until the nineteenth century nutrition had only a limited role and that most of the current information is based on the discoveries which were made between the 19th and the 20th century (Table 1.1).

However, significant advances in the field of human nutrition have been made **over the past 50 years.** During this period, the **science of nutrition has** also **moved out of the laboratory** and **gained recognition as an independent scientific discipline.**

- **Importance of the food has now been well recognized in human health and disease.**
- **Several specific nutritional diseases,** such as protein energy malnutrition **(PEM), endemic goiter, nutritional anemia, nutritional blindness,** etc. **have been identified.**
- Also, **new technologies have been developed for their diagnosis and control.**

Table 1.1: History of nutrition discoveries

Year	*Scientist*	*Discovery*
1747	James Lind	Role of orange and lemon in the cure of scurvy
1794	Lavoisier	Energy metabolism and respiration
1816	Francois Magendie	Dietary significance of protein
1820	Coindet	Role of iodine in treatment of goiter
1824	Shutter	Role of cod liver oil in treatment of rickets
1849	Regnault	Determination of respiratory quotient
1880	Carl Voil	Studies on protein requirement and metabolism
1887	Takaki	Prevention of beriberi
1897	Eijkman	Role of polished rice in development of polyneuritis
1906	Willcock and Hopkins	Significance of tryptophan for life
1901	Hopkins	Vitamins as accessory food factors
1909	McCollum and Davis	Importance of fat-soluble substance for growth
1915	Goldberger	Discovery of pellagra-preventing factor
1916	McCollum	Importance of fat-soluble A for growth
1922	Evans and Bishops	Importance of vitamin E in reproduction
1934	Dam	Discovery of vitamin K
1935	Williams	Kwashiorkor, its cause and cure
1941	Food and Nutrition Board, NRC, USA	First RDA

- The **discipline of nutrition has also extended its influence in several other fields** such as **agriculture, animal husbandry, economics and sociology,** which, in turn, led to green revolution and white revolution, resulting in overall **increase in food production,** storage and utilization.

CONCEPTS OF NUTRITION

Nutrition, basically, involves the bodily requirement of energy and various nutrients in the desired quality and quantity for maintenance of physical and mental health.

Accordingly nutritional concepts include a number of factors which include:

- Energy (calorie)
- Dietary nutrients
  - Macronutrients
  - Micronutrients
- Health and well-being

In spite of the increase in food production, poorer sections of the population, however, have continued to suffer from malnutrition. It is due to the **association of nutrition with several other factors**, such as **infections and immunity, fertility, maternal and child health**, and family health, which is receiving further scientific attention.

Accordingly, greater emphasis is being laid on **integrating nutrition into primary health care system** towards the **formulation of national dietary goals to promote health.**

Recently, a great deal of interest has also been focused on the **role of dietary factors in the pathogenesis of non-communicable diseases** such as **coronary heart disease, diabetes and cancer**.

With the newer concepts and approaches, the science of nutrition is now becoming more dynamic.

ROLE OF NUTRITION IN MAINTAINING HEALTH

World Health Organization **(WHO) defined health as a state of complete physical, mental and social well-being, and not merely the absence of disease or infirmity.**

WHO made further clarifications in 1986 that health is a positive concept emphasizing social and personal resources as well as physical capacities. Accordingly, it includes both physical health and mental health.

Physical Health

A person who has good physical health is likely to have bodily functions and processes working at their peak. This is not only due to an absence of disease, but regular exercise, balanced nutrition and adequate rest, etc. all of which contribute to good health.

Mental Health

Mental health refers to a person's emotional, social and psychological well-being.

Both of these are important and related to each other. For example, if an individual is not physically healthy, he or she may not be mentally healthy also, and may suffer from stress and, subsequently, depression. Similarly, if a person is mentally ill such as under depression, the individual may suffer from weight loss which, in turn, may affect physical ability to perform work. Further, such an individual may not only be performing his/her own work well, but will affect his/her utility for the family as well as society.

Factors Affecting Physical and Mental Health

As discussed above, wellness **(good physical and mental health)** is a continuous process. It **is regulated by several factors,** which include:

- **Balanced diet:** One should consume a balanced diet, mostly from the natural sources, every day.
- **Physical activity:** The individual must perform some type of exercise, at least 30 minutes each day for 5 days a week.

- **Lifestyle:** Besides balanced diet and exercise, one must adopt a lifestyle to remain busy to lead a stress-free life with a positive outlook.
- **Routine check-up:** One must undergo routine laboratory and medical check-up periodically, particularly, for the life-threatening diseases such as weight gain, obesity and cardiovascular disease, or a chronic infection.
- **Social work:** One should contribute to the family and the society, to the best of his/her physical and mental health, and financial status.

Role of Nutrition in Maintaining Physical and Mental Health

Nutrition plays an important role in maintaining health, both physical health and mental health.

1. **Nutrition is** not only **a basic component of preventive medicine** but **also effective in corrective medicine** for many common health problems.
2. **Many common symptoms and diseases can often be prevented with better nutrition.** According to US Department of Health and Human Services (2000), **several leading causes of death, including cardiovascular diseases** (atherosclerotic heart disease and hypertension), **cerebrovascular disease** (stroke), **diabetes and some cancers, have a strong link with the type and amount of food consumed**.
3. **Nutrition knowledge of** both, **the general public as well as health professionals,** is critical, if we are **to succeed in reducing morbidity and mortality** from these killer diseases.
4. With the advancements in the fields of molecular biology, biochemistry and genetics, it is now well understood that a disease may be genetically biased, but **is influenced by environmental factors including nutrition.**
5. **Role of nutrients and other biologically active food components on gene expression is also the focus of exciting field of nutrition,** called nutritional genomics or **nutrigenomics.**

COMMON NUTRITIONAL PROBLEMS IN INDIA

India is in the phase of economic development. Accordingly, it is facing a dual burden of malnutrition which includes, both undernutrition and overnutrition.

Undernutrition

Pre-transition diseases like undernutrition (undernourishment) are persisting due to poverty, large family size, unhealthy life style and poor health care system, faulty feeding habits, inadequate sanitation (resulting in frequent infections), or migratory population (or people) living in rural areas or urban slums, particularly, those belonging to socially-backward groups and landless laborers.

Low birth-weight babies, preschool children, adolescent girls, pregnant and lactating women, and elderly socially-deprived persons are at high risk of developing undernutrition.

Undernutrition may be a result of intake of quantitatively as well as qualitatively inadequate diet. The diet may be either less in quantity or may be **lacking in one or more nutrients.** For example:

- **Protein-energy malnutrition (PEM),** which includes **marasmus** (reduced intake of total food, including calories) and **kwashiorkor**, a deficiency of protein, particularly, in infants and young children.
- **Iron deficiency anemia** (IDA), in pregnant women and children, particularly, those with helminthic infections.
- **Iodine deficiency disorders** (IDD).
- **Vitamin A deficiency (night blindness** and **Bitot's spots**, etc.).

- **Vitamin B-complex deficiencies,** particularly the deficiency of **riboflavin** (vitamin B_2), **folate** (folic acid) and **vitamin B_{12}** (cyanocobalamin).
- **Vitamin D and calcium deficiencies** leading to **osteoporosis.**

Overnutrition

Prevalence of overnutrition is emerging as a significant post-transitional problem, especially, in urban areas. Causative factors include:

- **Over consumption of energy-rich diets containing increased amounts of saturated fat and highly processed sugar**
- **Lack of dietary fiber** and complex carbohydrates, particularly, by the higher income group
- **Lack of physical activity** and **sedentary lifestyle**
- **Increased consumption of alcohol** (empty calories), and
- **Use of tobacco**

All these factors in turn lead to the prevalence of diet-related chronic degenerative noncommunicable diseases, such as:

- Obesity
- Diabetes
- Hypertension
- Cardiovascular diseases (CVD), and
- Various types of cancer.

FACTORS AFFECTING FOOD AND NUTRITION

Since we consume food, it is essential to advocate nutrition in terms of food, rather than nutrients. Apart from supplying nutrients, food provides a host of other components (non-nutrient phytochemicals) as well, which have a positive impact on our health.

Food consumption, which largely depends on production and distribution, determines health and nutritional status of the population. This is largely determined by the availability and palatability of food.

The food we eat says a lot about our character, personality and where we are from. Food also reflects family history, culture and religious background, economic status, how one feels, where one goes and what one does socially. Thus, a number of factors affect the availability and intake of food and nutrition. These include:

- **Socioeconomic factors:** Our social existence is, probably, one of the biggest contributors to what we eat. The people, we live with, work with and socialize with, have a great deal of influence over what we eat. Some of the foods are considered to be **only for those with low income,** yet these foods are just as nutritious and can be prepared in as many delicious ways as the more expensive foods.
- **Cultural factors:** Eating and choosing food is no longer just about feeding our body what it needs and what tastes good, but food practices are different and vary from culture to culture, and generation to generation. Whether our background is European or African, Asian or Latin American, cultural influences contribute to food, what we eat or bring home. These influences can blend into preparation and serving methods, too. For example, **Mexican dishes** often include abundance of beans, rice and cheese. **Middle Eastern menus** are known for their olives and olive oil, fruits, vegetables and spices. **Chinese foods** include many stir-fry and combination meals. **Indian foods** often are deep fried and high in fat, etc.
- **Traditions:** Dietary habits and eating patterns form our **family's traditions** make our food habit in our young age.
- **Production:** Each region of the country is known for its distinct type of foods produced in that area. For example, **North East region** is famous for its supply of **seafood and fresh-fishes;** in the **Western Coast** (with its warm weather and trendy lifestyle) one can often find

many **fresh and Asian/Pacific-type of foods,** etc.

- **System of distribution:** A public distribution shop, also known as **fair price shop**, is a part of India's public food distribution system established by the Government of India, which distributes rations at a subsidized price to the poor. Locally these are known as **ration shops** and **public distribution shops,** and **chiefly sell wheat, rice and sugar** at a price lower than the market price, called **Issue Price.** The basic objective of the public distribution system in India is to provide essential consumer goods **at cheap** and **subsidized** prices to the consumers so as to insulate them from the impact of rising prices of these commodities and maintain the minimum nutritional status of the population.
- **Lifestyle: Friends, peers and colleagues have a big influence over food** choices. Teens choose fast food, like pizza, French fries, hot dogs, shakes and soft drinks, because everyone else is eating these items. On the other hand, they might choose not to eat at all, in order to trim down, like their friends. Some of the foods have more prestigious value than others and we have to use them as **company foods,** to honor or impress our friends, clients or officers, though they may cost more, may be hard to get, take a lot of time to prepare or are unusual.
- **Food habits:** Food habits also have deep psychological roots and are associated with religious customs and beliefs. For example, even some vegetarians do not take onion and garlic; Muslims avoid pork while Hindus avoid beef, etc. Some persons like much salt; others only a little; some like very sweet food; others do not; some like spicy food while others prefer bland food, etc.

MEDICINAL VALUE OF FOOD

Next to air and water, food is the prime necessity for life. It contains various **organic and inorganic substances** referred to as nutrients that an organism eats or drinks, in order to maintain life and for growth. These include carbohydrates, lipids, proteins, vitamins, minerals and water, which are used in the body of an organism **to sustain growth, repair and vital processes, and to furnish energy.** The substance is ingested by an organism and assimilated by the organism's cell to provide energy, maintain life or stimulate growth. Daily intake of food has a direct influence on the health and well-being of an individual.

Dietary modifications based on the nutrients may include decreased calories intake for weight reduction or consuming extra calories for weight gain; balance the amount of carbohydrates, fat or proteins; high fiber diet; low fat and/or low cholesterol diet; decreased amount of a nutrient such as low sodium diet; or to exclude a particular food due to allergy or intolerance.

Recent knowledge in medicine and allied sciences has provided new insight and opened up new vistas in the science of nutrition. Researchers have provided information on dietary patterns and components of food that have added benefits for health, such as **phytonutrients, carotenoids, plant sterols, flavonoids, pre- and probiotics, and nutraceuticals.**

CLASSIFICATION OF FOODS

Foods may be grouped in many ways, though some foods can also be placed in more than one group. Since each food has a different nutritional profile, from the nutritional point of view foods can be grouped as:

- **Foods of plant origin** and **animal origin.**
- As **energy-yielding foods, body building foods** and **protective foods**.
- **According to chemical composition** in several groups such as cereals and pulses (which are rich in carbohydrates; etc. Chapter 15).

FOOD STANDARDS

Food standards refer to the **set of criteria that a food must meet,** if it is approved, to be suitable for human consumption, such as source, composition, appearance, freshness, permissible additives and bacterial content. Some Governments have imposed very strict quality parameters for ingredients and their storage practices. There are many **regulatory bodies** that **help maintain standards in the quality of food.** Each country has its own such agency (Chapter 14).

ELEMENTS OF NUTRITION

There are six elements of nutrition called carbohydrates, lipids, proteins, vitamins, minerals and water. These are essential to supply energy, build and maintain body cells, and regulate metabolic processes. These are classified as macronutrients and micronutrients (Chapter 3).

Macronutrients

Macronutrients include **carbohydrates (including dietary fiber), fat (lipids) and proteins.** These are required by the body in relatively large amounts and are also referred to as the **proximate principles of food.** Macronutrients are oxidized in the body to **provide energy** that is required for various activities of life. Together with water, these form bulk of the food.

- **Carbohydrates:** Carbohydrates are the cheapest source of energy and are easily available. These are the main sources of energy for the body, which provide about 55–60% of the daily calories requirement. In addition, carbohydrates also serve as the components of cell membrane and receptors.

  Carbohydrates are classified according to the number of sugar units as **monosaccharides** (such as glucose and fructose), **disaccharides** (such as sucrose and lactose) and **polysaccharides** (such as starch and glycogen; Chapter 5).
- **Dietary fiber:** Dietary fiber includes several **complex carbohydrates** which are resistant to digestion in the human digestive tract, e.g. **cellulose, gums and pectin, etc.** (Chapter 6).
- **Fats:** Fats or lipids include a group of substances which are poorly soluble, or nearly insoluble, in water but are soluble in organic solvents. Over 90% of the dietary fat includes **triacylglycerols** (triglycerides), which consist of a molecule of glycerol (glycerin) with 3 fatty acids.

  A fatty acid contains a –COOH group attached to the unbranched hydrocarbon chain, where different carbon atoms are connected to each other by the single bonds only **(saturated fatty acids)** or may also contain both single as well as double bonds, referred to as **unsaturated fatty acids.** Other types of dietary lipids include **cholesterol, phospholipids, sterols** and **carotenoids**.

  Fat may be obtained from two different sources, i.e. from plants (oilseeds) and **animals** (meat, egg, milk and dairy products). **Plant fats** are superior to animal fats because fat from plant sources **contains more polyunsaturated fatty acids (essential fatty acids)** and **no cholesterol**.

  Cholesterol in diet should be restricted because excess intake of cholesterol **leads to** its deposition in tissues, thereby causing **atherosclerosis** (Chapter 7).
- **Proteins:** Proteins are organic compounds that consist of amino acids which are joined by peptide bonds. Proteins are needed for their content of certain amino acids that are essential to human body for the biosynthesis of proteins, body repair in adult, and for body building and growth in children.

  Human body proteins are made up of only **20** standard **amino acids**, out of which nearly 10 amino acids can be synthesized in the body but the remaining 10 cannot be synthesized in the body, hence they have to be supplied through the diet. Therefore, these amino acids are referred to as **essential amino acids**. Through digestion, proteins are broken down by proteases into free amino acids.

According to their source, proteins may be of good quality or poor quality.

Good quality proteins are mainly obtained from animal sources (e.g. meat, fish, eggs and dairy products). These contain all the essential amino acids needed by the body. These proteins are also referred to as **proteins of high biological value**.

Poor quality proteins are obtained from plant sources. They have **low biological value,** since an individual protein may lack one or the other essential amino acid.

Vegans and vegetarians cannot get all the amino acids they need, from a single source. However, combining plant foods from different sources provide good quality protein, e.g. pulses and cereals (Chapter 8).

Micronutrients

Micronutrients include **vitamins and minerals.** These are required, comparatively, in small quantities and are also referred to as **protective foods.**

- **Vitamins:** Vitamins are a group of organic compounds and perform a variety of functions in the body. Every vitamin is chemically different from each other. Although they do not yield energy but vitamins enable the body to use other nutrients. Since body is generally unable to synthesize most of the vitamins, these must be provided through food.

  Vitamins are divided into the two groups as follows:

  Fat soluble vitamins, which include vitamins **A, D, E and K,** and **water soluble vitamins,** which include **B vitamins** and **vitamin C** (Chapter 9).

- **Minerals:** Minerals are th**e inorganic substances**. These are required by the body in small amounts. Our body requires different amounts of each mineral.

  All the minerals and trace elements are present in healthy tissues, where their concentration remains relatively constant. Besides, there are certain elements, like nickel, vanadium, tin, boron, etc., which have not been shown to have any function in human body, thus are not dietary essential (Chapter 10).

  Besides, vitamins and minerals, **antioxidants and phytochemicals,** too, may be referred to as micronutrients, since they are also required in small quantities and said to protect (or influence) some of the body systems. Their essentiality, however, has not been well established like that of vitamins and minerals.

ENERGY

Energy is a prime requisite for body functions and growth. Energy is also required for doing physical work. Body gets energy from the combustion of carbohydrates, fat and proteins. Energy, present in these macronutrients is locked in chemical bonds, and is released when food is metabolized. Thus, body converts chemical energy present in food to mechanical, electrical and heat energy.

CALORIE

The **unit of energy is calorie. A calorie is defined as the** quantity of heat required to raise the temperature of 1 g of water by 1°C, **more specifically from 14.5°C to 15.5°C. Its large unit is kilocalorie, which is equal to 1000 calories.** In the context of nutrition, the large unit, i.e. kilocalorie (kcal), is used. **The calorie value, we see on a food package is actually in kilocalories.** The SI unit of energy is joule (J). **One kcal is approximately 4.2 kJ.**

Energy requirement is defined as the **calories intake** that is **required to maintain**

energy balance in a healthy person of a defined age, gender, weight, height and level of physical activity consistent with good health.

BASAL METABOLIC RATE

Basal metabolic rate (BMR) is the **amount of energy expenditure** (per hour) **while at rest,** in a neutrally temperate environment and the post-absorptive state (meaning that the digestive system is inactive, i.e. about twelve hours of fasting in humans). The amount of energy at complete physical and mental rest **meets the requirement for the functioning of vital organs,** i.e. the heart, lungs, kidneys, nervous system, intestine, liver, sex organs, muscles and skin, etc. The BMR remains constant throughout the day under normal conditions and constitutes about 50–75% of the total energy expenditure by an individual. It is **expressed in terms of kcal/h** (Chapter 4).

SOME IMPORTANT QUESTIONS

1. **Define nutrition. Describe the role of nutrition in maintaining health.**
2. **What is a nutrient? Describe various dietary nutrients.**
3. **Describe factors affecting food and nutrition.**
4. **Write notes on:**
    i. Nutritional problems in India
    ii. Medicinal value of foods
    iii. Food standards
    iv. Undernutrition
    v. Overnutrition
    vi. Macronutrients
    vii. Micronutrients

CHAPTER

2

Common Nutritional Problems in India

As discussed in Chapter 1, India is in the phase of economic development and is facing a **dual burden of malnutrition** including **undernutrition** as well as **overnutrition**.

A **nutritional problem,** generally referred to as **malnutrition,** may be defined as a pathological state, resulting from a relative or absolute deficiency; or excess of one or more essential nutrient(s). Accordingly, a **nutritional problem may be** observed in any of the following forms:

- **Undernutrition:** Undernutrition, or undernourishment, is a result of **insufficient food,** consumed over the extended period of time.
- **Specific deficiency of a nutrient:** It is a state resulting from the relative or absolute **lack of a specific nutrient**.
- **Over-nutrition:** It is a pathological state resulting from the **consumption of excessive quantity of food over an extended time.** Overnutrition can result in overweight and obesity, which in turn can cause several non-communicable diseases such as diabetes, hypertension, cardiovascular diseases (CVD) and cancer.

UNDERNUTRITION

Undernutrition is, largely, **a result of dietary inadequacy** and unhealthy lifestyle. Other contributing factors include **poor purchasing power, faulty feeding habits, large family size, frequent infections, poor health care, inadequate sanitation and low agricultural production.**

Population, living in the backward and drought-prone rural areas and **urban slums,** and those belonging to the **socially-backward groups** are highly susceptible to undernutrition. Similarly, **landless labourers** and destitute are also at a higher risk. The most rational, sustainable and long-term solution to the problem of malnutrition is ensuring availability, accessibility and consumption of adequate amounts of foods.

Undernutrition starts during conception. Because of extensive **maternal undernutrition** (underweight, poor weight gain during pregnancy, nutritional anaemia and vitamin deficiencies), about 22% of the **infants are born with low birth-weight** (<2500 g), as compared to less than 10% in the developed countries. Besides, clinical and sub-clinical undernutrition are widely prevalent even during early childhood and adolescence.

National surveys indicate that about half of the children below 5 years of age suffer from subclinical undernutrition such as underweight (43%), and stunting and wasting (20%). Further, studies have also shown that there is a steep increase in the prevalence of underweight with increase of age, from 27% at 6 months of age to about 45% at 24 months of age. **ICMR-NIN (2020) Expert Group,** based on the last National Family Health Survey, **has reported a slight decline in undernutrition,** with a prevalence of stunting as 38.4% and wasting as 21.5%.

Undernutrition is attributable to **faulty infant and young child feeding practices,** prevailing in the community. Persistent undernutrition throughout the growing phase of childhood leads to short stature in adults.

Causes of Undernutrition

- **Socioeconomic status:** In general, those who are poor, are at risk for undernutrition, due to inadequate intake of food.
- **Lack of breastfeeding:** Lack of breastfeeding results in low birth weight of the baby. It may be a result of large family size, poor maternal health, failure of lactation or premature termination of breast feeding, delayed supplementary feeding or use of over diluted milk.
- **Infections:** Infections such as tuberculosis, gastroenteritis, measles, diarrhea, respiratory infections and intestinal worms cause malnutrition.
- **Food habits:** Being strictly vegan, sometimes, may also result in protein malnutrition. This is due to the reason that the type of protein present in cereals does not parallel to the protein found in animal products.
- **Communicable diseases:** Communicable diseases, such as hepatitis, tuberculosis and malaria, are attributed to poor sanitation and inadequate safe drinking water. These can also be a result of increased resistance to drugs.
- **Noncommunicable diseases:** Noncommunicable diseases (NCD) include cardiovascular diseases (CVD), diabetes, chronic obstructive pulmonary disease (COPD), cancer, mental health disorders and injuries. It may also be attributed to genetic predisposition, metabolic syndrome and adverse changes in coronary artery vasodilation.
- **Poor environment and hygiene:** Poor sanitation (may be due to open air defecation) leads to the spread of diseases through parasitic and bacterial infections, and malnutrition.

Several million people worldwide suffer from multiple episodes of diarrhea, or fall ill on account of Hepatitis A, enteric fever, intestinal worms, and eye and skin infections which are caused by poor hygiene and unsafe drinking water.

Insufficient maintenance of the environment around the drinking water sources, groundwater pollution, excessive arsenic and fluoride contents in drinking water also pose a major threat to health in many countries.

High Risk Groups

- **Low birth-weight babies:** A low birth weight newborn is any newborn with a **birth weight of less than 2.5 kg** regardless of gestational age. Nearly one-third of the babies born in low- and middle-income group countries are low birth weight babies (undernourished in the womb). They have a poor start of life cycle and are exposed to the increased risk of morbidity and mortality.

The problem of low-birth weight is widespread and multi-factorial:

- Low birth weight is **associated with poor growth during infancy,** and thereafter, throughout the **childhood** period.
- Retrospectively, low birth weight reflects poor nutritional and health status of women during pregnancy, childhood as well as during adolescence.

Causes of low birth weight:

- Illness/infections
- Short maternal stature
- Young age of women
- High parity

- Close birth intervals
- Intrauterine growth retardation
- Hard physical labor during pregnancy
- Maternal malnutrition
- Anemia
- Smoking

- **Preschool children:** Pre-school children are most vulnerable to the effect of undernutrition because of their rapid growth. A large population of children under five years of age has protein energy malnutrition (PEM) which is a major nutritional health problem in low- and middle-income group.
- **Adolescent girls:** Adolescence is a period of second decade of life (10–19 years). During this phase significant physical, physiological, psychological and emotional changes occur. In females, adolescence also marks beginning of the menstrual cycle. Adolescents gain 50% of their weight and more than 20% of their height during 10–19 years of age which is called growth spurt. Chronic deprivation of food, particularly, during this period of growth and development also leads to short stature.
- **Pregnant and lactating women:** During pregnancy and lactation nutritional requirements increase to support foetal and infant growth, and development as well as maternal metabolism and tissue development specific to reproduction.

  Maternal metabolism is adjusted through the elaboration of hormones that serve as mediators, redirecting nutrients to highly specialized maternal tissues specific for reproduction, i.e. placenta and mammary glands. Requirements for energy-yielding macronutrients increase modestly compared with several micronutrients that are unevenly distributed among foods. Altered nutrient utilization and mobilization of reserves often offset enhanced needs, but sometimes nutrient deficiencies are also precipitated by reproduction.

  Additional food is required to improve weight gain during pregnancy (10–12 kg) and birth weight of the infant (about 3 kg). Hence, it is important to ensure provision of extra food and healthcare to pregnant and lactating women.

  In low- and middle-income group population, it is observed that the diet of women from the low socioeconomic group is essentially similar during pre-pregnant, pregnant and lactating periods. Consequently, there is widespread maternal malnutrition leading to high prevalence of low-birth weight infants and very high maternal mortality.
- **Elderly socially-deprived persons:** Nearly one-third of the adult population has various grades of chronic energy deficiency. The effects of undernutrition during childhood are carried over to adolescents and adults. Work capacity of the adult goes down due to chronic malnutrition of long-standing. PEM may also occur in persons who are unable to absorb vital nutrients which are essential for healthy tissue formation and organ functions.

PROTEIN–ENERGY MALNUTRITION

Protein–energy malnutrition **(PEM)**, also referred to as **protein–calorie malnutrition** (PCM), is a form of malnutrition due to **inadequate intake of protein and/or energy** (calories). According to World Health Organization, PEM refers to an **imbalance between the supply of protein and energy,** and the **body's demand for the nutrients** to ensure optimal growth and function.

PEM affects, particularly, **the preschool children** (<6 years) with its dire consequences ranging from physical to cognitive growth and susceptibility to infections. So, PEM affects the child at the most crucial period of time of development that can lead to permanent impairment in later life. Although, normally, it is difficult to separate protein intake from the energy intake, since a diet adequate in energy, usually, has adequate protein. Similarly, a diet which lacks energy, also limits dietary protein which is essentially needed for the synthesis of various proteins required by the body.

PEM, though, **occurs in all parts of the world,** but is most common in South East Asia, Africa, South and Central America, and Middle East countries. It is also seen, most often, in population living in poverty, the elderly people and the hospitalized patients, particularly, those with some associated conditions such as anorexia nervosa, AIDS, cancer or malabsorption syndrome.

The findings about worldwide distribution of protein energy malnutrition, based on nationally representative cross-sectional data gathered between 1980 and 1992, in 79 developing countries in Africa, Asia, Latin America, and Oceania, confirm that more than one-third of the world's children are affected by PEM.

PEM is also a major public health problem in India. Estimates indicate that the prevalence of stunting among under five is about 62% (moderate and severe), wasting is nearly 20% (moderate and severe) and with an underweight prevalence of around 64% (moderate and severe).

Classification of PEM

Classification of PEM is **based on deficit in body weight for age** and the **presence or absence of edema.**

Two main clinical syndromes of the extreme forms of PEM are referred to as **kwashiorkor** and **marasmus,** although a mixed picture is also seen frequently. These two are differentiated on the basis of clinical findings, with the primary distinction between kwashiorkor and marasmus, being the **presence of edema in kwashiorkor**.

KWASHIORKOR

The term kwashiorkor (means the **sickness of the weaning**) comes from a word used in Ghana, which means **"a disease of a baby deposed from the breast when the next one is born"**. It is most serious and prevalent form of malnutrition in the world, especially, in industrially-underdeveloped countries. Kwashiorkor usually develops in children between 18 and 24 months of age, at the time when weaning occurs and that the diet is low in protein (Fig. 2.1).

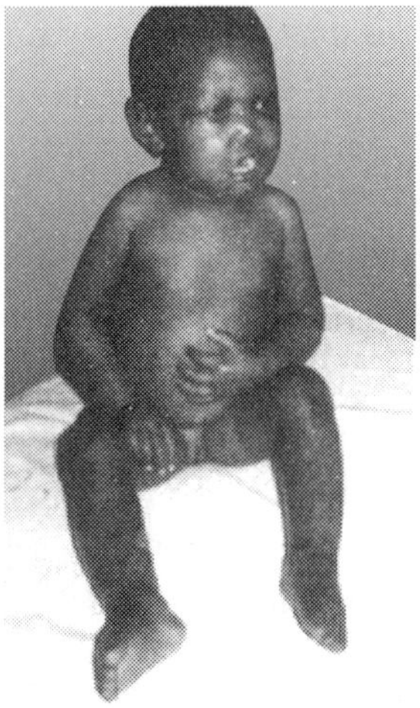

Fig. 2.1: Kwashiorkor

Causes of Kwashiorkor

It is said that **kwashiorkor,** usually, **develops when a baby is weaned from the protein-rich breast milk** and **switched to a protein-poor food.** It tends to occur mainly in older infants and young children, and results from a diet with inadequate protein but reasonably normal calorie intake, often exacerbated by superimposed infections. A common scenario is when the older infant or toddler is displaced from breastfeeding, by the birth of a younger sibling and has to wean rapidly, but is unable to increase protein intake adequately. The term **sugar baby** also has been used to describe these children, as their typical **diet is low in protein** but **high in carbohydrates.**

Signs and Symptoms of Kwashiorkor

Symptoms include **edema** (swelling of body tissues due to accumulation of fluid), usually, in feet and legs. Belly becomes bloated **(pot belly)**, due to accumulation of fat in the liver **(fatty liver)**. Other features include growth retardation **(stunted weight and height)**, increased susceptibility to infections, **dry and fleshy skin, dry and brittle hair,** and changes in skin color **(pigmentation)**. Protein deficiency also **impairs digestion and absorption of other nutrients.**

Common signs and symptoms of kwashiorkor include:

- Edema with swollen legs
- Pot belly (enlarged liver)
- Muscle atrophy
- Mild to moderate growth retardation
- Some weight loss and low subcutaneous fat
- Round face (moon-like face)
- Dry, flaky peeling skin
- Thin, dry and easily plucked hair

MARASMUS

Marasmus results from the **body's physiologic adaptation to starvation** in response to **severe deprivation of calories and all the other nutrients**, i.e. protein, energy, vitamins and minerals (total food). Intakes of all these are grossly inadequate, depleting body fat reserves and severely wasting muscle tissue. Growth slows and children are, both short and thin for their age. Their hairs are sparse and fall easily. It also reduces brain development and leads to learning disabilities. Marasmus occurs, most often in infants and children between 6 and 18 months of age, particularly, in those who are given diluted milk (Fig. 2.2).

Causes of Marasmus

Marasmus is a form of undernutrition caused by inadequate intake of energy.

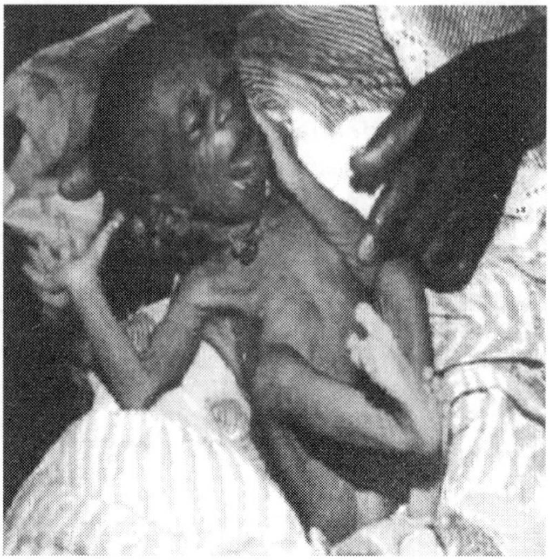

Fig. 2.2: Marasmus

It affects infants as a result of failure of breastfeeding or a debilitating condition, such as chronic diarrhea.

Signs and Symptoms of Marasmus

Common signs and symptoms of marasmus include:

- Severe weight loss
- No edema
- Severe growth failure
- Severe loss of subcutaneous fat
- Weight loss (up to 40%)
- Severe muscle atrophy
- Wrinkled face, like old man's face
- Rare skin changes
- Common hair changes

Differences Between Kwashiorkor and Marasmus

Marasmus can be distinguished from **kwashiorkor in the way that, kwashiorkor is a protein deficiency with adequate energy intake,** whereas **marasmus is due to inadequate intake of energy and protein.** Besides, there are other differences between the two conditions, as shown in Table 2.1.

Table 2.1: Differences between kwashiorkor and marasmus

Kwashiorkor	*Marasmus*
• Scaly skin • Distended abdomen (pot belly) • Swollen ankles (oedema)	• Wrinkled (dry and loose) skin • Severe muscle wasting (particularly, loss of fat from the buttocks and thighs) • Old person's face • Hair loss

PROBLEMS RELATED TO SPECIFIC DEFICIENCY OF A NUTRIENT

A nutritional problem may also be a result of the **deficiency** of some specific nutrient such as **vitamin A, iron, iodine,** some **B-vitamin, vitamin D** and **calcium.**

VITAMIN A DEFICIENCY

Vitamin A deficiency (VAD) is a **lack of vitamin A,** which, in humans, **produces night blindness, delayed dark adaptation, lowers resistance to infections** and may produce **blindness** as a permanent disability (Chapter 9).

Vitamin A deficiency (VAD) is the leading **cause of preventable childhood blindness,** afflicting 2,50,000–5,00,000 malnourished children in the developing world. Young children (below the age of 3 years), and pregnant and lactating women are most vulnerable to vitamin A deficiency. It also increases the risk of other diseases and may cause death. Its deficiency is more prevalent in vegetarian and often occurs along with the deficiency of zinc.

Risk Factors for Vitamin A Deficiency

- Faulty feeding practices and early weaning
- Recurrent infections, particularly, infectious diarrhea
- Use of the skimmed milk, which is devoid of vitamin A, and
- Poor dietary intake of vitamin A along with the deficiency of protein and zinc (as commonly observed in PEM).

Prevention of Vitamin A Deficiency

National Nutrition Policy has suggested certain preventive actions for vitamin A deficiency. These include:

- **Short-term action:** Oral administration of large dose of vitamin A (Retinol-palmitate)
- **Medium-term action:** Food fortification with vitamin A, e.g. milk, ghee, etc.
- **Long-term actions:** Consumption of dark-green leafy vegetables, promotion of breast feeding, improvement in environment, health and immunization against measles.

NUTRITIONAL ANEMIA

Nutritional anaemia is a condition, where hemoglobin content of blood is lower than normal (below 8 g/dl), may be a result of the deficiency of iron or some other essential nutrient such as folate and vitamin B_{12}.

Iron is required by the body for the synthesis of hemoglobin which is present in red blood cells.

Main function of hemoglobin is to transport oxygen from lungs to the various parts of the body (Chapter 10).

In India, among children between the age of 6 months and 5 years, a majority (70%) are found to be anaemic. Nearly, 75% of these children suffer from anaemia due to iron deficiency while about 22% have been reported to have vitamin B_{12} deficiency.

Nearly, three-fourths (75%) of the women have been reported to be anemic, with the prevalence of moderate to severe anaemia being highest (50%) among pregnant women. According to ICMR-NIN (2020), the problem is further aggravated with helminthic infections.

It is estimated that nutritional anaemia contributes to nearly 24% of the maternal deaths every year. It has also been shown to be one of the major causes of low birth weight.

Nutritional anaemia is most commonly observed in pregnant women and lactating mothers, infants, preschool children and adolescent girls.

Risk Factors for Anemia

- Infants and children
- Pregnant women
- Pre-menopausal women
- Adolescent girls
- Older adults
- Alcoholism
- Chronic/critical illness
- Excessive exercise
- Reduced intake
- Excessive blood loss in menstruation

Prevention Measures for Anemia

- Routine estimation of hemoglobin to assess the degree of anaemia
- Blood transfusion in severe cases of anaemia (<8 g/dl)
- Dietary supplementation of iron and folic acid to the pregnant women, lactating mothers and children under 12 years of age
- Fortification of salt and food with iron
- Change in dietary habits
- Control of parasite infection
- Nutrition education and awareness about anaemia

IODINE DEFICIENCY DISORDERS

Iodine deficiency is due to the dietary deficiency of trace element iodine but is an environment problem. Lack of dietary iodine leads to a wide range of disorders collectively referred to as **iodine deficiency disorders (IDD)** which affect health of humans from fetal stage to adulthood.

Iodine deficiency is prevalent worldwide. In India, it is very common among large section of the population in several parts of the country and that the classical goitre belt has been reported to be from North in J&K and HP to east in West Bengal and NE states. It is estimated that about 167 million of people are living in IDD endemic areas.

According to the ICMR Task Force study in 1989, prevalence of goitre varies from 6.2% in the Mirzapur District of UP to 65.8% in Dibrugarh (Assam). The prevalence of cretinism has been reported to vary from 0.15% in Gorakhpur (UP) to 6.1% in Central Manipur.

About 90,000 stillbirths and neonatal deaths occur every year due to maternal iodine deficiency. Around 54 million persons are estimated to have goitre, 2.2 million have cretinism and 6.6 million suffer from mild psycho-motor handicaps.

As per ICMR-NIN (2020) report, though the problem of the severe forms of IDD has been considerably reduced after universalization of the iodized salt; the milder forms of IDD exist in several parts of the country.

Iodine deficiency has serious health and social implications. It may result in abortion or stillbirth, goitre (enlargement of thyroid gland, termed endemic goitre in the neck), neonatal hypothyroidism, cretinism (among newborns), mental retardation, delayed motor development, stunting, deaf-mutism and neuromuscular disorders (Chapter 10).

Causes of Iodine Deficiency

- The main **cause of iodine deficiency is** its **environmental deficiency** such as due to soil erosions, as a result of deforestation, which, in turn, reduces iodine content of the soil and cause low iodine content of the crops that are grown on the iodine depleted soil.
- Increased demand for iodine by the body such as during infancy, puberty, pregnancy and lactation.
- Loss of iodine during cooking
- **Presence of goitrogens** (goiter producing substances), which are naturally present in some foods like cabbage, cauliflower, etc. These substances interfere with iodine utilization and metabolism.

Prevention of Iodine Deficiency

- For the prevention of IDD, **Government of India** (GOI) **launched National Goiter Control Program in 1962.**
- **To promote the consumption of the iodized salt,** GOI started **Universal Salt Iodization Program in 1984.**
- **For iodine monitoring and surveillance GOI** also amended the Prevention of Food Adulteration **(PFA) Act in 1988,** to specify the iodine content of 30 ppm in the iodized salt at the production level.
- Government of India also **banned the sale of non-iodized salt for human consumption from May 2006.**
- Besides these, GOI also launched programs for **public awareness and education** for the prevention of IDD
- Also promoted the **consumption of** seafoods and green-leafy vegetables, etc., the **foods which are rich in iodine.**

VITAMIN B DEFICIENCIES

Recent studies have reported deficiencies of several B-vitamins, particularly of thiamin, riboflavin, niacin, pyridoxine, folate and vitamin B_{12}.

Deficiency of some of these vitamins (thiamine, riboflavin and niacin, etc.) may be due to the increased consumption of junk foods, which are rich in energy, since dietary requirement of these vitamins is directly related to the intake of energy (Chapter 9).

Thiamin

Thiamin is also referred to as **vitamin B_1**. It is also designated as **anti-beriberi factor** due to its role in the prevention of peripheral nervous system disease called beriberi.

As per ICMR-NIN (2020) Expert Group report **inadequate intake is the major cause of thiamine deficiency in India.** Besides, thiamine deficiency has also been shown to be correlated with the **consumption of raw fish** which contains thiaminase that destroys thiamine. Its deficiency also occurs in **chronic alcoholics,** particularly, in those who also consume poor quality of diet with low thiamine content.

Riboflavin

Riboflavin is also referred to as **vitamin B_2**. It is also designated as **lactoflavin** due to its **occurrence in milk.** It is required for normal structure and function of the mucous membrane and skin.

Riboflavin deficiency may be observed due to **inadequate dietary intake, malabsorption, respiratory infections** and **prolonged fever, hyperthyroidism, exercise** and **negative nitrogen balance, pregnancy** and **malignancy.**

Niacin

Niacin is also referred to as **vitamin B_3**. It is also designated as **pellagra-preventive factor** due to its role in the prevention of pellagra.

Niacin deficiency is **common in persons whose staple food is maize and jowar** (called millets). Such individuals develop pellagra-like symptoms, since **maize and jowar are deficient in tryptophan.** At the same time, these millets are rich in **isoleucine.** The amino acid imbalance due to low tryptophan and high isoleucine, in turn, reduces the biosynthesis of niacin in the body.

Pyridoxine

Pyridoxine is also referred to as vitamin B_6. Its deficiency is observed along with the deficiency of other water-soluble vitamins.

Vitamin B_6 deficiency is observed in people who are heavy smokers and consuming alcohol. Its deficiency is also commonly observed in persons using antitubercular drugs (isoniazide, INH) and in women taking oral contraceptives (estrogens).

Folate and Vitamin B_{12} Deficiency

Folate and vitamin B_{12} deficiency is commonly observed due to dietary inadequacy and is associated with elevated homocysteine level. Deficiency of these vitamins is also observed in vegans and during pregnancy.

- **Folic acid deficiency** is seen in stressful conditions, intestinal malabsorption such as steatorrhea and during antibiotic therapy.
- **Vitamin B_{12} deficiency** is seen in geriatric persons, particularly, in those who are strict vegetarians, and in patients with malabsorption, atrophy of the gastric mucosa, and in those with deficiency of the intrinsic factor such as in pernicious anaemia.

VITAMIN D DEFICIENCY

Vitamin D is a **sterol**, also called **sunshine vitamin,** since it is **synthesized in the skin**. Due to its role in the prevention of rickets, vitamin D is also referred to as **antirachitic factor**.

Vitamin D deficiency may be a result of its poor synthesis in skin due to increased pollution, use of sunscreen, increasing age and indoor sedentary behavior.

PROBLEMS RELATED TO EXCESSIVE INTAKE OF SPECIFIC NUTRIENTS

ENDEMIC FLUOROSIS

Endemic fluorosis is due to excess intake of fluoride in drinking water. It has been observed in many parts of the world, where drinking water contains excessive amounts of fluoride (3–5 mg/L). It occurs, when excess fluoride is ingested during the years of tooth calcification, i.e. first 7 years of life. It is characterized by molting of dental enamel, particularly, on the incisors of upper jaw (Chapter 10).

Prevention

- Keep the drinking water fluoride level below 1 mg/L.
- Prevent use of fluoride toothpaste in areas of endemic flurosis. Fluoride supplements not prescribed for children consuming fluorinated water.
- Change the water source.
- Chemical defluorination.

PROBLEMS RELATED TO OVERNUTRITION

With increasing urbanization, **energy-rich diets** containing **higher amount of fat and sugar,** which also provide **less dietary fiber** and complex carbohydrates, are being frequently consumed, particularly, by high income groups. In addition, the urban population is turning to be more **sedentary** with a **little physical activity. Consumption of alcohol,** providing empty calories, and **use of tobacco** is also common among them. Hence, prevalence of **noncommunicable diseases** like obesity, heart disease, hypertension (high blood pressure), diabetes and certain types of cancer is on the increase and account for 60% of all deaths.

The prevalence of diabetes mellitus and coronary heart disease (CHD) is higher in urban areas as compared to their rural counterparts. The incidence rate of cancer is comparatively higher among women (123) compared to men (113 for 100,000).

OVERWEIGHT AND OBESITY

Excess intake of energy is stored in the body as fat, which over the time results in an individual becoming overweight and obese (Fig. 2.3).

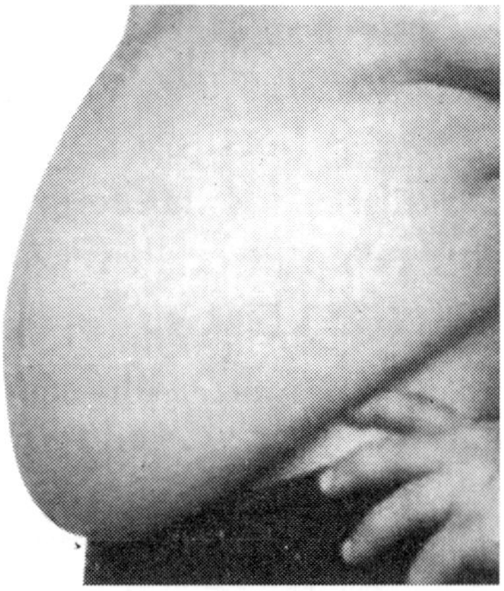

Fig. 2.3: Obesity

- **Overweight** is defined as abnormal or **excessive fat accumulation** that presents a risk to health.
- **Obesity** is defined as **increase in body weight by more than 20%** of the desirable weight. It is one of the most prevalent overnutrition problems, nowadays.

Obesity is a serious medical condition where excess body fat, negatively affects children and adolescent's health and well-being. **The problems is global** and is steadily **affecting many low- and middle-income groups,** particularly, in urban settings. In addition, childhood obesity is one of the most serious public health challenges of the 21st century and its prevalence has increased at an alarming rate. Globally, in 2016, the number of overweight children, under the age of five, was estimated to be over 41 million. Almost half of these lived in Asia.

Obesity is a multi-factorial problem and there are several health consequences of it (Fig. 2.4).

- Excessive body weight **increases the risk of heart disease, hypertension, diabetes, gallstones, certain types of cancer** and **osteoarthritis.**
- Obesity invariably predisposes to **reduced** levels of high-density lipoproteins (**HDL** or **good cholesterol**) and to **increased** levels of low-density lipoproteins (**LDL** or **bad cholesterol**), and **triglycerides,** besides an **abnormal increase in glucose** and **insulin** levels in blood.

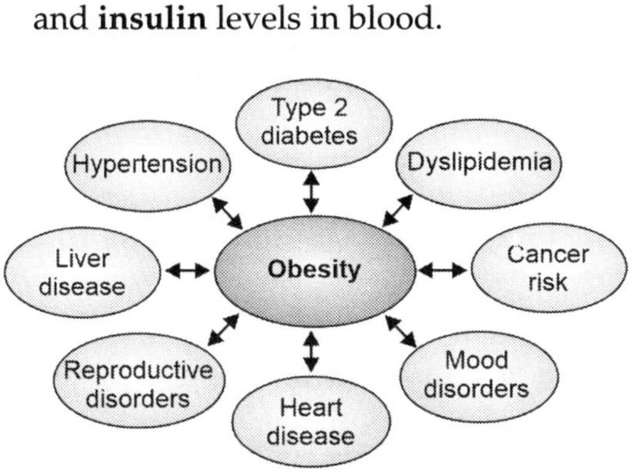

Fig. 2.4: Health problems associated with obesity

- Besides, it may also **predispose to liver and renal diseases,** and **reproductive dysfunctions.**

The most common causes are **genetic factors,** lack of physical activity and **sedentary behavior,** unhealthy eating patterns such as **increased intake of energy-dense foods** which are high in fat and sugar but low in vitamins, minerals and other micronutrients, or a combination of these factors.

DIABETES MELLITUS

Diabetes mellitus is a **chronic metabolic disease** characterized by **persistent hyperglycemia (high blood glucose concentration)** with or without glycosuria (glucosuria). This is the commonest endocrine disease caused by the **deficiency in secretion and/or action of insulin.** Besides insulin, several diabetogenic hormones also influence metabolism of glucose.

As per WHO, diabetes is a **worldwide problem** and that nearly 422 million people are suffering from the disease. A majority of these are living in low- and middle-income countries. Further about 1.5 million deaths are directly attributed to diabetes.

ICMR-NIN (2020) reported that **India has the second largest number of diabetics,** worldwide. According to an estimate, over 74 million Indians were diagnosed of diabetics in 2021 and the number is expected to rise to over 124 million by 2045.

Majority of the diabetic patients (over 80%) **suffer from type 2 diabetes mellitus,** also called **non-insulin dependent diabetes mellitus (NIDDM)**. It is also called maturity-onset-diabetes, since it usually occurs in the middle age group (usually more than 40 years of age), who are generally obese. It is **characterized by hyperglycemia,** often with **hypertriglyceridemia. Long-term complications** of the disease include **acute myocardial infarction** (diabetic patients often present with painless acute myocardial infarction, i.e. silent MI) due to accelerated **atherosclerosis** and **coronary heart disease, nephropathy, retinopathy, neuropathy, infections and delayed wound healing.**

Causes of Diabetes Mellitus

Diabetes mellitus is a **multifactorial disease.**

Genetic, environmental and **metabolic risk factors** contribute to the development of diabetes mellitus. Besides **age, obesity and physical inactivity** are also responsible for its causation.

HYPERTENSION

Hypertension refers to **high blood pressure,** a condition that **affects arteries.** It is a **result of lifestyle, age and environment.**

According to WHO estimates, 1.8 billion people aged 30–79 years, worldwide suffer from hypertension, majority living in low- and middle-income countries.

ICMR-NIN (2020) reported that prevalence rate of HT in India was 118 million in 2000 and expected to be doubled (213 million) in 2025.

Uncontrolled blood pressure is one of the **risk factors of CVD** such as heart attacks and stroke, and are responsible for one-third of total deaths in India.

Risk factors include **old age, high salt intake (as sodium chloride), physical inactivity, increased consumption of alcohol,** meat products, and processed (ready to eat) food, and **obesity and overweight.**

CARDIOVASCULAR DISEASES

Cardiovascular diseases **(CVD)** refer to a **class of diseases** that includes **angina, heart attack, heart failure, cardiomyopathy,** etc., some of which also involve atherosclerosis.

CVD is the **number one cause of death** around the World. According to **American Heart Association** about 19 million deaths were attributed to CVD globally. The **highest mortality rates** were attributable **to Eastern Europe and Central Asia. It affects low- and middle-income countries** even more than high-income countries.

Public health estimates indicate that **India accounts for approximately 60% of the world's heart disease burden.**

Causes of CVD

CVD have been classified as one of the **food habit related illnesses.** These include:

- **Hypertension, diabetes mellitus, lack of physical exercise, obesity, smoking** and **excessive consumption of salt** and **alcohol.**
- **Frequent consumption of high-energy foods** such as processed foods, which are high in sugar and fat, **promote obesity and increase the risk of CVD.**
- **High dietary intake of saturated fat and trans-fat elevates blood levels of cholesterol** and low-density lipoprotein **(LDL).**
- **Low intake of fruits, vegetables and fish** are also linked to cardiovascular risk.
- **High fiber intake** has been shown to **reduce the risk of CHD.**

Majority of the **CVDs may be prevented by improving risk factors** through **exercise, healthy eating, restricting alcohol intake** and **giving up smoking.**

CANCER

Cancer is a **group of diseases** as a result of **abnormal growth** which has a **potential to invade and spread to other parts** of the body. It is a **multifactorial disease**. Besides **genetic factors,** cancer may be a result of the consumption of **tobacco** (in any form), **alcohol, ionizing radiation, environmental pollutants** and **poor diet,** etc.

The global burden of cancer has been estimated to have increased to more than 18 million new cases and over 9 million deaths in 2018.

Several studies have shown a **relationship between dietary factors and the risk of cancer:**

- **Artificial sweeteners** have been shown to **increase the risk of cancer.**

- **Increased consumption of alcohol** has been linked to the increased risk of **liver cancer.**
- Population surveys have shown a strong positive correlation between the dietary intake of fat, and colon and breast cancers.
- Studies have also shown that the **risk of colon cancer** is **inversely related to** the **consumption of dietary fiber.**
- People with **higher blood levels of vitamin D** have been shown to have **lower risk of** cancer, particularly the **colorectal cancer,** and the **overall cancer mortality.**
- **Cancers of the lungs and stomach** have been shown to be related to **low intake of vitamin A and vitamin C.**
- Some of the trace elements, e.g. **selenium** has also been implicated in the etiology of cancer.

SOME IMPORTANT QUESTIONS

1. **Describe common nutritional problems in India.**
2. **Describe protein energy malnutrition.**
3. **What is undernutrition? Describe causes and prevention of undernutrition.**
4. **Describe various nutritional problems related to the deficiency of a specific nutrient.**
5. **Describe various nutritional problems related to overnutrition.**
6. **Differentiate between:**
   i. Kwashiorkor and marasmus
   ii. Undernutrition and overnutrition
   iii. Overweight and obesity
7. **Write notes on:**
   i. Undernutrition
   ii. Low-birth weight babies
   iii. Protein energy malnutrition
   iv. Kwashiorkor
   v. Marasmus
   vi. Overweight
   vii. Obesity

CHAPTER

3

Elements of Nutrition

Elements of nutrition refer to all the **organic and inorganic substances** that are obtained from the food, which we eat. These are also referred to as **accessory food factors** or **nutrients.** These are essential to supply energy, build and maintain body cells, and regulate metabolic processes. These are, generally, divided into two groups, i.e. as **macronutrients** and **micronutrients** (Table 3.1).

Table 3.1: Elements of nutrition (macro and micronutrients) with their primary functions

Nutrients	*Functions*
Carbohydrates	Major sources of energy
Lipids	Provide large amount of energy, insulation, fat soluble vitamins and essential fatty acid
Proteins	Building and maintenace of tissues and synthesis of antibodies, enzymes, hormones and other compounds
Vitamins	Facilitate use of other nutrients, used in regulation of growth and several metabolites
Minerals	Help in building bones and teeth, maintenance of acid–base balance, muscle functions and nervous system activities
Water	Dissolves and carries nutrients, removes waste products and regulates body temperature

- **Macronutrients:** Macronutrients include **carbohydrates, fat** and **proteins.** These are **needed in** relatively **large amounts** and are also called the **proximate principles of food.** These are oxidized in the body, to provide energy which is required for various activities of life. **Dietary fiber,** i.e. non-digestible carbohydrates, such as cellulose, is required for mechanical as well as biochemical functions. Lipids are essential for the formation of cell membrane and signaling molecules. Proteins provide structural material. Macronutrients form bulk of the food, in a diet.
- **Micronutrients:** Micronutrients, mainly, include **vitamins** and **minerals.** These are **required in smaller quantities,** from milligrams to a few grams, and may also be referred to as **protective foods.**

Besides, vitamins and minerals, **anti-oxidants and phytochemicals,** too may be said as micronutrients, since these are also said to influence (or protect) some body systems. Their necessity, however, is not as well established as that of vitamins and minerals.

CARBOHYDRATES

Carbohydrates are the **cheapest source of energy** and are easily available. These are also the main sources of energy for the body. Carbohydrates, in addition to the supply of energy, also serve as the components of cell membrane and receptors.

Carbohydrates are **classified according to their number of sugar units** as **monosaccharides** (such as glucose and fructose), **disaccharides** (such as sucrose and lactose) and **polysaccharides** (such as starch, glycogen and cellulose).

- **Monosaccharides** include glucose and fructose (found in fruits, vegetables and honey).
- **Disaccharides** include sucrose (found in sugar, also called table sugar) and lactose (found in milk)

  Monosaccharides and disaccharides are also **referred to as simple carbohydrates.**
- **Polysaccharides** include **starch** (found in cereals, millets, pulses and root vegetables) and **glycogen** (found in animal foods). These are also referred to as **complex polysaccharides** (Chapter 5).

ICMR-NIN (2020) has recommended that **55–60% of the total dietary energy intake** should be derived from carbohydrates.

The **minimum requirement** for carbohydrate has been recommended to be **100 g/day.** The requirement **during pregnancy** has been recommended as **135 g/day** and **during lactation** as **155 g/day**.

Dietary free sugar should be restricted to 5–7% of energy intake.

DIETARY FIBER

Diet rich in dietary fiber is healthier than a low-fiber diet, which is generally based on the refined and processed foods. Dietary fiber has several health benefits, such as it delays and retards absorption of carbohydrates and fat, and increases the satiety value. Diets rich in fiber also reduce glucose and lipids in blood, and increase bulk of the stools (Chapter 6).

Dietary fiber comprises:

- **Insoluble fiber,** also called **crude fiber** or **roughage,** include **cellulose** and hemicellulose. Their functions include:
  - **Retention of water** during intestinal transit, thereby preventing constipation.
  - **Binding various dietary toxins,** thereby reducing the incidence of colon cancer.
  - Imparting a **sense of early satiety** (fullness of stomach), thereby helping to reduce calorie intake and thus, to control obesity and diabetes mellitus.

  Insoluble fibers are **abundant in vegetable grains.** It is worth mentioning that insoluble fibers also include some nonpolysaccharides, e.g., lignins (carrots, strawberry seeds), cutins and tannins.
- **Soluble fiber,** e.g. **gums and pectins,** is found in legumes, fruits and oats. Their functions include:
  - **Binding of cholesterol** and bile salts, thereby reducing their enterohepatic circulation and enhancing the conversion of cholesterol into bile salts, thereby lowering plasma cholesterol level.
  - **Reducing gastric emptying,** thereby delaying the postprandial rise of blood glucose, particularly, in diabetic patients.

ICMR-NIN (2020) Expert Group has suggested **15 g of dietary fiber per 1000 kcal per day,** as its adequate intake.

LIPIDS

Lipids or fat include a group of substances, which are poorly soluble, or nearly insoluble, in water but are soluble in organic solvents. Over 90% of the dietary fat includes **triacylglycerols** (triglycerides). Other types of dietary lipids include **fatty acids, cholesterol, phospholipids, sterols** and **carotenoids** (Chapter 7).

Fatty acids are the molecules which contain a –COOH group attached to a long hydrocarbon chain, where several carbon atoms are linked together either through the single bonds alone (saturated fatty acids) or with both double bonds as well as single bonds (unsaturated fatty acids). Other types of dietary lipids include cholesterol, phospholipids, sterols and carotenoids.

Essential Fatty Acids

Essential fatty acids are those which cannot be synthesized in our body; hence, these should be supplied through the diet. These include **linoleic acid** and **linolenic acid.**

ICMR-NIN (2020) Expert Group has recommended that dietary fat **should not contribute more than 20–30% of the energy requirements.** Further, it is suggested that not more than **10% of energy** should be available **from visible fat.**

On an average, **an adult moderate worker female** can consume **25 g of visible fat per day** while a **moderate worker male** can consume **30 g of visible fat per day.** The **diet of the pregnant and lactating women may contain 30 g of visible fat.**

Minimum intake level for essential fatty acids to prevent deficiency symptoms should be **2.5% energy intake of linoleic acid** plus 0.5% **α-linolenic acid**.

While a minimum amount of fat should be included in the diet, to meet the requirement of EFA, excess of fat is harmful.

PROTEINS

Proteins have more physiological roles than any other nutrient. Like carbohydrates and fat, proteins can **provide energy**, when necessary, but it also helps in maintaining **water and pH balance.** Protein also keeps the **immune system** strong (Chapter 8).

Proteins are in a constant state of flux in the body, with **continuously being synthesized and degraded.**

These are the organic compounds that **consist of amino acids,** which are joined by peptide bonds.

Proteins are needed for their content of amino acids that are essential to human body for the biosynthesis of proteins, body repair in adults, and for body building and body repair in children.

Essential Amino Acids

As discussed in Chapter 8, all the proteins are **made up of** only **20 amino acids,** out of which, nearly, **10 amino acids can be synthesized** in the body but most of the remaining once **cannot be synthesized,** hence, must be supplied in the diet. Therefore, these are known as **essential amino acids.**

An adult human body can maintain its nitrogen equilibrium on a mixture of 8 amino acids as the sole source of nitrogen, which are called essential amino acids. These include **isoleucine, leucine, lysine, methionine, phenylalanine, threonine, tryptophan and valine.** Besides, **histidine and arginine** are also needed in extra amounts by infants during growth and by females during pregnancy and lactation.

Foods rich in proteins include meat, poultry, fishes, nuts, eggs, milk and milk products.

According to ICMR-NIN (2020) protein should contribute to, approximately, 10–15% of the total energy intake. Accordingly, women should aim to consume, nearly, 46 grams of protein daily, while men should consume about 55 grams per day. Proteins are in a constant state of flux in the body, with continuously being synthesized and degraded.

Different foods contain different amounts and combinations of amino acids (the building blocks of proteins). Accordingly, proteins are said to be the:

- **High quality proteins,** which are, mainly, obtained from **animals** (e.g. meat, fish, eggs and dairy products). These proteins contain full range of essential amino acids, needed by the body. These are also referred to as the proteins of high biological value.
- **Low quality proteins** are obtained from plant sources. These proteins have low biological value, since an

individual protein may lack one or the other essential amino acid. **Vegans and vegetarians** cannot get all the amino acids they need, from a single source. However, combining the plant foods from different sources provide them good quality protein, e.g. pulses with cereals.

VITAMINS

Vitamins are a group of organic compounds and perform a variety of functions in the body. Every vitamin is chemically different from each other. Though they do not yield energy but enable the body to use other nutrients. Since body is, generally, unable to synthesize most of the vitamins, hence, they must be provided in food (Chapter 9).

Vitamins are divided into two groups, as:

i. **Fat soluble vitamins,** which include vitamins A, D, E and K.
ii. **Water soluble vitamins,** which include B vitamins and vitamin C.

Though recommended daily allowance for each vitamin differs, but it is important to consume all the vitamins, each day, to keep our body healthy.

- Vitamins are required by the body in small amounts, for a variety of essential processes.
- Most vitamins cannot be synthesized by the body, so these are to be provided in the diet.
- Vitamin D can be made by the body in the skin when it is exposed to sunlight.
- Requirements for vitamins change across life stages.

MINERALS

Minerals are the inorganic substances required by the body in small amounts, for a variety of functions (Chapter 10).

Various functions of minerals include:

- Formation of bones and teeth
- As essential constituents of body fluids and tissues
- As components of enzyme systems, and
- For normal nerve functions.

Our body requires different amounts of each mineral; accordingly, minerals are divided into two classes as minerals and trace elements (Table 3.2).

Table 3.2: Essential minerals and trace elements required by human body

Minerals	*Trace elements*
Calcium	Copper
Phosphorus	Chromium
Magnesium	Managanese
Sodium	Molybdenum
Potassium	Selenium
Iron	Iodine
Zinc	Fluoride

- **Minerals,** such as sodium, potassium, calcium, phosphorus, magnesium, sulfur and chloride, which are required in large amounts (grams or milligrams).
- **Trace minerals,** like copper, fluoride, zinc, iron, chromium, selenium, iodine, molybdenum and manganese, which are needed in small amounts (microgram to milligrams). All minerals and trace elements are present in healthy tissues, where their concentration remains relatively constant. Besides, there are certain elements, like nickel, vanadium, tin, boron, etc. which have not been shown to have any function in human body, are not dietary essential.

WATER

Water is essential for life. Although human can survive for a number of weeks without food, one cannot live without fluid for more than two or three days. On an average, water makes up nearly 60% of body weight and is essential for normal functioning of all the cells in the body. Amount of fluid needed varies according to age, time of the year, climate conditions, diet and level of physical activity.

According to ICMR-NIN (2020) 1500 ml water from beverages should be consumed by a sedentary adult woman and 2050 ml by a sedentary adult man.

Water helps to:

- Regulate body temperature
- Lubricate joints
- Protect major organs and tissues
- Transport important substances.

We can obtain our fluid requirements from a number of sources, such as water and other drinks, as well as the food we eat. Dehydration can impair physiological responses, and, in extreme cases, can be fatal. At the same time, it can be dangerous to drink too much water, as water intoxication can lead to hyponatremia (Chapter 11).

SOME IMPORTANT QUESTIONS

1. **Describe various elements of nutrition.**
2. **Write notes on:**
   i. Accessory food factors
   ii. Macronutrients
   iii. Micronutrients

CHAPTER

4

Energy

Energy is a prime requisite for body functions and growth. Energy is also required for doing physical work.

Our body gets energy from the combustion of carbohydrates, fat and proteins. In these macromolecules, energy is **locked in the form of chemical bonds** and is **released when the food is metabolized.** Thus, **during combustion of food,** body converts **chemical energy** (present in food) to heat, mechanical and electrical energy.

UNIT OF ENERGY

The unit of energy is calorie.

A calorie is defined as the **quantity of heat required to raise the temperature of 1 g of water by 1°C,** more specifically from 14.5°C to 15.5°C.

In the context of **nutrition,** unit of energy is referred in terms of **kilocalories or kcal** (1000 calories).

The value of calories **mentioned on food packets** is in terms of kilocalories.

The **international unit of energy** (SI unit) adopted by the International Union of Nutritional Sciences is referred to as **joule**.

One kcal is equal to 4.184 kJ (kilo joules).

SIGNIFICANCE OF DIETARY ENERGY

Dietary energy is required for performing several functions in the body. These include:

- The **maintenance of body temperature**
- **Growth**
- Performing **metabolic activities** such as digestion of food, absorption of the dietary nutrients, etc.
- Performing daily **physical activities.**

ENERGY INTAKE AND ENERGY OUTPUT

Energy requirement (need) of an individual is defined as the **level of energy intake in relation to energy expenditure (output).** Energy intake and energy output of normal healthy individuals are **finely balanced.**

- **Energy intake:** Energy intake refers to the total **amount of energy** (calorie) **consumed** from the diet.
- **Energy output:** Energy output refers to the **amount of energy** (calorie) **used** (expenditure) by the body to meet its requirements.

ENERGY BALANCE

To maintain a steady state, stable body weight, and physical and mental health, **energy intake** should be **equal to energy output.** This is referred to as energy balance or energy equilibrium.

- **Positive energy balance:** When **energy intake is more than the output,** i.e. the body's requirement, it is referred to as **positive energy balance.** Under these conditions, **surplus of the energy is stored in the body as fat.** Thus, a **positive energy balance** leads to **overweight, obesity** and **several non-communicable diseases.** Positive energy balance is, however, essential under certain conditions such as growth and pregnancy.
- **Negative energy balance:** When **energy intake is less than the output,** it is referred to as **negative energy balance.** It **results in weight loss.** Negative nitrogen balance is observed in protein catabolic states such as prolonged illness and high-grade fever, tuberculosis and malignancy, and reduced food intake **during pregnancy and lactation** where it results in **undernutrition and growth retardation** of the infant.

FACTORS AFFECTING ENERGY REQUIREMENT

As discussed above, energy requirement is determined in terms of energy expenditure. Several factors affect energy requirements. These include:

- Age
- Sex
- Physiological state such as pregnancy or lactation
- Level and duration of physical activities.

COMPONENTS OF ENERGY REQUIREMENT

Total energy requirement, for different categories of people, is made up of three components, which include:

1. BASAL REQUIREMENT

The total amount of energy used over the period of 24 hours in the state of complete physical and mental rest at comfortable environment (temperature and humidity) is referred to as **basal energy requirement** or **energy requirement during resting.** Since energy requirement is defined in terms of energy expenditure, it is also called **basal energy expenditure.**

It is the **amount of energy spent by the body** for performing various routine metabolic activities which are necessary to sustain normal body functions and homeostasis such as **respiration, blood circulation, synthesis of several substances for use in the body, pumping of ions across the membranes** as well as **maintenance of body temperature.**

Basal energy expenditure is expressed in terms of the basal metabolic rate **(BMR).**

BASAL METABOLIC RATE

Basal metabolic rate (BMR) is the **amount of energy expenditure at rest** in a neutral temperate environment, in the post-absorptive state, i.e. it is the amount of energy expenditure at complete physical and mental rest. It is used to meet the requirement of energy for the functioning of vital organs, i.e. the heart, lungs, kidneys, nervous system, intestine, liver, sex organs, muscles and skin, etc.

Determination of BMR

BMR is measured, by indirect calorimetry in the laboratory settings, when a person is lying **at complete rest but awaken after** a normal overnight sleep, **10 to 12 hours after the last meal** and **performing no physical activity.**

BMR remains constant throughout the day under normal conditions and constitutes about 50–75% of the total energy expenditure by an individual. BMR value is **expressed in terms of kcal/hr.**

Factors Affecting BMR

Several factors affect BMR (Table 4.1).

- **Body mass:** Lean body mass refers to the portion of the body, exclusive of the stored fat, i.e. the fat-free mass (metabolically active tissue). Muscles, various other organs, bones and body

Table 4.1: Factors affecting BMR

Factors that increase BMR	*Factors that decrease BMR*
Total body weight	Increasing age towards elderly
Increased lean body mass	Female gender
Large body surface area	Starvation
Rapid growth	Hypothyroidism
Hot and cold temperature Stress Hyperthyroidism Caffeine Pregnancy and lactation Smoking Fever	Sleep

fluids, make up most of the lean body mass. An individual, with a **large lean body mass,** has **higher resting energy expenditure** than the one with same weight but having higher proportion of body fat.

- **Age:** BMR is the **highest** during the period of rapid growth, mainly **within first two years of life.** It is reduced thereafter, but again **reaches a peak during puberty and adolescence.** BMR is further **reduced,** by about 2 to 3% per decade, **in adults.** This is due to the reason that whereas lean body mass tends to decrease, fat content increases with age.
- **Sex:** Metabolic rate is **higher in men** (by about 50 kcal per day) **than women.** This is due to the reason that women have less active muscle mass, for each kg of body weight. Women generally have less lean body mass. Resting metabolic rate also varies during menstrual cycle. It fluctuates from the low point from about one week before ovulation to the high point, just before the onset of menstruation.
- **Other factors:** These factors, however, may be less consistent, of shorter duration and limited to individual situations:
  - BMR **falls** by about 10% **during sleep.**
  - It **rises during the period of rapid growth,** such as in infancy and adolescence.
  - Hormones, especially **thyroxin and norepinephrine,** also **regulate BMR.** It has been shown that BMR is reduced in **hypothyroidism,** while it is increased in hyperthyroidism.
  - **Excitement and stress** which cause **release of epinephrine, increase** cellular activity and, thus, **BMR.**
  - BMR is decreased in early stages of pregnancy, whereas **later, in pregnancy, BMR is increased,** because of uterine, placental and fetal growth.
  - **Fever increases BMR** by about 7% for each degree increase in body temperature (above 98.4°F).
  - Environment temperature also affects BMR. It is known that during **exposure to cold BMR is increased,** as people living in tropical climate, usually have higher BMR than those living in the temperate areas.
  - **BMR is reduced during starvation.** It is due to the reason that body slows basic functions to conserve energy.
  - Some unknown **genetic factors** have also been attributed to the variations in BMR.

2. REQUIREMENT FOR PHYSICAL ACTIVITY

It is the most variable component of energy expenditure. Energy expenditure for physical activities varies from 30 to 100% of the basal requirement. It depends upon the duration, type and intensity of physical activity, including the energy expenditure for occupational work. According to the type of occupational work, individuals have been classified into 3 categories, as:

- **Light workers** (such as those doing office work)
- **Moderate workers** (like a student)
- **Heavy workers** (such as those performing manual physical labor, rickshaw pullers, etc.).

Amounts of energy expenditure for different types of physical activities, as per National Institute of Nutrition, Indian Council of Medical Research (NIN–ICMR, 2011) are shown in Table 4.2.

ICMR-NIN (2020), while defining the **energy expenditure using physical activity estimations,** have **suggested three terms** which include:

- **Physical Activity Ratio (PAR):** It is expressed as the **ratio of the energy cost of an individual activity per minute to the cost of BMR per minute.**
- **Physical Activity Level (PAL): PAR** values **calculated** as above, **for the various activities performed in a day** can be aggregated to a 24-hour period to get the physical activity level. It is actually the **ratio of the energy expenditure for 24 hours and the value of BMR for 24 hours.**

PAL value is proposed as 1.4, 1.8 and 2.3 for the sedentary, moderate and heavy work, respectively.

- **Total Energy Expenditure (TEE):** TEE is **calculated based on a multiplication of basal metabolic rate (BMR) to the physical activity level** (PAL), i.e.:

$$\textbf{TEE} = \text{BMR} \times \text{PAL}$$

TEE values are particularly **given for infants.**

3. REQUIREMENT ON ACCOUNT OF SPECIFIC DYNAMIC ACTION OF FOOD

Specific dynamic action **(SDA)** is also referred to as **diet-induced thermogenesis** or **thermogenic effect of food.** It is the amount of energy expenditure **associated with the consumption of food.** It actually refers to the **amount of energy our body spends to digest, absorb and metabolize dietary nutrients** which depends upon the type and amount of nutrients consumed. As fat is metabolized more efficiently compared to carbohydrates and proteins,

Table 4.2: Energy expenditure for different types of physical activities

Activity zones	*Type of activities*	*Energy expenditure* (kcal/min)*
1	Sleeping, resting or relaxing	1.0
2	Sitting (light activities); eating, reading, writing, listening or talking	1.5
3	Standing (light activity); washing face, shaving, combing, or watering plants	2.3
4	Walking (slow), driving, dusting, bathing, dressing, marketing or childcare	2.8
5	Light manual work, sweeping, cleaning utensils, washing clothes or other house chores	3.3
6	Warm-up and recreational activities, walking upstairs/downstairs, cycling or fetching water	4.8
7	Manual work (moderate pace), loading/unloading, walking with load, harvesting, carpentry or plumbing	5.6
8	Practice of non-competitive sports/games, cycling (15 kmph), gymnastics, swimming or digging	6.0
9	High intense manual work and sports activities–tournaments, wood cutting, carrying heavy loads, running or jogging	7.8

* NIN–ICMR (2011).

SDA values are more for carbohydrates and proteins than the fat.

For a mixed diet, SDA value is considered as **10% of the total energy expenditure.**

DIETARY SOURCES OF ENERGY

Main dietary sources of energy in our diets include **carbohydrates, fat and proteins.**

Recently, ICMR-NIN (2020) in its report has also emphasized the importance of **dietary fiber** and has suggested that dietary fiber, both soluble and insoluble, undergo fermentation in the large intestine and in turn produces short chain fatty acids. These fatty acids are used by the cells of the colon and the liver, as a source of energy, and thus, dietary fiber also provides **2 kcal per gram.** Hence, the **metabolizable energy available from the dietary components** (macronutrients) should be accounted for as shown in Table 4.3.

Table 4.3: Amount of metabolizable energy available from different dietary components

Dietary component	*Metabolizable energy available (kcal/g)*
Carbohydrates	4
Fat	9
Proteins	4
Dietary fiber	2

ENERGY REQUIREMENT FOR DIFFERENT CATEGORIES OF PEOPLE

As discussed above, several factors determine energy requirement such as basal metabolic rate, level and duration of physical activity, age and physiological state (pregnancy and lactation), and SDA (processes involved in the extraction of energy from food). Besides, it also depends upon the source of energy.

- Energy requirements have been laid down by various expert groups of the FAO/WHO and these standards are revised from time to time in light of the newer knowledge.
- For Indian people, ICMR-NIN (2020) Expert Group has assessed the energy requirement in terms of energy expenditure instead of energy intake.
- The Committee has recommended dietary intake of energy for a healthy, well-nourished and active population.
- The Committee has further suggested that while computing the requirement of energy, the source of energy should also be considered. In Indian diets, major sources of energy are, mainly, the plant-based foods which consist of carbohydrates, fat and proteins.
- Energy requirement for adults with sedentary activity has been lowered, due to the lowered BMR.
- It has been recommended that, on an average, **a moderate male worker requires 2710 kcal/day** while a **female** performing the same type of work **needs 2130 kcal/day.**
- Further, it is also suggested that **55–60% of dietary energy should be derived from carbohydrates, 20–30% from fat** and **10–15% from proteins.**

Average daily energy requirement for people of different age groups and the type of work performed by them is shown in Table 4.4.

MEASUREMENT OF ENERGY EXPENDITURE

The amount of energy expenditure can be measured either **calculating the energy content of the food** or by measuring the **amount of the heat released in relation** to the amount of oxygen consumed.

- By calculating energy content of the food consumed

As we know, that all the foods and drinks provide energy (calories). Whereas, some foods such as vegetables and lettuce, etc. provide less energy (contain a few calories) while others like sugar and fat release a lot of energy (calories).

Table 4.4: Energy requirements for Indians (ICMR-NIN, 2020)

Population/ group	*Category of worker/ period*	*Body weight (kg)*	*Energy* (kcal)*
Adult men (19+)	Sedentary	65	2110
	Moderate		2710
	Heavy		3470
Adult women (19+)	Sedentary	55	1660
	Moderate		2130
	Heavy		2720
Pregnant women	2nd Trimester	(+) 10	(+) 350
	3rd Trimester		(+) 350
Lactating women	0–6 Months		(+) 600
	7–12 Months		(+) 520
Infants	0–6 Months**	5.8	530
	7–12 Months	8.5	680
Children	1–3 Years	12.9	1110
	4–6 Years	18.3	1360
	7–9 Years	25.3	1700
Adolescents	Boys 10–12 Years	34.9	2220
	Boys 13–15 Years	50.5	2860
	Boys 16–18 Years	64.4	3320
	Girls 10–12 Years	36.4	2050
	Girls 13–15 Years	49.6	2400
	Girls 16–18 Years	55.7	2500

* Estimated energy requirement (EER)
** Adequate intake (AI)

Accordingly, we can **compute** that how many **calories** are **present in the particular food.**

- **By determining the amount of heat given-off in relation to the amount of oxygen consumed**

Measurement of the **amount of heat given off by** an individual, i.e. the **total energy expenditure,** is called **calorimetry.** The amount of energy expenditure **in relation to the oxygen consumed** can be measured either directly or indirectly.

Direct Calorimetry

It **measures the amount of heat produced by the body,** which is proportional to the amount of the total energy used. For this purpose, the **subject is enclosed in a small insulated chamber** which is **surrounded by the circulating water.** Thereafter, rise in **temperature of water is measured,** which is directly related to the energy consumed by the subject. Though, direct calorimetry provides a measure of energy expenditure in the form of heat, it **does not provide any information on the kind of food consumed** (fuel oxidized). Further, it is a **very cumbersome procedure** and is **not commonly used.**

Indirect Calorimetry

It refers to determination of **energy expenditure by the body, indirectly,** i.e. without measuring heat production.

Indirect calorimetry estimates energy expenditure **by determining the amount of oxygen consumed in relation to the**

amount of carbon dioxide produced by an individual, **over a given period of time.**

It is, comparatively, easier and less expensive than direct calorimetry.

Data obtained from indirect calorimetry **are used for the calculation by respiratory quotient.**

RESPIRATORY QUOTIENT

Respiratory quotient (RQ) refers to the **moles of CO_2 expired in relation to the moles of O_2 consumed,** i.e.:

RQ = Moles of CO_2 expired/moles of O_2 consumed

The value, thereafter, is **converted into kcal** (heat produced) per square meter of body surface area/hour, and is **extrapolated to energy expenditure per 24 hours.**

RQ value depends upon the type of food consumed.

- **RQ for carbohydrates is 1.**

  It is due to the reason that the **number of moles of carbon dioxide produced from 1 gram of carbohydrate is equal to the number of moles of oxygen consumed.**
- **RQ for protein is 0.82.**
- **RQ for fat is 0.7.**

Energy output **for a mixed diet** is calculated by taking the **RQ value of 0.85.**

SOME IMPORTANT QUESTIONS

1. **What is the unit of measurement of energy? Describe various methods of measurement of energy.**
2. **Define basal metabolic rate (BMR). Describe various factors affecting BMR.**
3. **Describe various components of energy requirement of a person.**
4. **Discuss energy requirements of different categories of people.**
5. **Write notes on:**
   i. Direct calorimetry
   ii. Indirect calorimetry
   iii. Basal metabolic rate (BMR)
   iv. Specific dynamic action (SDA)
   v. Energy balance
   vi. Energy
   vii. Respiratory quotient (RQ)

CHAPTER

5

Carbohydrates

Carbohydrates (CHO), also called **saccharides** (Greek: Sakcharon, sugar), are the most abundant biological molecules containing C, H and O, which are combined in the ratio of 1:2:1, i.e. as $(CH_2O)n$, where n is 3 or more. For example, **glucose ($C_6H_{12}O_6$) contains 6 carbons, 12 hydrogen and 6 oxygen** $[(CH_2O)_6]$.

Carbohydrates are one of the **macronutrients** and are a **major source of energy in a diet.**

BIOLOGICAL IMPORTANCE OF CARBOHYDRATES

- Carbohydrates provide significant fraction of energy in the diet.
- These also act as the storage form of energy in the body.
- Carbohydrates also serve as component of a cell membrane that mediates intracellular communication.
- These also serve as structural component of many organisms, including cell wall of bacteria, exoskeleton of insects as well as the fibrous cellulose portion of the plants.

CLASSIFICATION OF CARBOHYDRATES

Carbohydrates are classified **based on chemistry (according to size of the molecule and their structure)** as well as **according to their nutritional significance.**

According to the size of the molecule and their structure.

According to the size of the molecule and their structure, carbohydrates are **classified into four groups,** i.e. as **monosaccharides, disaccharides, oligosaccharides and polysaccharides.**

- **Monosaccharides:** Monosaccharides are also called **simple sugars.** Common monosaccharides include **glucose, galactose and fructose.** These three share the same molecular formula, i.e. as $C_6H_{12}O_6$.

  Since each one of these contains six carbons, these are referred to as hexoses:
  - *Glucose:* The most important monosaccharide is glucose, due to its role in blood sugar. It is the immediate source of energy for cellular respiration.
  - *Galactose:* It is a sugar present in milk (and yogurt).
  - *Fructose:* It is a sugar found in honey.

  Monosaccharides, in a closed-chain, **can form glycosidic bonds with other monosaccharides,** creating **disaccharides** (such as sucrose), **oligosaccharides** (such as malto-triose) and polysaccharides which include structural **polysaccharides** such as **cellulose and pectin** important for cell wall construction, or **energy** reservoirs **(storage polysaccharides)** such as **starch and glycogen** (Fig. 5.1).

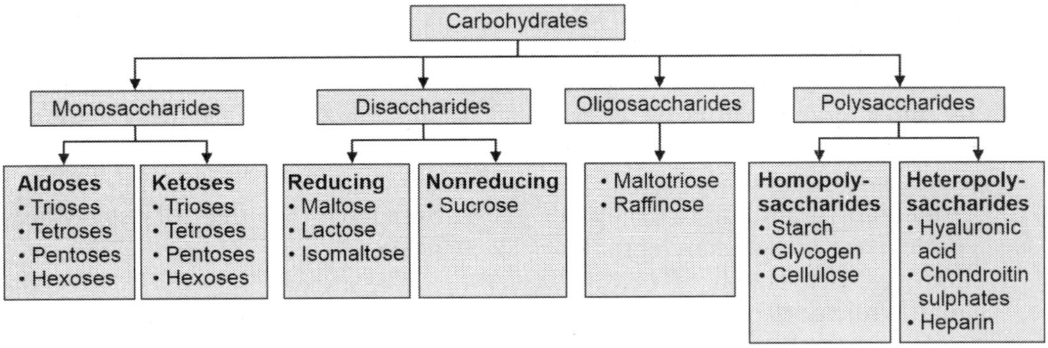

Fig. 5.1: Classification of carbohydrates

- **Disaccharides:** Disaccharides are formed by linking two monosaccharides with the removal of a molecule of water.

  Commonly available disaccharides include lactose, maltose and sucrose.

  - *Lactose:* It is **formed** when a molecule of **glucose** is linked to **galactose.** It is also called **milk sugar,** since it is found naturally in milk.

    Lactose is **synthesized in the mammary glands during lactation** and is secreted into the milk.

    During digestion, lactose is **hydrolyzed to** its monosaccharide units, i.e. **glucose and galactose by** the intestinal enzyme referred to as **lactase.**

  - *Maltose:* It is formed when a molecule of **glucose** is linked to another molecule of **glucose**.

    It is obtained during **hydrolysis of starch.**

    During digestion, **maltose is hydrolyzed to** its monosaccharide units, i.e. **glucose and glucose by** the intestinal enzyme referred to as **maltase.**

  - *Sucrose:* It is formed when a molecule of glucose is linked to fructose.

    It is also referred to as **table sugar** since it is commonly used on the table for routine use in home-made drinks. Sucrose is also referred to as **cane sugar** since it is obtained from the stems of sugarcane and roots of sugar beet.

    During digestion, **sucrose splits into** its constituent monosaccharides **glucose and fructose by** the enzyme sucrase (also called **invertase**).

    Sucrose is used by people as a **sweetener for foods** (e.g. toast and dessert) **and beverages** (e.g. coffee and tea).

- **Oligosaccharides:** Oligosaccharides are the carbohydrates built by the linking of more than two (generally **three to nine**) monosaccharide units that are linked by O-glycosidic bonds. These include malto-oligosaccharides (e.g. **malto-triose**) and non-digestible oligosaccharides (**raffinose,** etc.). Non-digestible oligosaccharides cannot be digested by the human beings, as we do not have enzymes that digest these oligosaccharides. So, these pass as such through the digestive tract and are metabolized by the bacteria in the gut.

- **Polysaccharides:** Polysaccharides are made up of **many monosaccharide molecules** (usually more than ten). Examples of polysaccharides are **starch, glycogen** (the form in which glucose is stored in the body), and **cellulose** and **pectin** (components classed as dietary fiber), etc.

  - *Starch:* Starch or **amylum** is a polymeric carbohydrate **con-**

sisting of numerous glucose units **joined by glycosidic bonds.** This polysaccharide is **produced by most green plants as energy storage.** Starch molecules arrange themselves in the plant in semi-crystalline granules. Each plant species has a unique starch granular size, e.g. rice starch is relatively small while potato starch has large granules. Starch content of different foods varies, e.g. potatoes 15%, wheat 55%, corn 65% and rice 75%.

Structurally, starch is a mixture of two polymers, i.e. **amylose and amylopectin.** Natural starches consist of about 10–30% amylose and 70–90% amylopectin.

- **Amylose** is a **linear polysaccharide, composed, entirely, of D-glucose units, which are joined by the α-1,4 glycosidic linkages.**
- **Amylopectin** is a **branched-chain polysaccharide,** composed of **glucose units linked** primarily by **α-1,4-glycosidic bonds** but with occasionally **α-1,6-glycosidic bonds,** which are responsible for the branching. A molecule of amylopectin may contain many thousands of glucose units with branch points occurring after about every 25–30 units.

In the human body, several enzymes collectively referred to as **amylases degrade starch** sequentially **into** usable **glucose** units. Amongst them, **α-amylases** are **found in plants and animals. Human saliva is rich in amylase** and the **pancreas** also secretes the enzyme. The **complete hydrolysis of starch yields,** in successive stages, **glucose,** i.e.:

$$\text{Starch} \rightarrow \text{Dextrin} \rightarrow \text{Maltose} \rightarrow \text{Glucose}$$

Starch is the **most common carbohydrate in the human diet** and is contained in many staple foods. The **major sources** of starch intake worldwide are the **cereals** (rice, wheat and maize) and the **root vegetables** (potatoes and cassava). Widely used prepared foods containing starch are **bread, pancakes, cereals, noodles and pasta.**

- *Glycogen:* Glycogen is the energy reserve carbohydrate of **animals including** humans, hence is also referred to as animal starch. Like starch in plants, glycogen is **found** as granules **in liver** (4–8% by weight of tissue) and in **skeletal muscle cells** (0.5–1.0%). When fasting, humans draw on these glycogen reserves during the first day without food to obtain the glucose needed to maintain metabolic balance.

  Glycogen is **structurally** quite **similar to amylopectin;** however, glycogen is more branched (8–12 glucose units between branches) and the branches are shorter.

  Enzyme **phosphorylase catalyzes the breakdown of glycogen** to glucose, when energy is needed, by a process called glycogenolysis.
- *Cellulose:* Cellulose is a polysaccharide (homopolysaccharide) like amylose, but it differs from amylose in the way that glucose molecules, in cellulose, are linked together by **β-1,4-glycosidic linkages** instead of α-1,4-glycosidic linkages present in amylose. Cellulose is found in **plants,** as a **structural component of** their **cell wall.**

  Cellulose cannot be digested by human beings because we lack cellulase, i.e. the enzyme which is required to hydrolyze β-1 → 4 linkages.

Classification of Carbohydrates According to Nutritional Significance

According to their significance in nutrition, carbohydrates are classified as simple sugars and complex carbohydrates including fiber.

Simple Sugars

- **Intrinsic sugars,** which are incorporated into the cellular structure of foods, e.g. **glucose, fructose, pentoses,** etc. i.e. the sugars found in whole fruits and vegetables.
- **Extrinsic sugars,** which are not bound into a cellular structure, e.g. **lactose** (milk sugar) found in dairy products, **sucrose** (table sugar) found in confectionery, etc.

Complex Carbohydrates

- **Starch:** It is found in potatoes, bread, rice and pasta.
- **Dietary fiber:** These are the carbohydrate polymers, which are neither digested nor absorbed in the small intestine, e.g. cellulose, pectin, etc.

CALORIC VALUE OF CARBOHYDRATES

Calorific value or **caloric value** of the food is the amount of heat produced by combustion of one gram of fuel.

Calorific value of carbohydrate is **4 kilocalories (kcal) per gram.**

RECOMMENDED DAILY ALLOWANCES

Considering the cultural aspects, physical activity level and the cost of carbohydrates, ICMR-NIN (2020) Expert Group has suggested that the dietary carbohydrates should provide 55 to 60 percent of total energy intake.

The minimum intake of carbohydrate, required for brain glucose utilization, has been suggested as 100 g per day. The suggested minimum requirement of carbohydrates for pregnant women is 135 g per day and during lactation it is 155 g per day.

DIETARY SOURCES OF CARBOHYDRATES

Main dietary sources of carbohydrates include grains, vegetables and fruits. Complex carbohydrates are present in whole grains (such as cereals and rice), bran, beans, bread and pasta. Milk and milk products provide lactose, while beverages, jams, jellies and candies provide refined sugar, such as glucose or fructose (Fig. 5.2).

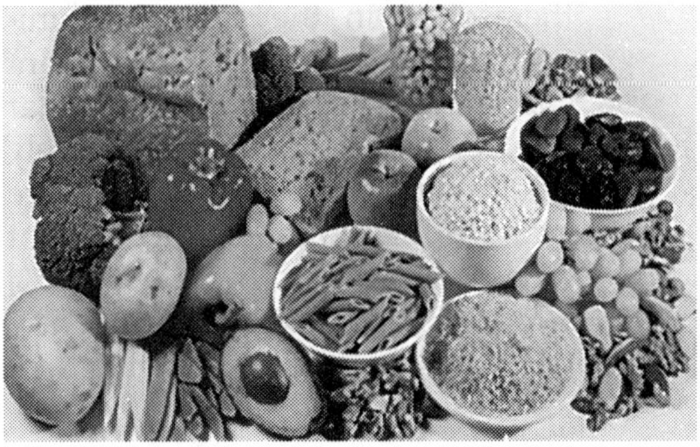

Fig. 5.2: Dietary sources of carbohydrates

Foods which are rich in carbohydrates include:

- **Dairy:** Milk, yogurt and ice cream
- **Fruits:** Whole fruits and fruit juice
- **Grains:** Cereal grains, bread and rice
- **Legumes:** Beans and pulses
- **Starchy vegetables:** Potatoes and corn
- **Sugary sweets:** Soda (when fluid intake is high), candy, cookies and other desserts.

Good Carbohydrates versus Bad Carbohydrates

Carbohydrates form the basis of most diets, making up half of total energy (calorie) intake. Dietary carbohydrates can be separated into two types, as complex (good) carbohydrates and simple (bad) carbohydrates.

- **Good carbohydrates:** Carbohydrates, usually, considered to be good include **complex carbohydrates** such as those **obtained from whole grains, fruits, vegetables, beans and legumes.** These contain large chains of sugar molecules and **take longer to digest** than processed grains. These are not only digested slowly, but **also contain a bounty of other nutrients** (Fig. 5.3).

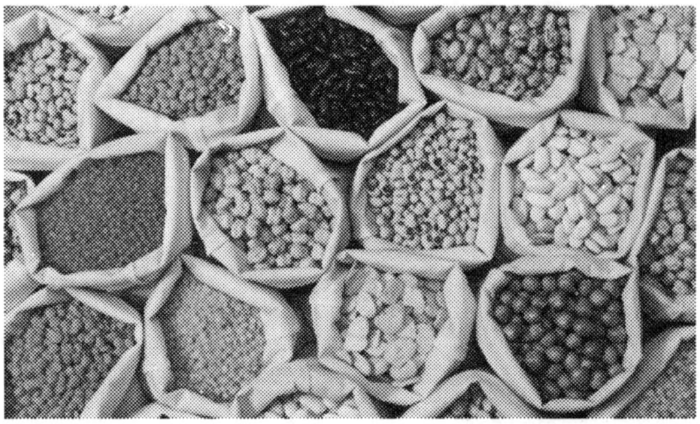

Fig. 5.3: Sources of good carbohydrates

Good carbohydrates are:

- Low or moderate in calories
- High in nutrients
- Devoid of refined grains and sugar
- High in naturally occurring fiber
- Low in sodium
- Low in saturated fat
- Very low in, or devoid of, cholesterol and trans-fat

Bad carbohydrates: Carbohydrates, usually, considered bad include **refined sugars**, such as those obtained from pastries, white sugar, honey, fruit juices and soda, **highly processed foods,** white rice, white bread and other white-flour foods (Fig. 5.4).

They are **digested more quickly** by the body. This makes them a **faster source of energy.** Also, these types of carbohydrates **do not offer as many additional nutrients.**

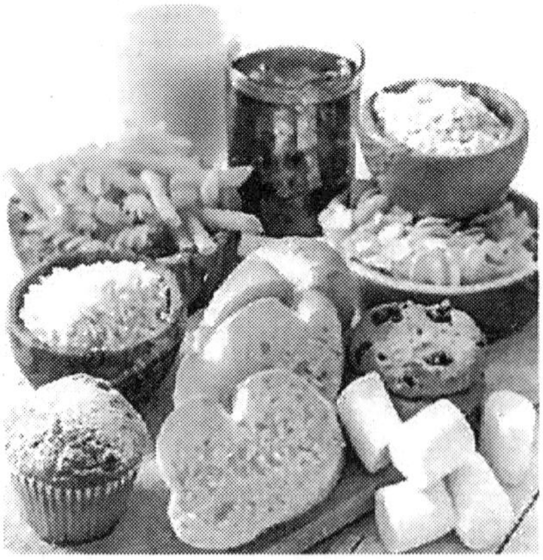

Fig. 5.4: Sources of bad carbohydrates

Bad carbohydrates are:

- High in calories
- Full of refined sugars
- Low in many nutrients
- Low in fiber
- High in sodium
- High in saturated fat, cholesterol and trans-fat

DIGESTION, ABSORPTION AND STORAGE OF CARBOHYDRATES

DIGESTION OF CARBOHYDRATES

- Digestion of carbohydrates begins in the **mouth,** where **salivary amylase** hydrolyses starch into smaller polysaccharides (dextrin) and maltose.
- Chewing stimulates production of saliva and mixes the enzyme salivary amylase with food. Only about **5% of the dietary starch is hydrolyzed in the mouth.**
- When dietary contents enter the stomach, HCl (present in the gastric juice) stops the action of salivary amylase.
- After the dietary contents enter **small intestine,** pancreas starts secreting **pancreatic amylase,** which **further hydrolyses starch,** and converts it to maltose, isomaltose, oligosaccharides and dextrin.
- Thereafter, **brush border disaccharidases hydrolyze disaccharides** into monosaccharides.
- Thus, disaccharides, oligosaccharides and polysaccharides are hydrolyzed to their monosaccharide constituents (Table 5.1).

ABSORPTION OF MONOSACCHARIDES

- After the enzymatic hydrolysis of dietary carbohydrates (polysaccharides and disaccharides) to monosaccharides, different monosaccharides are absorbed into the mucosal cells lining the small intestine, by two mechanisms:
  - **Fructose** is absorbed **by facilitated diffusion**

Table 5.1: Role of various enzymes in the digestion of carbohydrates

Enzyme	*Site of action*	*Catalytic action*
Salivary amylase	Mouth	Starch/glycogen → Partially hydrolyzed dextrins, oligosaccharides, isomaltose and maltose
Pancreatic amylase	Small intestine	Partially hydrolyzed dextrins/oligosaccharides → Dextrins, maltose, isomaltose, maltotriose
α-Dextrinase	Small intestine	α-Limit dextrins → Maltotriose, glucose
Disaccharidases	Small intestine	
Sucrase		Sucrose → Glucose and fructose
Lactase		Lactose → Glucose and galactose
Maltase		Maltose/maltotriose → Glucose
Isomaltase		Isomaltose → Glucose

- **Glucose and galactose** are absorbed **by** the process of **active transport,** with the help of **sodium-linked glucose transporter 1** (SLGT1).
- In the villi, absorbed monosaccharides pass through the intestinal mucosal cells and enter liver, via portal vein.
- In the liver, galactose and fructose are also converted to glucose.

Thereafter, glucose is either **stored in the liver** or is **oxidised for the production of energy.**

STORAGE OF GLUCOSE

Carbohydrates, mainly **glucose,** are **stored as glycogen in the liver and muscle.**

During fasting **liver glycogen is hydrolyzed to glucose to maintain blood glucose level,** whereas **muscle glycogen is used as a source of energy during exercise.**

Excess of dietary glucose is stored in the adipose tissue as fat (triacylglycerols).

METABOLISM OF CARBOHYDRATES

METABOLIC FATES OF GLUCOSE

As discussed above, after absorption monosaccharides are transported to the liver and enter systemic circulation (blood).

Increased concentration of glucose promotes insulin concentration. This in turn stimulates entry of glucose into different cells and tissues.

- **In the liver and muscle,** glucose is metabolized to produce energy, where firstly, it is **converted to pyruvate** by the process of **glycolysis.**
- **Pyruvate may be converted to acetyl-CoA,** aerobically, **or to lactic acid** anaerobically. Once it is converted to acetyl-CoA, it is not retrievable.
- **Acetyl-CoA** enters **citric acid cycle** (TCA cycle) and **produces** energy **(ATP)** through **electron transport chain** and **oxidative phosphorylation.**
- **Excess of dietary glucose is converted to glycogen** and is **stored in the liver and muscle by** the process of **glycogenesis,** which serves as a **source of energy.**
- When blood glucose level is low, glycogen is converted to glucose, by **glycogenolysis (Fig. 5.5).**

GLYCOLYSIS

Glycolysis, also called Embden-Meyerhof (or **Embden-Meyerhof-Parnas**) pathway,

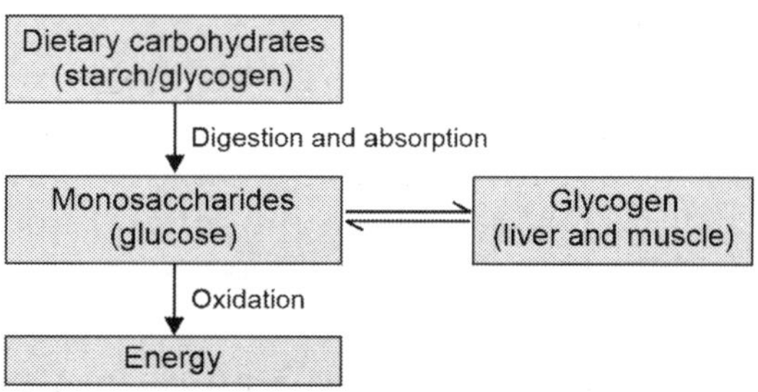

Fig. 5.5: Metabolic fates of glucose

is a process of utilization (catabolism) of glucose, mainly, in the **liver (aerobic glycolysis)** and **skeletal muscle (anaerobic glycolysis).**

Glycolytic enzymes are present in the extramitochondrial compartment of the cell to produce energy.

Biomedical Importance of Glycolysis

In the liver and other tissues, **aerobic glycolysis is the main source of ATP. In the muscle, anaerobic glycolysis** provides energy **during exercise.**

Outline of Glycolysis

Various reactions of the glycolytic pathway are outlined in Fig. 5.6.

1. **Glucose is** first **converted to glucose-6-phosphate.** This reaction is catalyzed by the **enzyme hexokinase,** which requires ATP and Mg. Hexokinase is present in all the tissues.

   In the fed state, this reaction is catalyzed by another enzyme, called **glucokinase.** This enzyme is found in the liver, where it is induced by high glucose concentration after meals.
2. In the next reaction, **glucose-6-phosphate is isomerized,** in a freely reversible reaction, **to fructose-6-phosphate,** by the enzyme **phosphohexose isomerase.**
3. **Fructose-6-phosphate** is then **phosphorylated** by an allosteric enzyme phosphofructokinase to form **fructose-1,6-bisphosphate.**

   This is an irreversible reaction and requires ATP.
4. Thereafter, **fructose-1,6-bisphosphate** (a hexose) is **cleaved by aldolase to** 3-phosphoglyceraldehyde **(glyceraldehyde-3-phosphate)** and **dihydroxyacetone phosphate,** two trioses.
5. Subsequently, only **3-phosphoglyceraldehyde enters the pathway.**

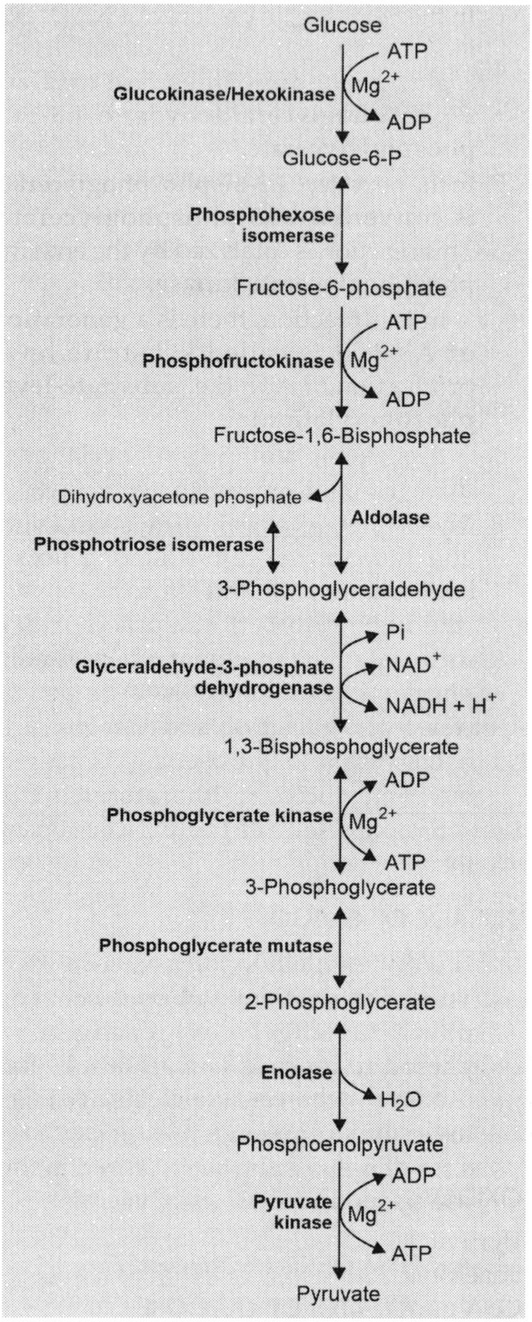

Fig. 5.6: Outline of glycolysis

So, **dihydroxyacetone phosphate** also gets **converted to 3-phosphoglyceraldehyde.** This reaction is catalyzed by the enzyme **phospho-triose isomerase.**

Glycerol also enters glycolytic pathway at this point.

6. In the next step, in presence of NAD^+ and inorganic phosphate (Pi), **glyceraldehyde-3-phosphate dehydrogenase oxidizes 3-phosphoglyceraldehyde to 1,3-bis-phosphoglycerate.**
7. In the next step, **1,3-bisphosphoglycerate is converted to 3-phosphoglycerate.** This reaction is catalyzed **by** the enzyme **phosphoglycerate kinase.**

   In this reaction, there is a **generation of ATP.** It is called substrate-level production of ATP (i.e. **substrate-level phosphorylation**).

   Arsenate inhibits phosphorylation at **this step** and, thus, ATP production.
8. Thereafter, **3-phosphoglycerate** is **converted to 2-phosphoglycerate** by the enzyme **phosphoglycerate mutase.**
9. In the next step, **enolase converts 2-phosphoglycerate to** a high-energy compound, called **phosphoenolpyruvate.**

   Enolase requires Mg^{2+} for its activity but **is inhibited by fluoride.**

   Since fluoride inhibits this reaction, therefore, **fluoride is added to the blood, as a preservative, in glucose estimation.**
10. Subsequently, **phosphoenolpyruvate is converted to pyruvate,** irreversibly. This reaction is catalyzed by the enzyme **pyruvate kinase,** which, in turn, phosphorylates ADP to ATP.

    Deficiency of pyruvate kinase leads to hemolytic anemia.

OXIDATION OF PYRUVIC ACID

Pyruvic acid is reduced to lactic acid under anaerobic conditions or is oxidized to acetyl-CoA under aerobic conditions.

- **Under anaerobic conditions: Pyruvate is reduced to lactate.** This reaction is catalyzed **by** the enzyme **lactate dehydrogenase,** which requires NADH.

  Tissues such as skeletal muscle, when function under hypoxic conditions, produce a large amount of lactic acid.
- **Under aerobic conditions: Pyruvate is** transported into mitochondria, where it is **oxidatively decarboxylated to acetyl-CoA by** the enzyme **pyruvate dehydrogenase complex** (Fig. 5.7).

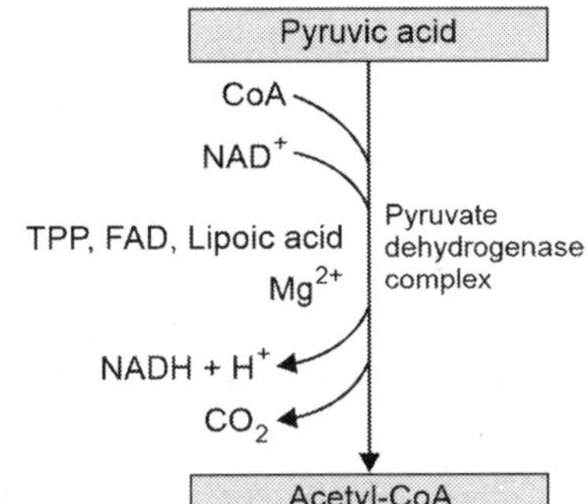

Fig. 5.7: Conversion of pyruvic acid to acetyl-CoA

ATP Production in Glycolysis

Number of ATP produced during glycolysis vary, depending upon the condition:

- **Under anaerobic condition,** conversion of 1,3-bisphosphoglycerate to 3-phosphoglycerate and phosphoenolpyruvate to pyruvate, each produces one ATP, thus, a total of 2 ATP are produced per molecule of a triose, or **4 molecules of ATP per molecule of hexose** (Fig. 5.8).

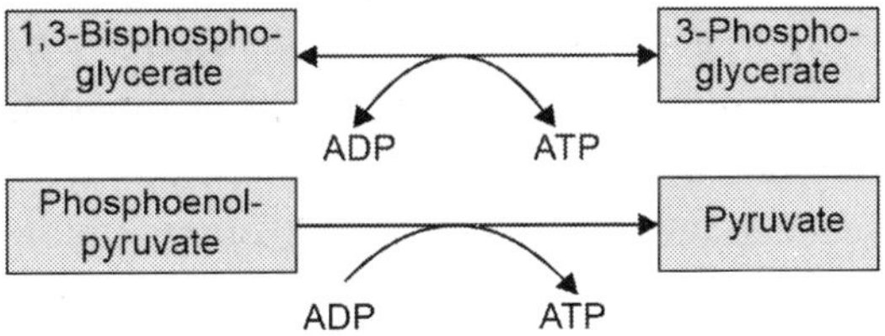

Fig. 5.8: ATP producing steps in anaerobic glycolysis

As 2 ATP are used in the initial two reactions of the process, i.e. in the conversion of glucose to glucose-6-phosphate and fructose-6-phosphate to fructose-1,6-bisphosphate, the **net energy yield** per molecule of glucose is only **2 ATP**.

- **Under aerobic conditions** NADH, which is produced during the conversion of 3-phosphoglycerate to 1,3-bisphosphoglycerate, enters the electron transport chain and releases 2.5 ATP, thus, additionally, 5 more ATP are produced per molecule of glucose. Therefore, a total yield under aerobic conditions is 9 ATP while the net yield is 7 ATP.

GLYCOGENESIS

Glycogenesis **(glycogen synthesis)** is the process of the synthesis of glycogen, wherein glucose is converted to glycogen. Although, it is operative in several tissues, liver and muscle are the main organs for the synthesis of glycogen. Glycogenesis is **stimulated by insulin.**

Though glycogen is synthesized from glucose, **excess intake of carbohydrate will not increase glycogen level in liver or muscle** due to the reason that:

- **Glycogen concentration is tightly regulated by hormones.**
- All the **dietary carbohydrates are digested and absorbed as glucose, which is mainly catabolized via glycolysis and is converted to pyruvate and finally to acetyl-CoA.**
- **Acetyl-CoA** has various metabolic fates, but **is primarily used in fatty acid synthesis and is finally converted to triacylglycerols** (Chapter 7).

Accordingly, **excess of dietary carbohydrate** is not converted to glycogen but to triacylglycerols and is **stored as fat**.

Various reactions of glycogenesis are described in Fig. 5.9.

1. Firstly, **glucose is activated** (phosphorylated) **to form glucose-6-phosphate.**
2. **Glucose-6-phosphate is isomerized to glucose-1-phosphate,** by the enzyme **phosphoglucomutase.**

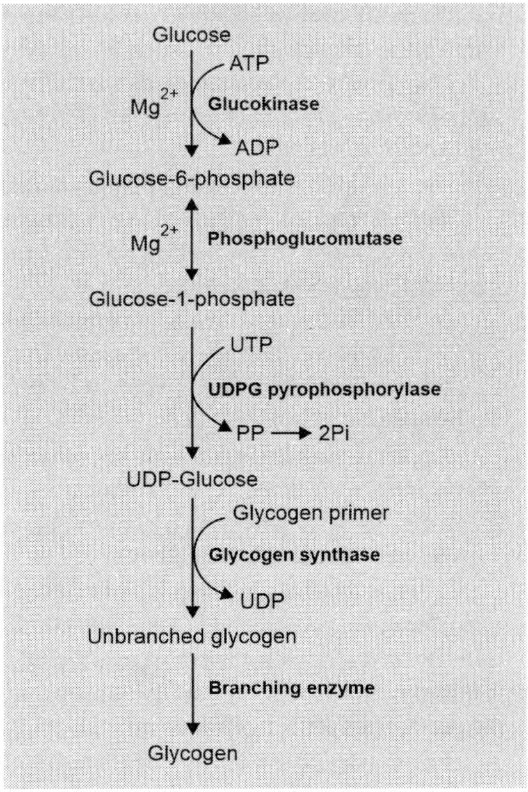

Fig. 5.9: Outline of glycogenesis

3. **Glucose-1-phosphate** reacts with UTP and gets **converted to** uridine-diphosphate glucose (**UDP-Glu** or UDPG). This reaction is catalyzed **by UDPG pyro-phosphorylase** (glucose-1-phosphate uridyl-transferase).
4. **From UDP-Glu, glucose is transferred to the glycogen** primer (i.e. the preformed oligosaccharide). This reaction is catalyzed by the enzyme **glycogen synthase.**

   The incoming glucose is linked to the primer at the non-reducing end by 1,4-α-glycosidic linkage and results in elongation of the pre-existing branch. This results in the formation of unbranched glycogen.
5. Once the straight chain containing nearly 11 glucose residues is formed, branching enzyme removes a block of 7–8 glycosyl residues from the growing

chain and transfers it to the neighboring chain.

The branch point again grows with the addition of more glucose molecules at the 1 → 4 linkage. This, in turn, results in the formation of a highly branched glycogen structure.

REGULATION OF BLOOD GLUCOSE LEVEL

Blood glucose level is maintained within the **normal** physiological **range** of **60–90 mg per 100 mL,** in the fasting (post-absorptive) state. If blood glucose level falls below the normal range, it is referred to as **hypoglycemia**. If blood glucose level rises above the normal range, it is referred to as **hyperglycemia.**

Blood glucose level is **regulated by several hormones.** Besides, some of the food stuffs also help in this process.

HORMONAL REGULATION OF BLOOD GLUCOSE

Several hormones regulate blood glucose concentration, as a result of which blood glucose level is maintained within the **normal range,** in the post-absorptive state.

Hormones which regulate blood glucose concentration are divided into two groups, i.e. (i) those which **lower blood glucose** level, and (ii) those which **increase blood glucose** level (Fig. 5.10).

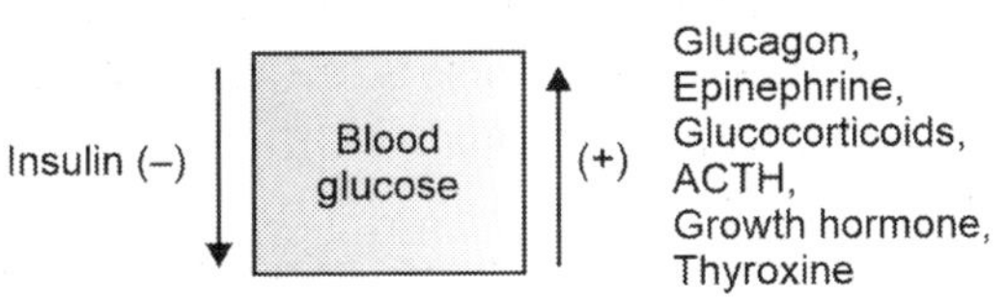

Fig. 5.10: Regulation of blood glucose by hormones

i. **Hormones which lower blood glucose level**

   Insulin is the only hormone which lowers blood glucose level, i.e. **has hypoglycemic action.**

   - Insulin is **released** into the blood stream **under the direct influence of hyperglycemia.**
   - Insulin is a **polypeptide containing 2 chains.**
   - It is **produced by the β-cells of the islets of Langerhans** of the pancreas.
   - Insulin **lowers blood glucose concentration** by various mechanisms:
     - Insulin **promotes uptake of glucose by the extrahepatic tissues.**
     - It also **promotes glycolysis and glycogenesis,** both **in the liver** and the **muscle.**
     - Insulin also **suppresses glycogenolysis in the liver** and the kidney.
     - It also **suppresses gluconeogenesis.**
     - Insulin also promotes transport of amino acids across the cell membrane and, thus, stimulates protein synthesis.
     - It also **inhibits ketogenesis** and **promotes lipogenesis.**

ii. **Hormones which increase blood glucose level**

   Several hormones are known to increase blood glucose level and are referred to as **hyperglycemic hormones** or **diabetogenic hormones.** These include **glucagon, epinephrine, glucocorticoids, growth hormone and thyroxine.**

   - **Glucagon:** Glucagon is **produced by the α-cells of the islets of Langerhans** of the pancreas.
     - Glucagon **synthesis is stimulated under the influence of hypoglycemia.**
     - It **acts only in the liver,** where it **promotes glycogenolysis.**
     - Glucagon also **promotes gluconeogenesis from amino acids and lactate.**
   - **Epinephrine:** Epinephrine, also called **adrenaline,** is a derivative of tyrosine. It is **secreted by the adrenal medulla.**
     - Epinephrine is a hormone in the **first line of defense against hypoglycemia.**

- It **promotes glycogenolysis,** both **in the liver and muscle.**
- Epinephrine also **promotes gluconeogenesis in the liver.**
- It also **inhibits the release of insulin from the pancreas,** which, in turn, reduces the **transport and utilization of glucose** in different tissues.
- At the same time, epinephrine also **stimulates secretion of glucagon.**

- **Glucocorticoids:** Glucocorticoids are **steroids, secreted by the adrenal cortex.**
  - Glucocorticoids are **antagonist to insulin.**
  - **Cortisol is a major glucocorticoid** present in blood.
  - Cortisol **stimulates protein catabolism in muscle** and **promotes gluconeogenesis in the liver.**
  - It also **stimulates lipolysis** and **inhibits glucose oxidation** by the liver.
  - Cortisol also **facilitates action of other hyperglycemic hormones** (permissive effects) such as glucagon, epinephrine, and growth hormone, **which further inhibit uptake and utilization of glucose** by the peripheral tissues.
- **Growth hormone:** Growth hormone is **secreted by the anterior pituitary.**
  - **Secretion** of growth hormone is **stimulated under the influence of hypoglycemia.**
  - Prolonged administration of the growth hormone also **stimulates the secretion of insulin.** As a result of which, **β-cells are exhausted,** thereby **producing a diabetes-like situation.**
  - Growth hormone also **decreases glucose uptake and utilization by muscles.**
  - It also **promotes lipolysis in the adipose tissue.**
- **Thyroxine:** Thyroxine is **secreted by the thyroid gland.**
  - Thyroxine **stimulates intestinal absorption of glucose.**
  - It also **promotes glycogenolysis** as well as **gluconeogenesis in the liver.**

EFFECT OF TYPE OF FOOD ON BLOOD GLUCOSE

Type of food also exhibits its effect on blood glucose level.

- **Foods** which are **rich in simple carbohydrates** or starch, but low in fiber and fat, **are digested and absorbed rapidly.** As a result of it, these **cause large and rapid rise in blood glucose concentration.** Body reacts to the rising blood glucose level and releases insulin, which in turn, lowers blood glucose level and stabilizes it.
- **Other foods,** especially, those, which are **rich in dietary fiber,** resistant starch or fat, **cause lesser response to blood glucose** with smaller alterations.

GLYCEMIC INDEX AND GLYCEMIC LOAD

Glycemic Index

Glycemic index (GI) refers to the **effect of a particular type of carbohydrate food on blood glucose level** in relation to carbohydrate-containing reference food such as glucose or white bread. It is a measure of how quickly the glucose is released into the bloodstream, after consuming a particular food.

Glycemic index, thus, measures how quickly, and how much, a carbohydrate raises blood sugar.

According to the glycemic index foods are categorised into **three groups** as:

Low GI foods—with a GI value below 55,

Moderate GI foods—GI value between 56 and 69, and

High GI foods—GI value of 70 and above.

High-glycemic foods, like pastries, raise blood sugar high and rapidly, whereas low-glycemic foods raise it gently and to a lesser degree.

Low GI foods, that are rich in fiber, should form an important component of a healthy diet.

Glycemic load

Glycemic load refers to the GI and the total amount of the available carbohydrate present in the consumed food.

Glycemic load (glucose load) value is categorized into three groups as:

Low: Below 10,

Moderate: Between 10 and 19, and

High: Above 20.

CARBOHYDRATE MALNUTRITION

Carbohydrate Deficiency

When a person is **on a carbohydrate-free diet,** proteins and fat are used as alternate sources of energy. Excessive breakdown of these substances, in turn, leads to excessive **formation of ketone bodies.**

Such individuals **exhibit symptoms,** similar to those seen during starvation, e.g. **abnormal fat metabolism, breakdown of tissue proteins, increased sodium excretion, loss of energy and fatigue.** Small amount of carbohydrates (50 to 100 g) prevents these symptoms.

Not getting enough dietary carbohydrate can cause problems, such as:

- Without sufficient fuel, **body gets no energy.**
- Additionally, without sufficient glucose, **central nervous system (CNS) suffers,** which may cause dizziness, and mental and physical weakness.
- If **body** has insufficient carbohydrate intake or stores, it will **consume protein as a source of fuel.** This is problematic because the body needs protein to make muscles. Using protein for fuel, instead of carbohydrates, also **puts stress on the kidneys,** leading to the passage of painful byproducts in the urine.
- People, who do not consume enough carbohydrates, may also **suffer from deficiency of dietary fiber,** which can cause **digestive problems and constipation.**

Overconsumption of Dietary Carbohydrates

Increased regular consumption of refined sugars has been shown to be associated with the **increased risk of weight gain** and body mass index **(obesity)**. This can also lead to **type 2 diabetes mellitus, cardiovascular diseases** (CVD) and **dental caries.**

- **Weight gain and Obesity:** Carbohydrates are the preferred source of energy for the body. When we eat any type of carbohydrate our body breaks it to glucose, which is released into bloodstream and causes a rise in blood glucose level. If we eat a moderate amount of carbohydrates, body's cells use what they need for energy and store excess of it as glycogen. However, glycogen stores are limited and once these are saturated, an **excess of glucose is stored as fat.** Thus, overconsumption of carbohydrates, for a long period, **results in weight gain and obesity.**
- **Poor appetite control:** Eating **too much of carbohydrates,** in one sitting, causes a large **increase in blood glucose level.** This, in turn, causes **pancreas to release large amount of insulin,** which leads to an equally **large decrease in blood glucose level.** When blood glucose level suddenly falls, brain sends hunger signals, meaning that one **demands more food.** Thus, the overall result is **poor appetite control,** as one is constantly craving for food, despite eating regularly.
- **Fatigue:** As overconsumption of carbohydrates causes a rapid surge and, thereafter, a rapid fall in blood glucose level, this has a direct effect on overall energy level. As a result of it, one will suddenly feel full of energy, and shortly the energy level will crash. **Fluctuating**

energy levels affect proper functioning of the body, since one will be constantly switching between feelings of too much energy and not enough energy.

- **Dental caries:** Dental caries is the **progressive destruction** (demineralization) **of teeth,** by the **acids produced by bacteria** acting on sugars and other fermentable carbohydrates on the tooth surface. Longer the sugar remains in the mouth, more likely it will promote dental caries. Foods that stick to the teeth, such as candies, cookies and beverages like cola, are more likely to cause dental caries. The most important way to protect against dental caries is regular (twice daily) brushing of teeth with a fluoride-containing toothpaste. Fluoride strengthens the tooth enamel, providing resistance to decay.
- **Risk of type 2 diabetes:** Level of glucose in blood is carefully monitored and kept within narrow limits by the action of the hormone insulin. **Overconsumption of carbohydrates** cause pancreas to produce and release increasing amount of insulin. Pushing the **pancreas to over exert** and, ultimately, interferes with its ability to produce insulin. Both, insulin resistance and pancreas failing to produce enough insulin are characteristics of **type 2 diabetes.** This, in turn, can also cause permanent damage to the body and may affect all the major organs and vessels, including heart, kidneys, eyes, nerves and blood vessels.
- **Risk of a cardiovascular disease (CVD):** As discussed above, high carbohydrate diet results in accumulation of fat. Increased concentration of lipids is also associated with an increased risk of CVD. Some forms of **complex carbohydrates,** such as pectin in fruit and β-glucan in oats, may slightly **reduce the level of cholesterol in blood.** These are the forms of soluble fiber. There is also some evidence that resistant starch may have a slight, beneficial effect on CVD risk. Regular consumption of wholegrain foods has been linked with heart health, possibly as a result of the breakdown products (e.g. short chain fatty acids) formed and absorbed in the large bowel.
- **Risk of cancer:** Some studies suggest that **populations with a high intake of fiber-rich foods** experience a **lower incidence of large bowel cancer** than populations with low intake of these foods.

SOME IMPORTANT QUESTIONS

1. **Define carbohydrate. Classify them.**
2. **Describe calorific value, recommended daily allowances, sources and biological functions of carbohydrates.**
3. **Describe various disorders due to carbohydrate overnutrition.**
4. **Define glycolysis. Outline the process of glycolysis.**
5. **Define glycogenolysis. Outline reactions of this pathway.**
6. **What is glycogenesis? Give reactions of glycogenesis.**
7. **Differentiate between**
   i. Simple sugars and complex carbohydrates
   ii. Good carbohydrates and bad carbohydrates
   iii. Anaerobic and aerobic glycolysis

8. Discuss briefly:

i. Digestion of carbohydrates
ii. Absorption of monosaccharides
iii. Hormonal regulation of blood glucose
iv. Gluconeogenesis

9. Write notes on:

i. Dietary fiber
ii. Calorific value of carbohydrates
iii. Dental caries
iv. Glycemic index

CHAPTER 6

Dietary Fiber

Dietary fiber refers to **indigestible carbohydrates** which include **resistant** or **nondigestible oligosaccharides, polysaccharides, lignin** and **similar plant products** such as cellulose and hemicelluloses, pectin, gums and mucilage. These are referred to as **indigestible carbohydrates** since these cannot be digested by human beings due to absence of the required digestive enzymes. Dietary fibers directly pass into the large intestine where some of these are **partially fermented while others are excreted as such in the large intestine.** However, dietary fiber forms an essential component of human diet, due to its several beneficial effects, and thus, is dietary essential.

BIOLOGICAL SIGNIFICANCE OF DIETARY FIBER

In recent years, dietary fiber is considered as an essential component for a healthy diet and has been shown to be beneficial not only for health maintenance but also for the prevention of several diseases including cardiovascular disease, diabetes, colon cancer.

High Intake of Dietary Fiber has many Health Benefits

- Dietary fiber has been shown to modulate ingestion, digestion, absorption and metabolism of macronutrients and thus reduces the risk of hyperlipidemia, hypercholesterolemia and hyperglycemia.
- Dietary fiber has also been shown to reduce contact time of various toxins including carcinogens within the intestinal lumen.
- It also promotes healthy bowel movement and reduces the risk of chronic diseases such as coronary heart disease and diabetes.
- The soluble fiber undergoing fermentation in the colon also provides 2 kcal per gram of fiber (ICMR-NIN, 2020).
- Diets rich in fiber forms bulk of the food, it takes longer to eat, and thus, gives a feeling of fullness. So, dietary fiber not only regulates body weight but also lowers the risk of obesity.
- Higher intake of soluble fiber also **delays stomach emptying** and, thus **regulates blood glucose level.** This in turn **reduces the risk of type 2 diabetes.**
- Diet rich in fiber also **lowers the risk of certain types of cancers.** It is due to the reason that food with large amounts of fruits and vegetables, **provides antioxidants,** which **protect our body against cell damage and cancer.**
- Soluble dietary fiber has long water holding capacity. It also **lowers serum**

cholesterol and thus, **reduces the risk of a cardiovascular disease.**

- Diet rich in insoluble fiber **adds bulk to feces and softens stool for its easy passage.** Thus, dietary fiber **helps in the prevention of** certain conditions such as constipation, hemorrhoids and diverticulitis, particularly when fluid intake is high.

However, excess of dietary fiber in the diet has been shown to inhibit the absorption of micronutrients (some of the vitamins and minerals). This in turn results in deficiency of some minerals, **such as zinc, calcium, magnesium and iron.**

CLASSIFICATION OF DIETARY FIBER

Dietary fiber can be classified in different ways, **according to their chemical structure, water solubility and fermentability**.

- **According to their chemical structure** dietary fibers are classified as **oligosaccharides and polysaccharides:**
  - **Oligosaccharides:** These types of dietary fibers include **resistant oligosaccharides** which comprise of **3 to 9 monosaccharide units.**
  - **Polysaccharides:** These types of dietary fibers include **non-starch polysaccharides** and **resistant starch** which **have more than 10 monosaccharide units.**
- **According to their solubility** in water dietary fibers are classified as **soluble dietary fibers** and **insoluble dietary fibers:**
  - **Soluble dietary fibers:** Pectin, gums, mucilage and some of the hemicelluloses are soluble in water, and hence are referred to as soluble fibers. These are the **resistant oligosaccharides** which gets well-fermented in the large intestine. Besides, these also include certain non-starch linear polysaccharides such as β-glucan and high molecular weight guar gum which have gel-forming nature. Due to their gel-forming nature in the intestinal tract, these influence the metabolism of glucose and lipids.
  - **Insoluble dietary fibers:** Cellulose, lignin, hemicelluloses and resistant starch are water insoluble, and hence are referred to as insoluble fibers. These are the branched polysaccharides which are less-fermentable in the large intestine and are excreted unchanged. These are also referred to as galactomannans and are predominantly found in cell walls of grains and vegetables.

CALORIFIC VALUE OF DIETARY FIBER

ICMR-NIN (2020) Expert Group has suggested that the soluble fiber undergoing fermentation in the colon provides 2 kcal per gram of fiber.

RECOMMENDED DIETARY INTAKE OF DIETARY FIBER

For the first time ICMR-NIN (2020) Group has considered recommendations for the dietary fiber, based on energy intake. **Safe intake of dietary fiber** has been suggested as 15 **g/1000 kcal**.

Adequate intake of dietary fiber has been suggested as **40 g/d for men performing moderate work** and **30 g/d for women performing moderate work.**

DIETARY SOURCES OF DIETARY FIBER

Dietary fibers are obtained from the edible, generally endogenous, portion of the plants. Common dietary sources include fruits, cereal grains (barley and oats, etc.), legumes and vegetables. The linear polysaccharides (β-glucan or mannans) are predominantly found in date, aloe vera and green coffee beans and mushrooms, etc.

Resistant starch is predominantly found in green banana while pectin in fruits and vegetables.

METABOLISM OF DIETARY FIBER

Unlike sugar and starch, dietary fiber is neither absorbed in the small intestine nor hydrolyzed to glucose, to release energy. Since these are resistant to digestion in human beings, they pass into the large intestine, relatively intact and directly reach the large intestine, where these are:

- Either, partially metabolized (fermented) by the bacteria in the large intestine to hydrogen, carbon dioxide and short chain fatty acids which are further metabolized to generate energy.
- Or, these are excreted as such in the stool.

Cellulose and stretch reflex: Cellulose (polysaccharide) materials present in the diet form the bulk of the food. It cannot be digested by human beings because of the absence of the enzyme cellulase. The cellulose helps in the movement of the food through the gastrointestinal tract. The cellulose material of the diet absorbs the waste from large intestine and while doing so it stretches the wall of the large intestine and as a result, defecation takes place. This is called stretch reflex.

SOME IMPORTANT QUESTIONS

1. **Define dietary fiber. Give its classification and explain the health benefits of dietary fiber.**
2. **Write notes on:**
   i. Sources and recommended dietary intake of dietary fiber
   ii. Significance of dietary fiber

CHAPTER

7

Lipids

Lipid (Greek: lipos, means fat) is a heterogeneous group of hydrophobic organic molecules found in cells. These are the molecules that yield high energy and have a chemical composition, mainly of **carbon, hydrogen** and **oxygen**.

Lipids, primarily, are composed of fats and oils, and include a family of organic compounds which are, mostly, **insoluble in water** but **soluble in organic solvents** such as alcohol, ether or acetone. These also occur throughout the living world, i.e. in all cell types including micro-organisms, higher plants and animals. Lipids contribute to cell structure, provide stored fuel and take part in many biological processes. They make up about 70% of dry weight of the nervous system and are crucial for the healthy functioning of nerve cells.

Dietary fat, mainly, consists of triacylglycerols (triglycerides). Besides, it includes a heterogenous group of compounds in small proportions, viz. phospholipids, glycolipids, monoacylglycerols, diacylglycerols and some non-glyceride components.

BIOLOGICAL IMPORTANCE OF DIETARY LIPIDS

- Dietary fat enhances texture, flavour, taste and palatability of food.
- Fats are essential for meeting some of the nutritional needs, like essential fatty acids, i.e. linoleic acid (ω-6 fatty acid) and α-linolenic acid (ω-3 fatty acid). EFAs are metabolized at various sites in the body, to generate a group of biologically active compounds, which perform several important physiological functions.
- Fat also serves as a rich source of energy, since it provides 9 kcal/g, compared to proteins or carbohydrates which provide 4 kcal/g.
- Fat also serves as a vehicle for fat-soluble vitamins (A, D, E and K) and thus helps in their absorption.
- Fat decreases its gastric emptying time and imparts a feeling of fullness and satiety.
- Fat, along with proteins, constitute major components of body fluids and cell membranes.
- Lipids also serve as structural components of cell membrane, function as energy storehouse, and provide insulation, cellular communication and protection.

CLASSIFICATION OF LIPIDS

Lipids exhibit great structural variability. They constitute a category of substances that are hydrophobic in nature and are soluble in nonpolar solvents. Lipids are classified into three groups (Fig. 7.1).

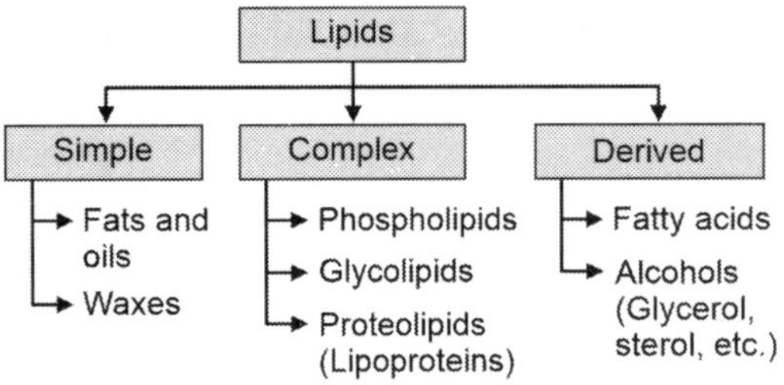

Fig. 7.1: Classification of lipids

1. Simple Lipids

Simple lipids are the **esters of fatty acids with alcohol.** These include **neutral fats, oils and waxes.** Neutral fats and oils are the mixtures of triacylglycerols (also called triglycerides) whose fatty acids composition may vary with the source. They differ from each other in the way that fats are solid while oils are liquid at room temperature.

i. **Neutral fats** are obtained from animal sources. They have, comparatively, a greater number of saturated fatty acids and have higher melting points.
ii. **Oils** are obtained from plant seeds. They are usually rich in unsaturated fatty acids and have low melting points.
iii. **Waxes** are the esters of long chain fatty acids with high molecular weight mono-hydroxy aliphatic alcohols. They are used in the manufacturing of wax-polish.

2. Complex Lipids

In addition to fatty acids and alcohol, complex lipids **also contain an amphipathic group.** For example, lipids conjugated with phosphoric acid are called **phospholipids,** lipids conjugated with sugars are referred to as **glycolipids,** etc.

3. Derived Lipids

Derived lipids are obtained after the hydrolysis of the simple and compound lipids. These include fatty acids, glycerol, monoglycerides and diglycerides, steroids, terpenes and carotenoids.

FAT AND FATTY ACIDS

Fat, mainly, comprises **triacylglycerols,** also called triglycerides or neutral lipids. These are the fatty acid tri-esters of glycerol (glycerin, a tri-hydric alcohol).

Glycerol with one molecule of fatty acid is called **monoacylglycerol,** with two molecules of fatty acids as **diacylglycerol** and with three molecules of fatty acids as **triacylglycerol** (Fig. 7.2).

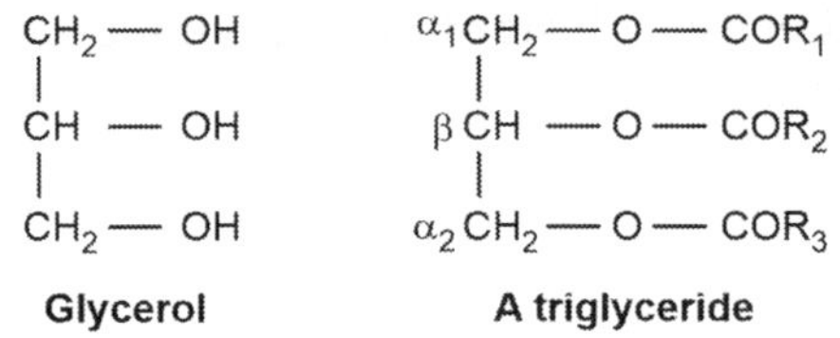

Fig. 7.2: Glycerol and a triacylglycerol

- A molecule of triacylglycerol may have **three similar or dissimilar fatty acids,** which **may be saturated and/or unsaturated.**
- All the natural fats and oils, generally, have three dissimilar fatty acids, both saturated as well as unsaturated. These are referred to as **mixed triacylglycerols.**
- **Plant oils are,** usually, **rich in unsaturated fatty acids.**
- **Triacylglycerols are transported in plasma, in chylomicrons** and very low-density lipoproteins **(VLDL).**
- **Nomenclature of triglycerides is done according to the presence of fatty acids** which are **attached to glycerol,** e.g. a triacylglycerol having palmitic acid at carbon-1, arachidonic acid at carbon-2 and stearic acid at carbon-3 of glycerol is called 1-palmitoyl-2-arachidonoyl-3-stearoyl-glycerol.
- Generally, **a saturated fatty acid is found at the primary alcoholic group,** i.e. **at α-position** of glycerol (position number 1 or 3) and an **unsaturated fatty acid** is found **at the β-position** (position number 2).

FATTY ACIDS

Fatty acids are the **carboxylic acids with a long hydrocarbon side chain** that may be **saturated or unsaturated** (having one or more double bonds). A fatty acid has a methyl group at one end and an acid group at the other.

Fatty acids are the building blocks of various lipids and are the primary constituents of all dietary fats.

- **Major source of the circulating free fatty acids is adipose tissue.**
- After **hydrolysis of the triacylglycerols** in chylomicrons and VLDL, **free fatty acids enter plasma** and serve an important source of energy for many tissues.
- Since free fatty acids have limited solubility in water, these are **transported in plasma, bound to albumin** which has specific binding sites for free fatty acids.
- Most of the naturally occurring fatty acids **have even number of carbon atoms,** since these are **synthesized from acetyl-CoA,** i.e. from two carbon units.
- According to their chain length, fatty acids are **divided into three groups,** referred to as:
  - **Short chain fatty acids,** which contain **4 to 8 carbon** atoms
  - **Medium chain fatty acids,** which contain **10 to 14 carbon** atoms, and
  - **Long chain fatty acids,** which contain **16 or more carbon** atoms.
- All types of fatty acids **have different physicochemical properties** and are metabolized in the body in different ways.
- In **plants and higher animals,** predominant fatty acids are those **containing 16 and 18 carbon atoms,** e.g. palmitic acid, oleic acid, linoleic acid, stearic acid, etc.

Biological Functions of Fatty Acids

Fatty acids perform several functions in the body:

- These are used in the body for the **generation of cellular energy and biosynthesis of membrane lipids.**
- Fatty acids are also essential for the **development of central nervous system** (CNS).
- These also **modulate lipoprotein metabolism** and risk for diet-related diseases such as coronary heart disease, diabetes and cancers.
- As **integral components of cell membranes,** fatty acids **affect membrane fluidity** and **lipid protein interactions,** which in turn **alters membrane-bound transport systems, ion channels, membrane-bound enzymes, cellular receptors for hormones** and **neurotransmitters.**
- α-Linolenic acid (AA) and eicosa-pentaenoic acid (EPA) of the membrane bound phospholipids also **give rise to bioactive eicosanoids** such as thromboxanes, leukotrienes and prostacyclins, which have strong proinflammatory, pro-aggregatory and vasoconstricting effects.
- During the fetal and early infant development, there is rapid accretion of AA and DHA in infant brain.

Classification of Fatty Acids

Based on their chemical nature, the fatty acids are broadly grouped as **saturated** (SFA), **monounsaturated** (MUFA) and **polyunsaturated** (PUFA). There are several fatty acids in each group.

Saturated Fatty Acids

Saturated fatty acids have a **suffix '-anoic'** after the name of the hydrocarbon chain, e.g. **octadecanoic acid,** a saturated fatty acid **having 18 carbon atoms.**

- Saturated fatty acids are highly flexible molecules and can assume a wide range of conformations because there is relatively free rotation around the C–C bond.
- These are commonly found in fat, which is obtained from the animal source, such as butter.

Saturated fatty acids of common biological significance are listed in Table 7.1.

Table 7.1: Saturated fatty acids

Fatty acids	*Number of carbons*	*Formula*	*Sources*
Acetic acid	2	CH_3–COOH	Fermentation of carbohydrates
Butyric acid	4	CH_3–$(CH2)_2$–COOH	Butter
Caproic acid	6	CH_3–$(CH2)_4$–COOH	Butter, fat from plant sources
Caprylic acid	8	CH_3–$(CH2)_6$–COOH	-do-
Capric acid	10	CH_3–$(CH2)_8$–COOH	-do-
Lauric acid	12	CH_3–$(CH2)_{10}$–COOH	Coconut oil
Myristic acid	14	CH_3–$(CH2)_{12}$–COOH	-do-
Palmitic acid	16	CH_3–$(CH2)_{14}$–COOH	Animal and plant fats
Stearic acid	18	CH_3–$(CH2)_{16}$–COOH	-do-
Arachidic acid	20	CH_3–$(CH2)_{18}$–COOH	Peanut oil

Most of the saturated fatty acids (SFAs) consist of **straight, even-numbered chains** of 4–24 carbon atoms. These are classified as **short chain** (SCFA: C <10), **medium chain** (MCFA: C12 and C14) and **long chain** (LCFA: C16–C24) fatty acids. These fatty acids **do not have a double bond,** e.g. arachidic acid, palmitic acid, etc.

- Fats from coconut oil, vanaspati, ghee and butter, and animal foods (milk and milk products, and meat) provide saturated fatty acids.
- The short and medium chain saturated fatty acids, present in ghee, butter and coconut oil, are easily digested and absorbed, and are therefore, good for infants and young children.
- High intake of saturated fatty acids is known to increase serum total and LDL-cholesterol levels, reduce insulin sensitivity, enhance thrombogenicity and increase CVD risk. Thus, their intake should be limited in adults.

Unsaturated Fatty Acids

Unsaturated fatty acids have a **suffix '-enoic'** after the name of the hydrocarbon chain, e.g. **octadecanoic acid,** an **unsaturated fatty acid having 18 carbon atoms** and **one double bond.** It is also called **oleic acid.**

Unsaturated fatty acids may have one **(monounsaturated: MUFA)** or more **(polyunsaturated: PUFA)** double bonds.

Double bonds in the unsaturated fatty acids **may be** either ***cis* or *trans*** relative to the plane of the acyl chain. Fatty acids of **nutritional significance** have ***cis* configuration.**

Unsaturated fatty acids having double bond in the *trans* configuration are called ***trans* fatty acids.**

Humans Can Synthesize SFA and MUFA Besides Obtaining them from the Diet

- **Monounsaturated fatty acids:** Monounsaturated fatty acids have one double bond. They are, usually, liquid at room temperature. Oils from palm, groundnut, cottonseed, sesame and olive, are rich in monounsaturated fatty acids as compared to other oils.
- **Polyunsaturated fatty acids:** These have more than one double bond in the molecule and are liquid at room temperature. Polyunsaturated fatty acids help reduce cholesterol, and lower the risk of a heart disease. Soybean oil, corn oil, safflower oil, walnuts and sunflower seeds are good sources of polyunsaturated fatty acids, i.e. these are present only in plant foods.

Polyunsaturated (PUFA) are grouped into two series (ω-3 or ω-6), depending upon whether the double bond closest to the methyl end is located at C3 or C6 position.

Humans however **cannot synthesize the parent PUFA,** i.e. linoleic acid (C18:2, ω-6) and α-linolenic acid (C18:3, ω-3) which are dietary essential fatty acids. These are metabolized by consecutive chain elongase and desaturase enzymes to other long chain fatty acids, such as arachidonic acid (C20:4, ω-6), eicosapentaenoic acid (EPA, 20:5) and docosahexaenoic acid (DHA, 22:6), which are incorporated into the membrane lipids.

Nomenclature of Unsaturated Fatty Acids

Widely used convention to represent an unsaturated fatty acid, is to indicate the **number of carbon atoms,** followed by the **number of double bonds with their positions** in the hydrocarbon chain. For example, **octadecanoic acid,** a fatty acid with **18 carbon atoms and one double bond** present **after carbon atom number 9** (i.e. between carbon atoms number 9 and 10), is represented as **18:1; 9** (Fig. 7.3).

$$\overset{18}{CH_3}-(CH_2)_7-\overset{10}{CH}=\overset{9}{CH}-(CH_2)_7-\overset{1}{COOH}$$

Fig. 7.3: Oleic acid—an unsaturated fatty acid

An unsaturated fatty acid **may be identified either by the delta or the omega system of nomenclature.**

Delta System of Nomenclature of a Fatty Acid

According to the delta (δ) system of nomenclature, carbon atoms in the fatty acid chain are **numbered from the carboxy-terminal end.** This carbon atom (–COOH) is labeled carbon atom number 1. The carbon atom next to the carboxyl group, i.e. **the α-carbon atom,** is referred to as carbon atom **number 2,** and so on.

Accordingly, an unsaturated fatty acid is represented by:

- A **number showing the number of carbon atoms,** followed by the **symbol colon (:)** and **another number,** which represents the **number of double bonds.**
- This is **followed by the symbol 'Δ'** and some **other numbers as superscript,** which indicate **positions of the double bonds.**

For example, **linoleic acid,** a **fatty acid with 18 carbon** atoms and **two double bonds,** which are present **after carbon atom numbers 9 and 12,** is represented as **18:2 $\Delta^{9,12}$** (Fig. 7.4).

Omega System of Nomenclature of a Fatty Acid

According to the omega (ω) system of nomenclature, carbon atoms are numbered from the methyl end. This carbon is referred to as omega (ω) carbon. Accordingly, an unsaturated fatty acid is represented by the **omega symbol** (ω), **followed by a number** represents the **number of the carbon atom** immediately after which the first double bond appears from the methyl end.

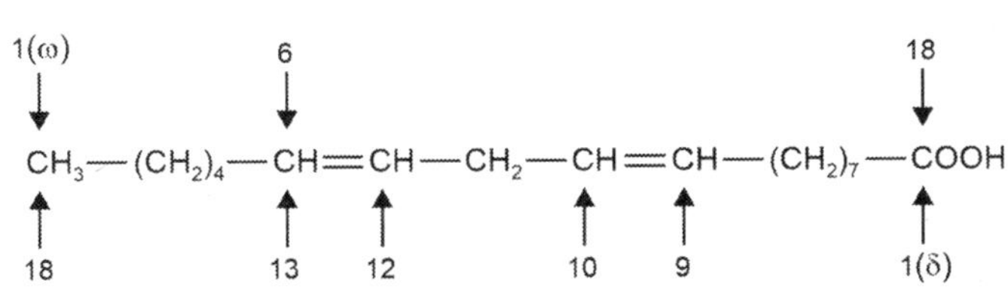

18:2 $\Delta^{9,12}$ (Delta system)
or ω-6 Fatty acid (Omega system)

Fig. 7.4: Linoleic acid

For example, in **linoleic acid,** since the **first double bond from the ω-end is present after the sixth carbon atom,** it is, thus, referred to as **ω-6 fatty acid** (Fig. 7.5).

Linolenic (ω-3 or n-3) and linoleic (ω-6 or n-6) acids are the simple PUFA.

- **Omega-3 fatty acid:** α-Linolenic acid is referred to as ω-3 fatty acid. It is beneficial for our body. The body cannot make omega-3 fatty acids and we have to get them from food. Soyabean, rapeseed and mustard oils contribute significant proportion of α-linolenic (n-3) acid. Legumes/pulses mustard and fenugreek seeds, and green leafy vegetables are also good sources of α-linolenic acid. On the other hand, fish and fish oils provide long chain n-3 fatty acids, which are biologically more active than α-linolenic acid present in plant foods. It helps to reduce inflammation (redness, swelling and irritation), which, in turn, can help with a wide range of diseases, including arthritis and heart disease. If this type of fat is missing in our diet, we might experience fatigue, poor memory, dry skin, depression, heart problems and poor circulation.
- **Omega-6 fatty acid:** Linoleic acid is referred to as ω-6 fatty acid, since the first double bond, from the ω-end, is present after the sixth carbon atom. Elongation and desaturation of linoleic acid can form arachidonic acid, which acts as a precursor for a series of 20-carbon compounds, called eicosanoids. Oilseeds, nuts and common vegetable oils are good sources of linoleic acid.

Polyunsaturated Fatty Acids

Unsaturated fatty acids having **two or more double bonds** are referred to as polyunsaturated fatty acids **(PUFA)**. They are obtained from plant seed oils, e.g. **soybean oil, sunflower oil, groundnut oil,** etc. PUFA perform various **functions**:

- PUFA form an important **constituent of biological membranes.**
- These are essentially required for the **esterification of cholesterol,** and, thus, help in its transport and metabolism. Particularly, consumption of fat containing **ω-6 fatty acids helps in lowering plasma cholesterol level.**
- Diet rich in **ω-3 fatty acids helps in lowering plasma level of triacylglycerols.**
- **Arachidonic acid** also **acts as a precursor** of some pharmacologically important compounds, such as **prostaglandins, thromboxanes and leukotrienes.** These are referred to as **eicosanoids.**

ESSENTIAL FATTY ACIDS

Linoleic acid (omega-6 fatty acid) and **linolenic acid** (omega-3 fatty acid) are referred to as **essential fatty acids, since these form an essential component of the diet and are necessary for growth and normal health.** These helps control inflammation, blood clotting and brain development (Fig. 7.6).

These are **not synthesized in our body** and serve a number of important functions, like:

i. Synthesis of prostaglandins.
ii. Serve as structural element of mitochondrial membrane.
iii. Help in the prevention of fatty liver.
iv. Play an important role in vision.

Biological Significance of Essential Fatty Acids

- Essential fatty acids (EFA) are **essential components of cell membranes.**

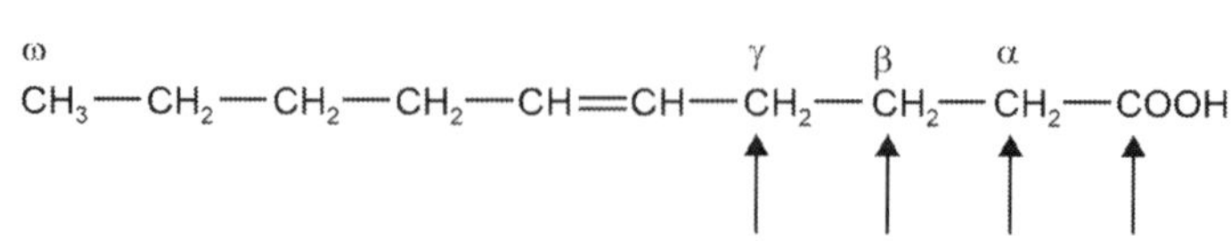

Fig. 7.5: Omega system of nomenclature of a fatty acid

$$\overset{1}{CH_3}—(CH_2)_7—\overset{9}{CH}=CH—(CH_2)_7—COOH$$

Oleic acid
(ω-9 Fatty acid, a nonessential fatty acid)

$$\overset{1}{CH_3}—(CH_2)_4—\overset{6}{CH}=CH—CH_2—CH=CH—(CH_2)_7—COOH$$

Linoleic acid
(ω-6 Fatty acid, an essential fatty acid)

$$\overset{1}{CH_3}—\overset{2}{CH_2}—\overset{3}{CH}=CH—CH_2—CH=CH—CH_2—CH=CH—(CH_2)_7—COOH$$

α-Linolenic acid
(ω-3 Fatty acid, an essential fatty acid)

Fig. 7.6: Essential and nonessential fatty acids

- While ω-6 PUFAs are predominant in all cells, the nerve tissue has high levels of long chain ω-3 PUFA.
- An appropriate balance of the two PUFAs, namely linoleic and α-linolenic acids in the diets, is **essential for the functioning of vascular, immune, nervous and renal systems and for early human development.**
- The lipid lowering and other physiological effects of individual members of the PUFAs vary widely. As compared to linoleic acid, **α-linolenic (ω-3) acid** is more beneficial **for prevention of inflammation** and accumulation of fatty material in blood vessels **(altherosclerosis)** and clotting of blood **(thrombosis).** The long chain ω-3 PUFA of fish oils and micro algae have greater antiatherogenic, antithrombotic and anti-inflammatory effects than α-linolenic (ω-3) acid of plant foods.
- These are **important for vision and brain growth.** Therefore, pregnant women should consume foods that are rich in α-linolenic acid and other long chain ω-3 PUFA from fish and fish oils.
- PUFAs, particularly ω**-3 PUFA, increase insulin sensitivity, increase peripheral glucose utilization** and **decrease adiposity,** and, hence, are anti-atherogenic.
- The **ω-6 PUFA decreases plasma cholesterol** as well as **HDL cholesterol** level (only at high intake).

CHOLESTEROL

Cholesterol is a **derivative of** the **cyclopentano-perhydro-phenanthrene ring,** also called **steroid nucleus,** which consists of four fused, nonpolar rings which are labeled A, B, C and D.

Cholesterol **has 27 carbon atoms** with a **hydroxyl group on carbon number 3,** a **double bond between carbon numbers 5 and 6, two methyl groups** attached to **carbon numbers 18 and 19,** and a **side chain** that is attached to **carbon number 17.**

Cholesterol, also referred to as free cholesterol, is hydrophilic in nature and thus, is not soluble in water. Due to this reason, it cannot be transported in plasma in free form.

An adult man contains about 1 g cholesterol/kg body weight. Cholesterol content in **normal** human **blood varies between 130 and 220 mg/100 mL,** which is equally distributed between plasma and erythrocytes. About 30% of the circulating cholesterol occurs free, while the remaining of it exists in the form of cholesterol esters.

Free cholesterol is **present** in abundance, **in bile.** It is also present in large amount in the **myelin structure of the brain and in biological membranes.**

Cholesterol is also used in the biosynthesis of **bile acids, steroid hormones and vitamin D** (Fig. 7.7).

Cholesterol is found in all body cells and plays a key role in the formation of brain, nerve tissue and is a precursor for some

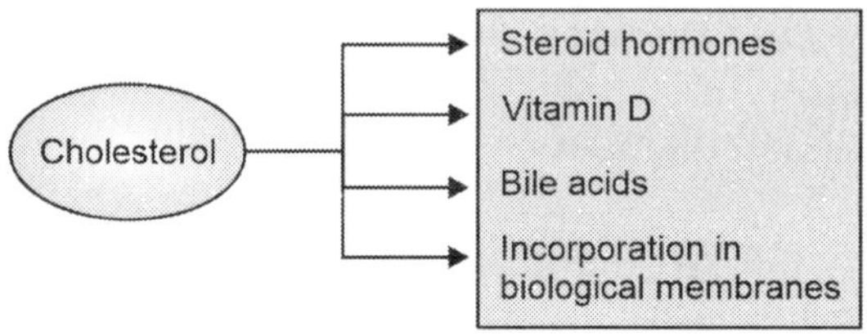

Fig. 7.7: Uses of cholesterol in the body

hormones and vitamin D. It is synthesized in the body and, hence, it is not an essential dietary component.

- Cholesterol is present only in foods of animal origin, such as milk, meat and prawn, but not in plant foods. Vegetable oils do not contain cholesterol. Egg yolk and organ meats, such as liver, kidney and brain contain very high amounts of cholesterol.
- High dietary cholesterol increases blood cholesterol. The blood cholesterol elevating effect of dietary saturated fat increases, when cholesterol consumption is high. Therefore, cholesterol intake should be maintained below 200 mg/day.
- One can reduce both saturated fat and cholesterol intake by limiting the consumption of high fat-containing animal foods, like butter, ghee, meat, egg and organ meats and consuming low fat (skimmed) milk instead of whole milk.

CALORIC VALUE OF FAT

Fat is a concentrated source of energy and provides 9 kcal/g.

RECOMMENDED DAILY ALLOWANCES OF LIPIDS

ICMR-NIN (2020) Expert Group has suggested that the requirement of fat should be based on the level of physical activity. It is also suggested that we should **consume correct combination of vegetable oils.**

- The Committee further recommended that a minimum of 20% energy should come from dietary fat (visible and invisible), with a maximum of 30–35%.
- Out of this, 10% of energy fat should come from all foods (invisible fats).
- A minimum of **10% of total energy requirement should be derived from visible fat.** Accordingly, the visible fat intake in the adult's diet should range between 20–40 g/person/d.
- Adults with sedentary lifestyle should consume about 25 g of visible fat, while individuals involved in hard physical work require 30–40 g of visible fat.
- Visible fat intake should be increased during pregnancy and lactation to at least 30 g. The higher fat and EFA requirements during pregnancy and lactation are to meet the requirements of the fetus and young infants, in view of their crucial role in physical and neuronal growth and development.
- Diets of the young children and adolescents should contain about 30–50 g of visible fat per day.
- Visible fat should include various types, viz. saturated, monounsaturated and polyunsaturated fat.
- **Saturated fat (SFA) should be limited to less than 10% of our daily calorie intake** since these are the biggest dietary cause of high LDL level (bad cholesterol). Replacing SFA with PUFA decreases LDL cholesterol concentration.
- Replacing SFA with carbohydrates decreases both LDL and HDL cholesterol concentrations.
- Replacing SFA with trans-fat decreases HDL cholesterol concentration.
- The remaining requirement should be divided, evenly, between the monounsaturated and polyunsaturated fats.
- To get a good proportion of all the classes of fatty acids, it is advisable to consume more than one type of vegetable oils.
- Minimum energy intake of ω-6 fatty acid (linoleic acid) to prevent deficiency symptoms is estimated to be 2.5% energy.

- Minimum energy intake of ω-3 fatty acid (α-linolenic acid) to prevent deficiency symptoms is estimated to be 0.5% energy.
- Recommended value for cholesterol is 200–300 mg/day.

DIETARY SOURCES OF LIPIDS

Dietary fats are derived from two sources, viz. the visible fat and invisible fat. The total fat (both visible and invisible) in the diet comes from three groups of foods, i.e. fats and oils; meat, poultry and fish; and dairy foods (Fig. 7.8).

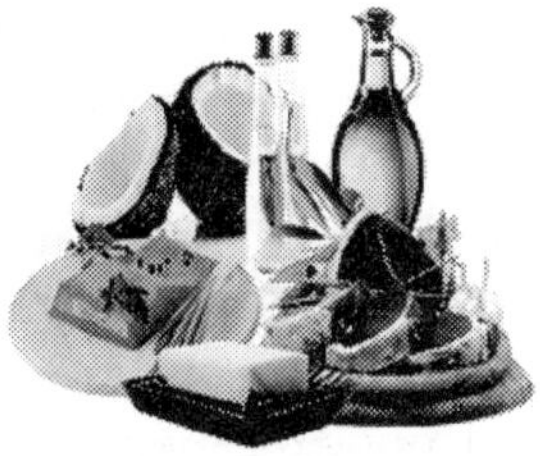

Fig. 7.8: Dietary sources of lipids

Visible fats: Fats and oils, such as vegetable oils, ghee, butter and vanaspati, which are used for cooking, contribute to visible fat, because these are easily seen and can be identified.

Invisible fats: The other group contains invisible fats, because these cannot be easily separated from the food. A small amount of invisible fat is present in almost every food such as cereals, millets, legumes, pulses.

Difference between visible and invisible fat can be described by looking at meat, as an example. After trimming the outer layer of the visible fat from the meat, we can still get 20 to 40 percent of its calories from the invisible fat, which is present in the lean portion of the meat. Other examples of invisible fat include the fat found in baked goods, nuts, peanut butter, processed meats and deep-fried foods such as potato chips, etc.

- **Saturated fats** are found in animal products, such as butter, cheese, whole milk, ice cream, cream and meat. These are also found in some vegetable oils, such as coconut oil and palm oil.
- **Unsaturated fats** are found in most vegetable oils (with the exceptions of coconut and palm oils). Out of these, **monounsaturated** fatty acids are found in olive oil and canola oil, whereas **polyunsaturated fatty acids** are found in safflower oil, sunflower oil, corn oil and soybean oil, and fish.
- Oilseeds and nuts are rich in **ω-3 fatty acids,** whereas vegetable oils, such as soybean oil and canola oil, are good sources of both ω-3 and **ω-6 fatty** acids.

Choice of Cooking Oil

Use of more than one source of fat/oil has the advantage of providing a variety of minor components in the diet. Ideally, part of visible fat and/or invisible fat from animal foods may be substituted by whole nuts and legumes with good proportion of α-linolenic (ω-3) acid. These are also good sources of protein, fiber, vitamins and minerals.

The plant oils, in addition, contain certain useful substances, such as lignans (sesame oil), sterols, tocopherols (vitamin E), oryzanole (rice bran oil), carotenoids, all of which reduce cholesterol and oxidant damage due to ageing, and during inflammation which occurs in chronic diseases.

Vanaspati

Vanaspati is prepared by hydrogenation of vegetable oils. During hydrogenation, the liquid oils become solid because the mono and polyunsaturated fatty acids are converted into saturated fatty acids called **trans** fatty acids.

Vanaspati is used as a substitute for ghee in cooking and the preparation of bakery products, sweets and snack foods. Since, saturated fats are resistant to oxidation, foods prepared in vanaspati keep fresh for a longer period.

Trans Fat

Trans fat is **found in commercially fried** and **processed foods,** partially hydrogenated vegetable oils, vanaspati, bakery products and margarines, etc. Current evidence indicates that saturated fatty acids and a high intake of trans fatty acids increase the risk of coronary heart disease (CHD). Trans-fat is **even more hazardous than the dietary cholesterol.**

Sources of trans-fat are shown in Fig. 7.9.

- Trans fat is formed from the chemical process, by hydrogenation, which converts liquid oils into semi-solid form.
- Our body is unable to metabolize trans fat, causing it to accumulate.
- While saturated fat (found in butter, cheese, red meat, and coconut and palm oils) raises serum cholesterol level, trans fat is still more harmful, since it **increases LDL cholesterol** (bad cholesterol) and **lowers HDL cholesterol** (good cholesterol).
- Though WHO recommends that trans-fat **should not be consumed,** the intake of trans fatty acids, however, should not exceed 1% of energy intake.

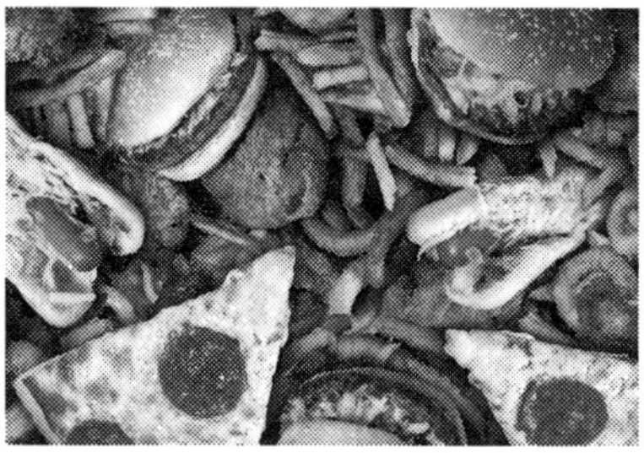

Fig. 7.9: Source of trans fats

DIGESTION, ABSORPTION AND STORAGE OF DIETARY FAT

DIGESTION OF DIETARY LIPIDS

- Dietary lipids mainly include triacylglycerols. Digestion of triglycerides is **initiated in the mouth** with the chewing of food as well as by the action of the **lingual lipase.**
- Thereafter, with the action of **gastric lipase,** and **churning and contraction by the stomach,** nearly 30% of the dietary triglycerides get degraded to diglycerides and free fatty acids, within 2 to 3 hours.
- Contents from the stomach **pass into the small intestine.** Presence of fat in the small intestine, **stimulates the release of** two hormones, i.e. **cholecystokinin** (CCK) **and secretin,** from the duodenal cells.
- **CCK signals** the **gallbladder** to contract and **release bile,** down the bile duct and **into the duodenum.** Bile contains large quantity of bile salts and lecithin.
- **Secretin signals the pancreas to release pancreatic juice,** which is rich in pancreatic lipase.
- **Bile emulsifies fat and breaks fat globules** (clumps of triglycerides) into small pieces and **keep them suspended in solution.** This, in turn, increases total surface area for the action of **pancreatic lipase.**
- **Pancreatic lipase hydrolyses** all the accessible **triglycerides,** within minutes, **into monoglycerides** and **free fatty acids.**
- **Bile salts** surround the hydrolyzed products of fat digestion and **form water-soluble globules** with a fatty core called **micelles.**
- **Micelles transport monoglycerides and free fatty acids** through the watery intestinal environment **to the brush border of the intestinal mucosal cells** for absorption.
- Similarly, **phospholipases hydrolyze phospholipids** and release monoglycerides, free fatty acids, phosphate, and a nitrogenous substance (Table 7.2).

ABSORPTION OF THE HYDROLYZED PRODUCTS OF LIPIDS

Most of the triacylglycerols are absorbed **in the duodenum or jejunum of the small intestine.**

- **Micelles** carry monoglycerides and long chain fatty acids to the surface of the microvilli in the brush border and **diffuse into the intestinal cells.**
- The **unabsorbed bile salts return** to the interior of the small intestine for the transport of more monoglycerides and fatty acids.

Table 7.2: Digestion of dietary lipids		
Enzyme	*Site of action*	*Action of the enzyme*
Lingual lipase (important in neonates)	Mouth	Triglycerides → Fatty acids, monoglycerides, glycerol
Lipase/colipase	Pancreas	Triglycerides → Fatty acids, monoglycerides, glycerol
Phospholipase A/B	Pancreas	Lecithin → Fatty acid, lysolecithin
Cholesterol esterase	Pancreas	Cholesterol esters → Cholesterol, fatty acids
Retinyl ester hydrolase	Pancreas	Retinyl esters → Retinol, fatty acids
Monoglyceride lipase	Small intestine	Monoglycerides → Glycerol, fatty acids
Lecithinase	Small intestine	Lecithin → Fatty acids, glycerol, phosphoric acid, choline

- **Bile salts are absorbed in the ileum and return,** via the portal vein, **to the liver,** where they are **again secreted into the bile.** This recycling pathway for bile, i.e. from the liver to the intestine and from the intestine to the liver is called **enterohepatic circulation.**
- As **monoglycerides and fatty acids** pass into the intestinal cells, they **reform triglycerides.**
- Most of the **triglycerides** as well as **cholesterol and phospholipids combine with apoproteins** and **form chylomicrons.**
- Chylomicrons make their way **to the central lacteal of the villi** where they **enter the lymph system** to be propelled through the thoracic duct and **emptied into vein, in the neck** (Fig. 7.10).
- **Glycerol, and medium and short chain fatty acids are absorbed directly into the blood stream.**
- Absorption of fat is drastically reduced in the absence of bile salts. As a result of it, bulk of the unabsorbed fat is excreted in the stool.

The production of stool with an abnormally high amount of fat is referred to as **steatorrhea**. Steatorrhea may follow diseases of malabsorption, such as **cystic fibrosis,** radiation therapy or digestive tract surgery. In such conditions triglycerides with medium chain fatty acids are often given in the diet. This is due to the reason that medium chain fatty acids are comparatively more water-soluble than long-chain fatty acids and thus can be emulsified more readily.

LIPOPROTEINS

Lipoproteins or proteolipids are the lipid–protein complexes. Since, lipids are **not soluble in** the aqueous **plasma,** hence, these are **transported** in the body in **association with proteins in the form of** coated-capsules, called **lipoproteins**. These are **globular micelle-like particles,** consisting of **nonpolar core of triacylglycerols and cholesterol esters,** which are **surrounded by the amphiphilic coating** that consists of **proteins, cholesterol and phospholipids.**

Lipoproteins are classified into four groups:

- **Chylomicrons**
- **Very low-density lipoproteins**
- **Low density lipoproteins**
- **High density lipoproteins**

Chylomicrons

Chylomicrons are triglyceride-rich particles which are assembled in the intestinal mucosal cells. They **carry dietary triacylglycerols, cholesterol and cholesteryl esters to peripheral** (extrahepatic) **tissues.**

- **Intestinal mucosal cells** release **nascent chylomicrons.** These particles, contain **apo B-48,** which is synthesized in the intestine.
- Thereafter, these **nascent chylomicrons receive apo E and apo C from the**

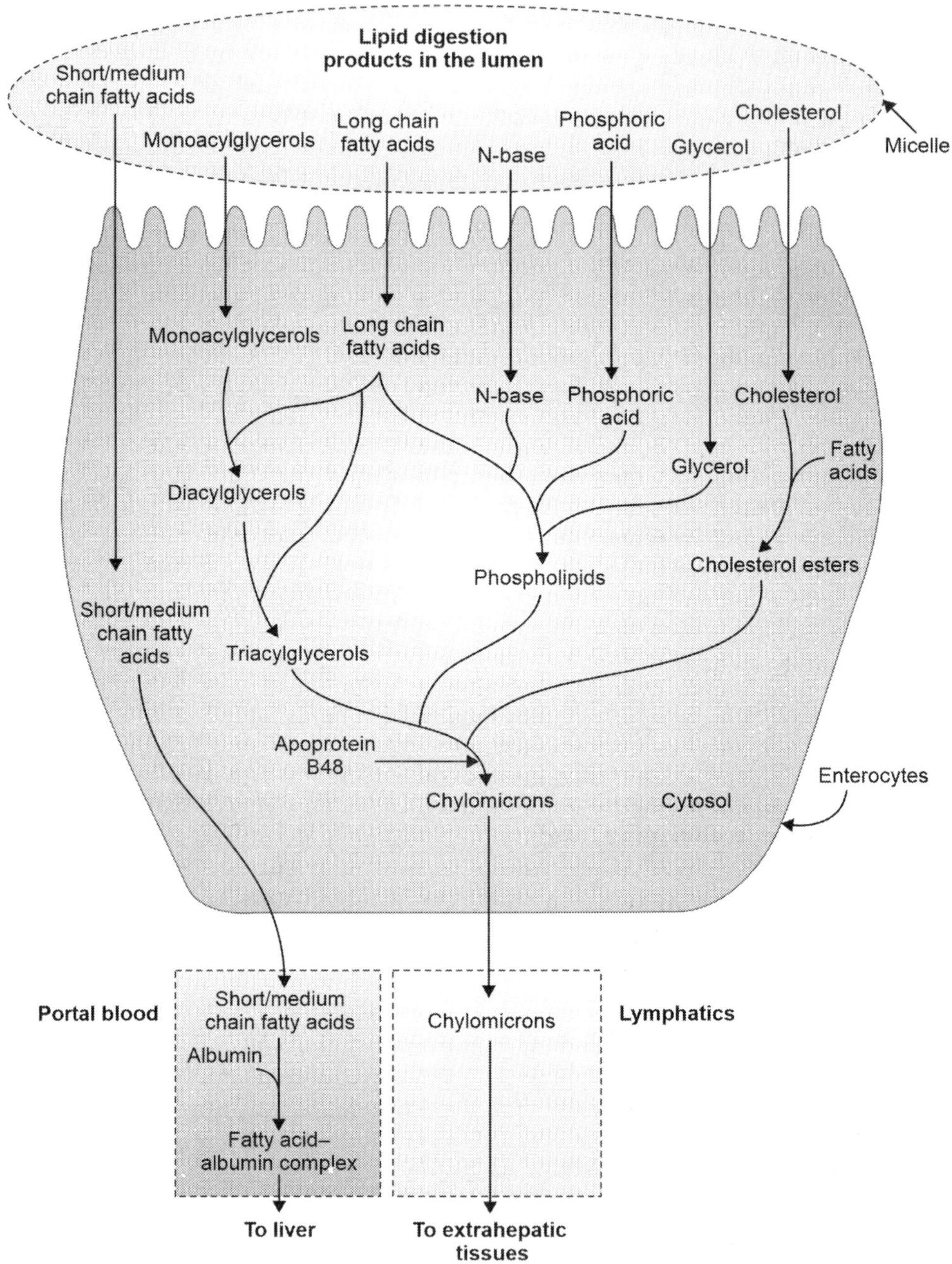

Fig. 7.10: Absorption of the hydrolyzed products of lipids in the intestine

circulating HDL and are **converted to chylomicrons.**

- **Apo C-II,** in turn, **activates lipoprotein lipase** and **hydrolyzes triacylglycerols** (present in chylomicrons) to mono-acylglycerols, free fatty acids and glycerol.
- As a result of **hydrolysis of triacylglycerols,** chylomicrons decrease in size and increase in density.
- Thereafter, **apo C is returned to HDL** and the leftover particles are called **chylomicron remnants.**

- Chylomicron remnants **bind to apo E receptors on the hepatocytes.**
- These are then **internalized** and **their lipids,** including cholesteryl esters, **are** either **utilized or stored,** intracellularly.
- A small amount of the released **free fatty acids enters the circulation** and contributes to plasma free fatty acids pool.

Very Low-Density Lipoproteins

Very low-density lipoproteins **(VLDL),** also called **pre β-lipoproteins,** are **composed of triacylglycerols,** like chylomicrons, but their function is to **transport lipids from the liver to the peripheral tissues.**

- VLDL is released from the **liver as nascent VLDL,** similar to the release of nascent chylomicrons from the intestinal mucosa. Nascent VLDL particles contain **apo B-100 and apo A-1.**
- Subsequently, nascent VLDL **acquires apo C-II and apo E from** the circulating HDL and are **converted** to **VLDL.**
- During circulation, **lipoprotein lipase hydrolyses triacylglycerols** and releases **free fatty acids,** which **are taken-up by the peripheral tissues.**
- **At the same time, apo C and apo E are also transferred to HDL.**
- In addition, **cholesteryl esters,** which are synthesized in the plasma as a result of the action of lecithin cholesterol acyltransferase (LCAT), are **transferred from HDL to VLDL,** via cholesteryl ester transfer protein (CETP).
- As a result of it, their particle size is reduced and density is increased. VLDL particles are, hence, converted to **VLDL remnants,** which are also designated as intermediate density lipoproteins (IDL).
- IDL particles are removed by the liver and converted to the LDL.

Low-Density Lipoproteins

Low density lipoproteins (LDL) **contain high concentration of cholesterol.** They retain apo B-100 and lose other apoproteins to HDL. **Primary function** of LDL **is to transport cholesterol from liver to the extrahepatic tissues.**

- LDL **binds to its receptors,** which are present in the cell membrane. The LDL receptors are negatively charged glycoproteins which are clustered in the pit on the cell membrane and **recognize apo B-100,** that in turn, acts as a ligand between LDL and its receptors. The intracellular side of the pits is coated with a protein, called clathrin, which stabilizes shape of the pit. Ability of the tissues to take up LDL depends upon the rate of transcapillary transport as well as the number of receptors. The number of these receptors is regulated by cholesterol content of the cell.
- After binding, **LDL particles are internalized by endocytosis,** in the form of vesicles. These vesicles rapidly **loose clathrin coat, fuse with the other vesicles and form endosomes** (large vesicles). This, in turn, results in **separation of LDL particles from their receptors.**
- **Receptors are recycled,** whereas **endosome contents are degraded,** resulting in release of cholesterol, free fatty acids, phospholipids and amino acids.
- **Free cholesterol is used for membrane biosynthesis or converted to steroid hormones.** Excess of the cholesterol, however, is re-esterified by acylcholesterol acyltransferase (ACAT) and is stored.
- In man, 70–80% of LDL is removed by LDL receptors while rest of it is removed by the nonspecific endocytosis via the scavenger pathway. The later is also a receptor-mediated process involving phagocytic cells in the reticuloendothelial system.

High-Density Lipoproteins

High density lipoprotein (HDL) particles are **synthesized in the liver** and are **released into the blood stream by exocytosis.**

- Secretory HDL particles are called **nascent HDL** and are discoid in shape.

Nascent HDL is composed of **apo A, apo E, phospholipids and free cholesterol.**

- There also occurs transfer of **apo C** from the chylomicrons and VLDL to nascent HDL, which is converted to **mature HDL**, also called HDL_3.
- From HDL_3, **cholesteryl esters** (produced by the action of LCAT) **are shifted to VLDL and IDL.**
- At the same time, HDL_3 **acquires triacylglycerols** and is converted to HDL_2.

Metabolism of various lipoproteins is outlined in Fig. 7.11.

As discussed above, though, there are several types of lipoproteins, but the most important of these are **h**igh **d**ensity lipoproteins **(HDL)** and **l**ow-**d**ensity lipoproteins **(LDL)**.

LDL transports cholesterol from liver to various tissues. High blood level of **LDL** cholesterol (referred to as **bad cholesterol**) results in accumulation of lipids in the cells and has atherogenic effect. On the other hand, **HDL** (also called **good cholesterol**) transports excess cholesterol from the tissues to the liver for degradation, and are therefore, anti-atherogenic.

STORAGE OF FAT

Fat is stored in the liver and adipose tissue, as follows:

- Chylomicrons travel through bloodstream into the lymphatic capillaries called lacteals.
- Lacteals absorb fat molecules and transport them from the digestive tract to the circulatory system.

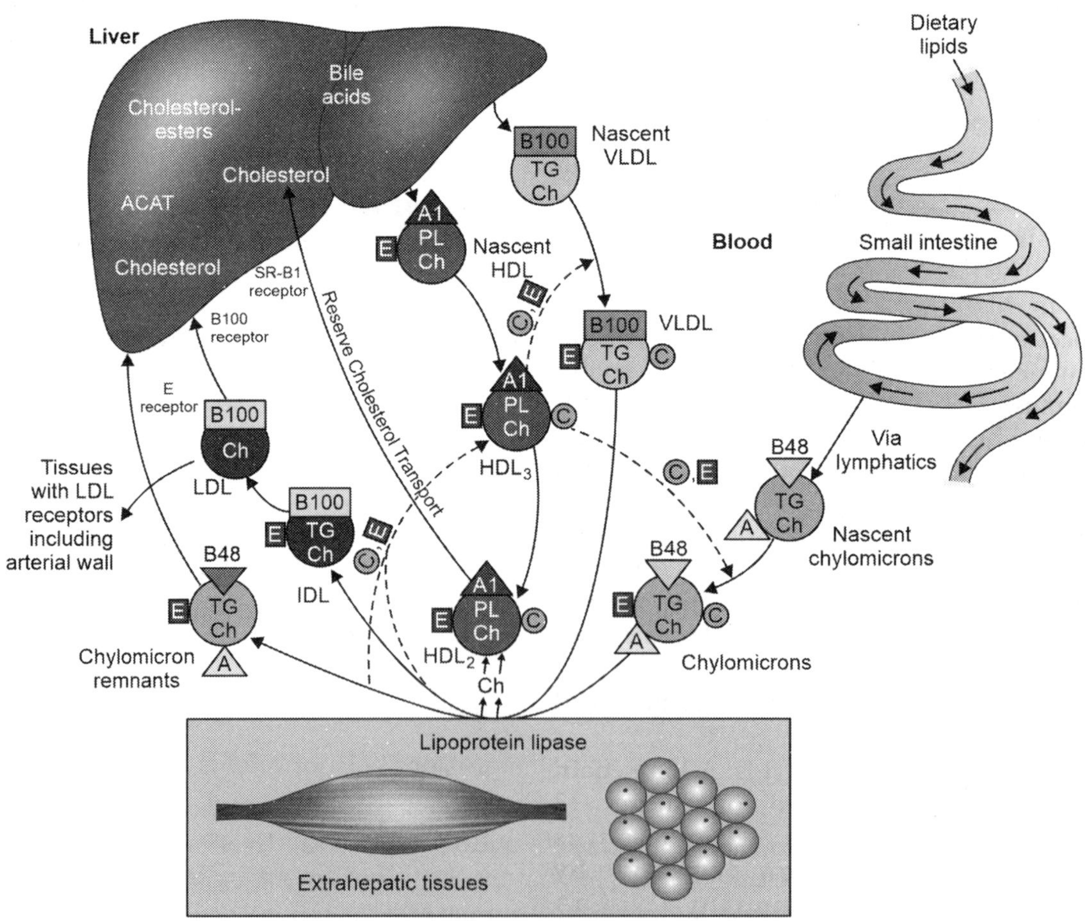

Fig. 7.11: Outline of lipoproteins metabolism

- Adipose tissue and liver release lipoprotein lipase, which hydrolyzes chylomicrons into monoglycerides and fatty acids.
- These molecules diffuse into adipocytes and liver cells where these are converted back to triglycerides and are stored.
- Fat depot, called adipose tissue (white adipose tissue) is utilized during prolonged starvation.

METABOLISM OF DIETARY FAT

Fatty acids, after absorption, bind with serum albumin and are transported to different tissues, for oxidation and release of energy. Glycerol, in turn, returns to the liver, where it is converted to dihydroxyacetone-phosphate, which either enters the glycolytic pathway or is converted to glucose, via gluconeogenesis. Fatty acids are either oxidized or used for the synthesis of triglycerides, which are incorporated in lipoproteins.

OXIDATION OF FATTY ACIDS

Major pathway for the oxidation of fatty acids occurs **in mitochondria.** This pathway is called β-oxidation of fatty acids and was proposed by Knoop.

In this process, **oxidation** of fatty acids **occurs at the β-carbon atom** (carbon-3) and **two-carbon fragments are successively removed** from the carboxyl end of fatty acyl-CoA. This, in turn, results in the elimination of two terminal carbon atoms **as acetyl-CoA,** thereby leaving fatty acyl-CoA that has two carbon atoms less than the original fatty acid.

β-Oxidation of a fatty acid involves activation of fatty acid, its transport into mitochondria and oxidation of the fatty acid within the mitochondria.

The process of β-oxidation of a fatty acid is outlined in Fig. 7.12.

- **Activation of Fatty Acids:** A **long chain fatty acid** (fatty acid containing >12 carbons) enters the cell, where it is **converted to its CoA derivative by** the enzyme **long chain fatty acyl-CoA synthetase (thio-kinase) in the cytosol.**

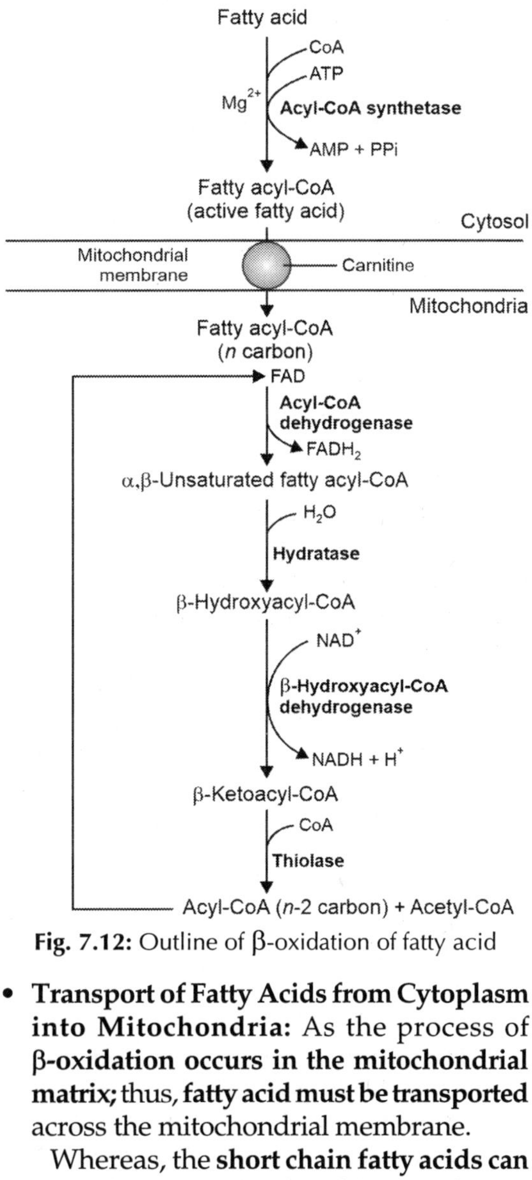

Fig. 7.12: Outline of β-oxidation of fatty acid

- **Transport of Fatty Acids from Cytoplasm into Mitochondria:** As the process of **β-oxidation occurs in the mitochondrial matrix;** thus, **fatty acid must be transported** across the mitochondrial membrane.

  Whereas, the **short chain fatty acids can cross the inner mitochondrial membrane,** it is, however, impermeable to **long chain fatty acids.** So, long chain fatty acids are to be transported from cytosol to the mitochondrial matrix. **Long chain fatty acids are transported with the help of** a carrier referred to as **carnitine.** This process is called **carnitine shuttle.**
  - During this process, firstly, an **acyl group is transferred from the cytosolic CoA to carnitine, by** the enzyme **carnitine palmitoyl**

transferase-I (CPT-I). This enzyme is associated with the outer mitochondrial membrane and is also referred to as carnitine acyltransferase-I (or CAT-I). As a result of it, acyl-CoA is **converted to acylcarnitine** and CoA is released.
- Thereafter, acylcarnitine is **transported into the mitochondrial matrix by** a protein called **carnitine acyl-translocase.**
- Finally, **CPT-II** (also called CAT-II, which is present in the inner mitochondrial membrane) catalyzes the **transfer** of the acyl group from **acylcarnitine** which is converted to acyl-CoA in the mitochondrial matrix and carnitine is released.

- **Oxidation of fatty acids:** The process of β-oxidation consists of four reactions, which result in shortening of the fatty acid chain by two carbons.
  1. **Oxidation:** After activation of the fatty acid, such as palmitic acid, and its entry into the mitochondrial matrix, flavoprotein containing acyl-CoA dehydrogenase removes two hydrogens from the α- and β-positions of the fatty acyl-CoA and produces $FADH_2$. The α-fatty acyl-CoA is changed to α,β-unsaturated fatty acyl-CoA (also called enoyl-CoA).
  2. **Hydration:** In the next reaction, enoyl-CoA hydratase adds a molecule of water at the double bond and converts the enoyl-CoA to β-hydroxy-acyl-CoA.
  3. **Oxidation:** Thereafter, β-hydroxyacyl-CoA dehydrogenase oxidizes β-hydroxyacyl-CoA to β-ketoacyl-CoA.
  4. **Cleavage:** In the fourth reaction, acyl-CoA: acyltransferase, also called thiolase, in the presence of CoA, results in the thiolytic cleavage of the β-ketoacyl-CoA into acetyl-CoA and fatty acyl-CoA (which has two carbons less than the original fatty acyl-CoA).

These four reactions are repeated, i.e. the fatty acyl-CoA (the end product after cleavage) again undergoes the above four reactions, starting with acyl-CoA dehydrogenase, and each cycle, in turn, produces acetyl-CoA, $FADH_2$ and NADH. The cycle continues, till the fatty acid is sequentially degraded to the acetyl-CoA, the final end product.

A molecule of **palmitic acid** ($C_{15}H_{31}COOH$), when undergoes β-oxidation, **releases 8 molecules of acetyl-CoA** in seven rounds.

ATP Production During β-Oxidation of Fatty Acids

As mentioned above, **in every round, one molecule each of $FADH_2$ and NADH + H^+ are produced,** which, enter mitochondrial electron transport chain (ETC) and, in turn, release 1.5 and 2.5 ATP, respectively. Thus, a total of 28 ATP molecules are produced during this process. In addition, each molecule of acetyl-CoA, when oxidizes via the citric acid cycle, produces 10 ATP. Therefore, additionally, 80 ATP are produced from 8 molecules of acetyl-CoA. Hence, **a total of 108 ATP molecules are produced from one molecule of palmitic acid.** As two high-energy phosphate bonds are hydrolyzed from one molecule of ATP, which is changed to AMP, thus, a total of 2 ATP are used during the activation of a fatty acid. Therefore, there is a **net yield of 106 ATP** when one molecule of palmitic acid (fatty acid with 16 carbons) is completely oxidized.

LIPOGENESIS

Triacylglycerols, as mentioned above, are the principle dietary lipids as well as lipids of the fat depot in the body. Excessive amounts of dietary carbohydrates are also stored as triacylglycerols in the adipose tissue. The process of biosynthesis of triacylglycerols is referred to as lipogenesis, which, though, mainly, occurs in the liver and adipose tissue; but also occurs in lactating mammary glands, kidneys and epithelial cells of the intestinal mucosa.

Lipogenesis involves **synthesis of glycerol-phosphate, activation of fatty acid and synthesis of triacylglycerol** (Fig. 7.13).

- **Synthesis of L-α-glycerol phosphate**: L-α-glycerol phosphate can be synthesized in two ways:
  - **In most of the tissues** which contain **glycerol kinase, glycerol is converted to L-α-glycerol phosphate.**
  - Alternatively, **in muscle and adipose tissue,** which lack glycerol kinase, L-α-glycerol phosphate is formed from **dihydroxyacetone phosphate,** an intermediate of glycolysis. The reaction is catalyzed **by glycerol-3-phosphate dehydrogenase.**
- **Activation of fatty acids:** Free **fatty acids,** in the presence of ATP and CoA, are activated **to acyl-CoA, by thio-kinase** (fatty acyl-CoA synthetase).
- **Synthesis of triacylglycerols:** After the synthesis of L-α-glycerol phosphate and activation of fatty acids, triacylglycerols are synthesized by sequential additions of the fatty acyl-CoA molecules, as follows:
  - Firstly, **a molecule of acyl-CoA combines with α-glycerol phosphate** and **forms 1-acylglycerol-3- phosphate** (lysophosphatidic acid). The reaction is catalyzed **by glycerol-3-phosphate acyltransferase.**
  - Thereafter, L-acylglycerol 3-phosphate **acyltransferase** (lysophosphatidyl-acyltransferase) **converts 1-acylglycerol-3-phosphate to 1, 2-diacylglycerol phosphate (phosphatidic acid).**
  - In the next step, **phosphatase** (phosphatidic acid phosphohydrolase) **hydrolyzes phosphatidic acid and forms 1,2-diacylglycerol.**

In many tissues, especially, in the intestinal mucosa, 1,2-diacylglycerol is

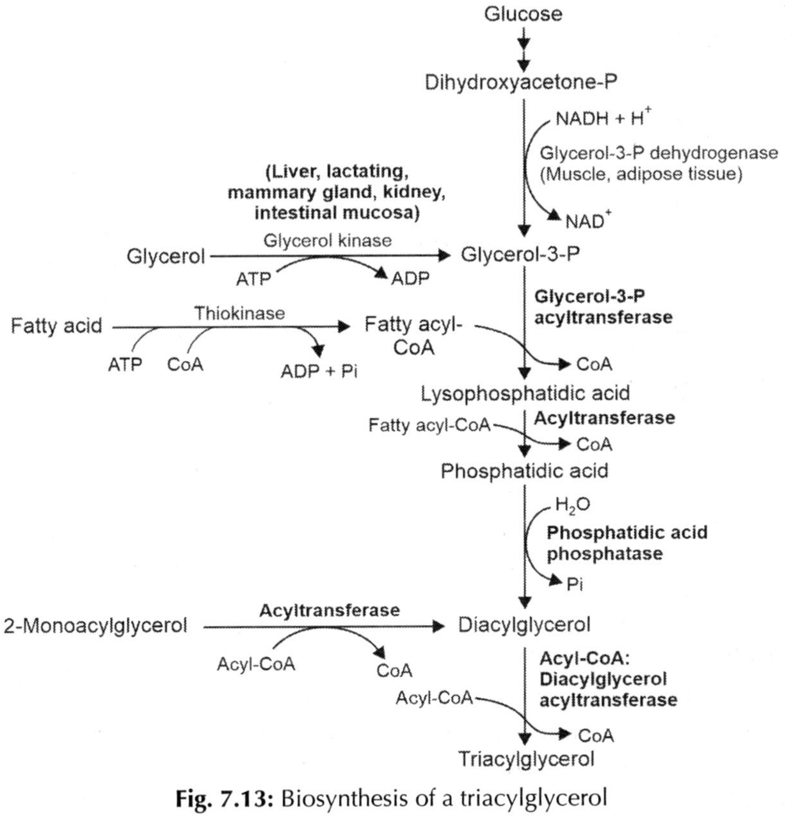

Fig. 7.13: Biosynthesis of a triacylglycerol

also formed from 2-monoacylglycerols, since monoacylglycerols are directly absorbed in the intestinal mucosa. The reaction involves the transfer of an acyl group by the enzyme monoacylglycerol acyltransferase.

DAG is a common intermediate for the biosynthesis of, both triacylglycerols as well as phospholipids.

– Finally, diacylglycerol **acyltransferase** esterifies diacylglycerol and **forms triacylglycerol.**

Generally, palmitic acid is present at positions 1 and 3 while oleic acid at position 2 of a triacylglycerol in the human adipose tissue.

LIPID MALNUTRITION

As mentioned above, fat is an essential component of diet for various body functions. At least a small amount of fat in our diet is necessary **to provide essential fatty acids** (omega-3 and omega-6 fatty acids, which our body cannot make) and to help in the **absorption of fat-soluble vitamins.** If we do not get at least 15 percent of our calories from fat, we may develop an essential fatty acid deficiency or a deficiency of one or more of the fat-soluble vitamins (vitamins A, D, E and K, because our body can only absorb these nutrients in the presence of fat).

LIPID DEFICIENCY DISORDERS

Inadequate Intake of Lipids

A low-fat diet reduces the performance of the nerve. It can cause psychological and neurological disorders, such as depression and behavioural changes (like anxiety, low moods and irritability), which can be due to serotonin dysfunction.

Deficiency of Essential Fatty Acids

Deficiency of essential fatty acids results in signs, such as scaly dermatitis, alopecia, thrombocytopenia, and, in children, intellectual disability.

- **Skin problems:** Essential fatty acids are required for keeping our skin healthy. An essential fatty acid deficiency increases the loss of water from the skin, which results in a dry, scaly rash. This type of deficiency can also make it harder for the wounds to heal.
- **Cardiovascular diseases:** Decreased levels of omega-3 fatty acids in the blood can lead to cardiovascular diseases, like coronary heart disease, hypertension, stroke, cardiac arrest and atherosclerosis.
- **Auto-immunity and chronic inflammation:** Chronic inflammation like chronic obstructive pulmonary disease (COPD), Crohn's disease, rheumatoid arthritis, multiple sclerosis, systemic lupus erythematosus, ulcerative colitis and immunoglobulin A nephropathy are also associated with depleted levels of omega-3 fatty acids.
- **Cancer:** Decreased levels of omega-3 fatty acids increase the risk of prostate and colon cancers.
- **Affects pregnancy and lactation:** Low blood levels of essential omega-3 fatty acids during pregnancy increases the risk of increase in blood pressure, pre-eclampsia and subsequent premature birth. Two types of omega-3 fatty acids, i.e. **eicosapentaenoic acid (EPA)** and **docosahexaenoic acid (DHA)**, are essential for brain development. DHA is very essential for the development of fetus and infants. Low DHA intake during pregnancy results in postpartum depression and low IQ.
- **Cognitive problems:** DHA deficiency may result in learning deficits and increases the risk for certain types of dementia, including Alzheimer's disease. The omega-6 fat (arachidonic acid) is also an important component of brain tissue.
- **Vision:** EPA and DHA are also important components of the retina. DHA helps form the pigment rhodopsin, which

we need for our brain, to turn the light hitting the retina into the images we see. Omega-3 fatty acid also helps to lower the risk for dry eyes and age-related macular degeneration.

Deficiency of Fat-soluble Vitamins

- Vitamin A deficiency symptoms include dry skin, night blindness, increased susceptibility to infections, and problems with bone and tooth development.
- Vitamin D deficiency can cause soft and weak bones.
- Vitamin K deficiency can lead to increased bleeding.

FAT OVERCONSUMPTION

Overconsumption of fat, particularly, the saturated fat increases blood cholesterol and leads to various health problems, such as obesity and atherosclerosis.

Coronary Heart Disease (CHD)

A high fat intake, in particular, a high intake of saturated fatty acids has been associated with a raised blood cholesterol level, which is one of the risk factors for coronary heart disease. Diets rich in saturated fatty acids are associated with the development of insulin resistance and dyslipidemia (abnormal blood fat levels) as part of the **metabolic syndrome** (a cluster of risk factors for cardiovascular disease), that is associated with increased risk of type 2 diabetes. On the other hand, mono and polyunsaturated fatty acids are associated with reduced blood cholesterol levels and a particular role in heart health has been established for dietary sources of the long chain omega-3 fatty acids present in oily fish.

Obesity

Fat is a concentrated source of energy and foods that are high in fat provide a lot of energy. Also, fat may have a less satiating (filling) effect than other food components (e.g. protein and fiber). This means, it is easier to consume an excess of energy when eating a high fat diet. If energy intake and expenditure are unbalanced, then the excess energy is stored in the body as fat, which may over time result in an individual becoming overweight and obese.

Obesity is a complex disorder with multiple contributing factors:

- **Genetic factors:** When both the parents are obese, it is likely that their children may also be obese.
- **Social influences:** Social factors have important influence on the development of obesity. Abundance of calories, highly palatable food and social enjoyment of eating, create pressure to overeat and lead to obesity.
- **Age and lifestyle:** People gain most of the body weight between 25 and 35 years of age. Exercise patterns also influence development of obesity, which is associated with reduced physical activity.
- **Sex:** Obesity is more prevalent in women than men. Women often develop obesity after pregnancy and menopause.

Besides race, ethnicity, socioeconomic status, psychological factors also contribute to obesity. Obesity is highly associated with the increasing risk of type II diabetes, diseases of the gallbladder, cardiovascular disease, hypertension and osteoarthritis (Chapter 2).

Atherosclerosis

Atherosclerosis (arteriosclerosis) is a disease of arterial wall. It is characterized by the accumulation **of cholesterol** and its esters in cells, which are derived from monocyte-macrophage line smooth muscle cells. This, in turn, results in the formation of **atherosclerotic plaque, which narrows the blood vessels** and serves as the site of thrombus formation (Fig. 7.14).

Risk of developing the disease is directly related to the concentration of the LDL-

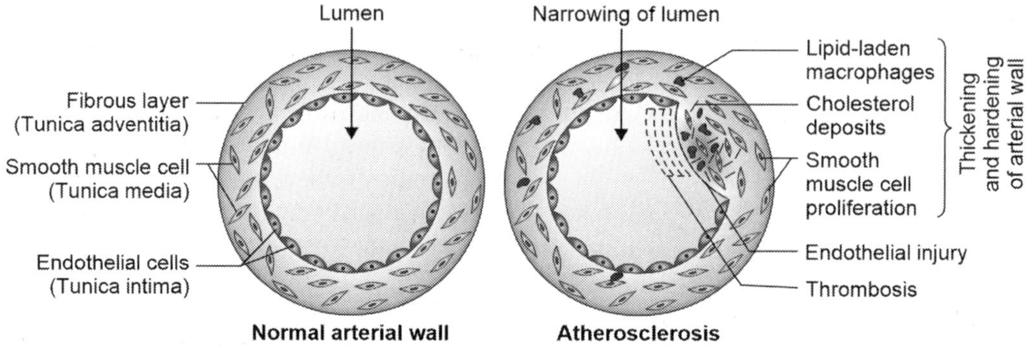

Fig. 7.14: Atherosclerosis

cholesterol, in plasma. It is also inversely related to the plasma concentration of HDL-cholesterol.

High calories diet, particularly, the diet rich in saturated fat and cholesterol, hypercholesterolemia, sedentary lifestyle, stress and strain, obesity, hypertension, and smoking are important contributory factors, favorable in the development of atherosclerosis.

SOME IMPORTANT QUESTIONS

1. **What are lipids? How do you classify lipids?**
2. **Define fatty acids. How do you classify fatty acids?**
3. **Describe significance, calorific value, recommended daily allowances and sources of dietary lipids.**
4. **Differentiate between:**
   i. Visible and invisible fat
   ii. Saturated and unsaturated fatty acids
   iii. Omega-3 and omega-6 fatty acids
5. **Describe briefly:**
   i. Significance of essential fatty acids
   ii. Coronary heart disease
   iii. Nomenclature of unsaturated fatty acids
   iv. Lipolysis
   v. Lipogenesis
   vi. β-Oxidation of fatty acids
   vii. Digestion and absorption of lipids
   viii. Dietary significance of omega-3 and omega-6 fatty acids
6. **Write notes on:**
   i. Essential fatty acids
   ii. Polyunsaturated fatty acids
   iii. Omega-6 fatty acids
   iv. Omega-3 fatty acids
   v. Phospholipids
   vi. Trans fat
   vii. Cholesterol
   viii. Atherosclerosis
   ix. Obesity

CHAPTER

8

Proteins

Protein (Greek: proteios means primary) is the class of natural products, which **contains nitrogen** and forms an essential structural component of a cell. These are most abundant and functionally diverse molecules **present in all living systems.**

Biochemical activities of the various proteins are **characterized by their structure, size and shape.** These factors are determined by the sequence and characteristics of the constituent amino acids which are defined by the sequence of gene, encoded by the genetic code. Thus,

- All **proteins,** from whatever source it may be, **are** the **polymers of amino acids.**
- **Amino acids are the hydrolyzed products of proteins;** these are also **used in protein synthesis.**
- Though a large number of amino acids may be found in the body, only **twenty** amino acids **commonly occur in all mammalian proteins.**

BIOLOGICAL IMPORTANCE OF PROTEINS

Proteins serve a variety of functions (Table 8.1).

Table 8.1: Biological functions of proteins

Biological function	*Examples of proteins*
As structural proteins	Collagen, keratins, etc.
As enzymes	Pepsin, amylase, etc.
As hormones	Insulin
As transporters	Hemoglobin
As receptors	Hormone receptors
As storage molecules	Ferritin
In immune response	γ-Globulin

- **Structural proteins:** Some of the proteins, e.g. **collagens** (found in bone and cartilage), **keratins** (found in hair and nail), etc., form an essential part of the particular structure within the body.
- **Enzymes:** Some of the proteins, such as **pepsin,** catalyze biological reactions and act as enzymes.
- **Hormones:** Some of the proteins act as hormones, e.g. **insulin.** Hormones regulate metabolic processes within the cell.
- **Transporters:** Several proteins serve as a carrier for the transport of a substance within the body. For example, **hemoglobin** is important for the transport of oxygen, ceruloplasmin transports copper, etc.
- **Protein receptors:** Some of the proteins, such as **hormone receptors,** act as receptors for certain hormones and play an important role in signal transduction.
- **Storage of substances:** Some of the proteins bind to a substance for its storage in different tissues in the body, e.g. **ferritin,** which stores Fe^{3+}.

- **Antibodies:** Some proteins, such as **γ-globulin,** act as antibodies and provide immunity.

AMINO ACIDS

As mentioned above, amino acids are the **hydrolyzed products of proteins.** These are also **used in the synthesis of proteins**. All the naturally occurring amino acids are designated as **α-amino acids,** because, both, the primary amino group ($-NH_2$), as well as the distinctive side chain (R–), are attached to the α-carbon atom, i.e. the carbon atom next to the carboxyl group (–COOH).

General structure of an amino acid is shown in Fig. 8.1.

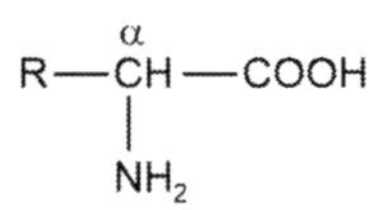

Fig. 8.1: General structure of an amino acid

CLASSIFICATION OF AMINO ACIDS

As mentioned above, there are 20 different amino acids which are commonly found in most of the proteins. These are classified into different groups according to the properties of the side chain such as **charge** and **polarity** as well as according to the **dietary requirement.**

According to Charge

According to the net ionic charge of their side chain (R-group), amino acids are classified as **neutral, acidic** or **basic** amino acids (Table 8.2).

According to Polarity

According to polarity amino acids are classified into different groups, as given in Table 8.3.

Table 8.2: Classification of amino acids according to charge

Amino acid	*Abbreviation**
NEUTRAL AMINO ACIDS	
Simple amino acids	
Glycine	Gly
Alanine	Ala
Branched chain amino acids	
Valine	Val
Leucine	Leu
Isoleucine	Ile
Hydroxy amino acids	
Serine	Ser
Threonine	Thr
Aromatic amino acids	
Phenylalanine	Phe
Tyrosine	Tyr
Tryptophan	Trp
Sulfur-containing amino acids	
Cysteine	Cys
Methionine	Met
ACIDIC AMINO ACIDS	
Aspartic acid	Asp
Glutamic acid	Glu
Amides of the acidic amino acids	
Asparagine	Asn
Glutamine	Gln
BASIC AMINO ACIDS	
Lysine	Lys
Arginine	Arg
Histidine	His
IMINO ACID	
Proline	Pro

* Three letters abbreviation is widely used. This, generally, includes first three letters of an amino acid.

According to Dietary Requirement

According to dietary requirement, i.e. **from the nutrition point of view,** amino acids are classified **into three groups,** referred to as essential **(indispensable)**, semi-essential **(conditionally indispensable)** and nonessential (**dispensable;** Table 8.4).

Table 8.3: Classification of amino acids according to polarity

Nonpolar side chain	*Polar side chain*	
	Uncharged	*Charged*
• Glycine	• Serine	• Lysine
• Alanine	• Threonine	• Arginine
• Valine	• Asparagine	• Histidine
• Leucine	• Glutamine	• Aspartate
• Isoleucine	• Tyrosine	• Glutamate
• Methionine	• Cysteine	
• Phenylalanine		
• Tryptophan		
• Proline		

Table 8.4: Classification of amino acids according to dietary requirement

Essential	*Semi-essential*	*Nonessential*
• Methionine	• Arginine	• Glycine
• Threonine	• Histidine	• Alanine
• Tryptophan		• Serine
• Valine		• Cysteine
• Isoleucine		• Tyrosine
• Leucine		• Aspartate
• Phenylalanine		• Glutamate
• Lysine		• Asparagine
		• Glutamine
		• Proline

Essential Amino Acids

Out of the 20 amino acids, commonly found in proteins, **eight amino acids,** i.e. **methionine, threonine, tryptophan, valine, isoleucine, leucine, phenylalanine** and **lysine** cannot be synthesized in human beings. These are **indispensable** and are called **essential amino acids.** These amino acids have to be supplied in the diet.

Semi-essential Amino Acids

Besides the above eight amino acids, there are **two amino acids,** i.e. **arginine** and **histidine,** which are **not essential for a normal adult human being** but **become dietary essential under certain conditions** when either their demand is increased (such as during growth, pregnancy or lactation) or in hypercatabolic states (like high grade fever and chronic infections). Hence, these two amino acids are referred to as **conditionally indispensable** or semi-essential **amino acids.** Since these **amino acids can be synthesized by an adult under normal healthy conditions. However, under other circumstances,** when either they cannot be synthesized or synthesized in insufficient amounts due to their increased demand, **these become dietary essential,** as given in the examples below.

- **In infants and children:** Arginine and histidine are considered to be essential (indispensable) amino acids, since infants and children cannot synthesize these two amino acids. **In premature infants tyrosine,** and in **preterm and term infants cysteine** is dietary essential.
- **In certain disease states:** There are certain disease states during adult life when demand of a particular amino acid is increased by the body, and thus, it becomes dietary essential, e.g.:
  - **In a liver disease** cysteine requirement cannot be met by the body, due to diminished trans-sulfuration capacity of the liver. Thus, cysteine becomes dietary essential.
  - **In chronic renal failure** concentration of tyrosine and its ratio to phenylalanine becomes consistently low, owing to reduced oxidation of tyrosine from phenylalanine. Thus, under these circumstances, tyrosine becomes dietary essential.
  - **During episodes of infections, inflammation** and **malnutrition, glutamine** is considered to be conditionally essential.
  - **During conditions of catabolic stress and uremia, taurine** has been shown as an indispensable substrate and potent antioxidant.

Nonessential Amino Acids

All the **other amino acids** are referred to as **nonessential amino acids** since these can be synthesized in the body, to meet the demand.

PROTEINS

Proteins are biologically occurring **long chains of amino acids,** which are **linked by peptide bonds.**

When two amino acids join together, it forms a peptide bond (–CO–NH–). During this process, carboxyl group of one amino acid reacts with the amino group of the other amino acid. This is a condensation reaction and results in the formation of amide linkage called peptide bond (Fig. 8.2).

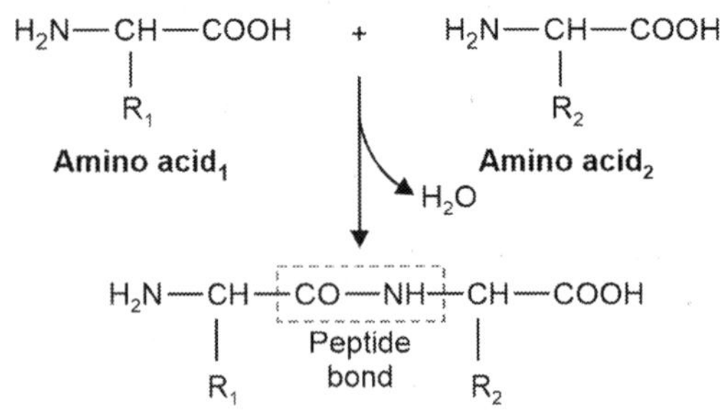

Fig. 8.2: Formation of a peptide bond

When several amino acids join to each other, it forms a polypeptide or protein where one end of the peptide chain has a free carboxyl group (referred to as C-terminus) while the other end has a free amino group (referred to as N-terminus; Fig. 8.3).

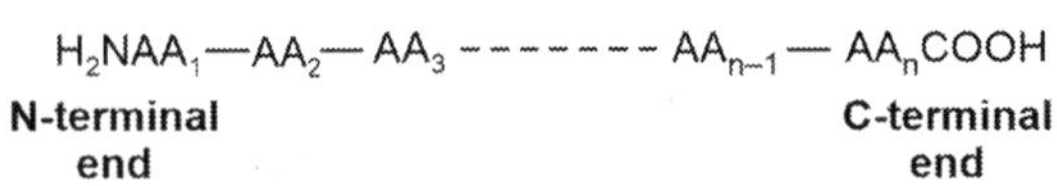

Fig. 8.3: A polypeptide

DIETARY SIGNIFICANCE OF PROTEINS

Dietary proteins provide amino acids for the synthesis of body proteins, several structural and biologically active compounds (enzymes and hormones), and various nitrogenous substances.

- Dietary proteins are the main **source of nitrogen** and **essential (indispensable) amino acids** which are necessarily required by the body for protein synthesis, growth and maintenance.
- Proteins are also essential as fundamental **structural and functional elements** within every cell of the body and are involved in a wide range of metabolic interactions.
- Proteins provide, approximately, 10 to 15% of dietary **energy** and is the second most abundant compound present in the body.
- Dietary proteins also provide amino acids for the **synthesis** of new tissue **proteins during growth, replacement** of the degraded proteins **during wear and tear in adults, synthesis of foetal, placental and maternal body proteins during pregnancy, and synthesis of breast milk proteins during lactation.**
- **Synthesis** of various **biologically active nitrogenous compounds,** such as **enzymes and hormones.**

PROTEIN QUALITY

For a healthy diet, it is important to consider not only the quantity but also the quality of a dietary protein, due to the **variable amounts** of different amino acids, especially the essential (indispensable) amino acids **(amino acid pattern of essential amino acids)** as well as its **digestibility pattern.**

Amino acid composition of a protein and the **requirement of essential amino acids** by the human body are expressed in terms of **per g of protein which has 100% digestibility.**

Various methods have been suggested to determine protein quality (amino acid pattern and digestibility).

Determination of Protein Quality

Various methods have been suggested to determine protein quality (amino acid pattern). These include:

- **Amino acid score:** Amino acid score (AAS) is a **comparison of the amino acid content of the test protein with the reference value.** It is expressed as a ratio to the recommended unit or on the percentage scale.
- **Protein efficiency ratio:** Protein efficiency ratio **(PER)** is the **ratio of weight gain and protein consumed by the test group over the control** (using the reference protein, generally casein).
- **Digestible indispensable amino acid score:** Digestible indispensable amino acid score (DIAAS) is expressed as the **ratio of the limiting indispensable amino acid in test protein compared to the reference protein corrected for ileal digestibility of the limiting indispensable amino acid.**

  DIAAS, thus, **calculates a score for each indispensable amino acid** (IAA) based on the concentration of each digestible IAA, which is calculated from the concentration of each IAA (per g protein) and its **ileal digestibility**. For each IAA, this value is then compared with a reference pattern for each age group and the **IAA with lowest score,** relative to the reference pattern, **is considered to be the first limiting amino acid.**
- **Protein digestibility corrected amino acid score:** Protein digestibility corrected amino acid score **(PDCAAS)** is expressed as the **ratio of the limiting essential amino acid of the test protein compared to the content of the same amino acid in the reference protein, corrected for fecal digestibility of the test protein.**

  PDCAAS, thus, **calculates a value for protein quality based on the first limiting amino acid, in relation to a reference pattern.** However, **digestibility** in the PDCAAS method is not determined at the ileal but **at the fecal level in test species,** and **also** it is determined **at a protein level,** and **not at the individual amino acid level.**

Protein Digestibility Methods

- **Biological value:** Biological value (BV) is defined as the **percentage of the absorbed N retained in the body over total nitrogen intake with the test protein** as the only source of N in the diet.
- **Net protein utilization:** Net protein utilization **(NPU)** refers to the **percentage of dietary N retained in the body over total nitrogen intake.**

CLASSIFICATION OF DIETARY PROTEINS

Dietary proteins are, generally, classified based on the **source** from which these are obtained and based on its **quality.**

According to Source

According to their source, dietary proteins are obtained either from the **animal sources** or the **plant sources.** These proteins also differ from each other with respect to their structures as well as functions.

Proteins from Animal Sources

Proteins from animal sources include albumins (egg albumin and lactalbumin), globulins (egg globulins and lactoglobulins), etc. These may be **globular** or **fibrous** in structure.

- **Globular proteins:** These are found in tissue fluids, e.g. **casein** in milk, **albumin** in egg white, and **albumin** and **globulins** in blood.
- **Fibrous proteins:** These are found in protective and supportive tissues, e.g. **keratin** (chief protein of hair), **collagen** (connective tissue), **fibrin** (blood clot), and **myosin** (muscle).

Proteins from Plant Sources

Proteins from plant sources include **glutelins** and **prolamines,** etc.

- **Glutelins:** These include **glutenin** from wheat, **hordenin** from barley, **orzynenin** from rice, etc.
- **Prolamines:** These include **gliadin** from wheat and **zein** from maize.

According to Quality

According to protein quality and digestibility, dietary proteins are divided into two groups as **high-quality proteins and poor-quality proteins.**

- **High quality proteins:** A high quality protein is the one that **provides all the essential amino acids** to meet human requirements. These are also referred to as the proteins with a **high biological value.** Generally, proteins from animal sources provide all the nutritionally essential amino acids in right proportions to meet the human requirements, e.g. proteins from meat, fish, egg, milk and cheese, etc. Hence, proteins **from animal sources** are, generally, referred to as high quality dietary proteins.
- **Poor quality proteins:** A poor quality dietary protein is the one that is **deficient in one or more essential amino acid, hence,** it may also be referred to as **incomplete protein.** Generally, **proteins form the plant-based foods,** e.g. whole grains, rice, corn, beans, legumes, oatmeal and peas, etc., do not supply all the nutritionally essential amino acids in the desired quantities, these proteins are therefore referred to as incomplete proteins or proteins with **poor biological value**.

  For example, **cereal proteins are,** generally, deficient in lysine while proteins from **pulses and legume have low amounts of methionine.**

  Besides quality, **proteins from plant sources also have low digestibility.**

  In the past, **proteins from the animal-based foods** were referred to as the **first-class proteins** while the proteins from the plant-based foods were referred to as the **second-class proteins.**

COMPLEMENTARY ACTION OF PROTEINS

Complementary **(supplementary)** action of proteins refers to the **pattern of amino acids from the combination of proteins from different plant-based food sources.** For example:

- **Cereals,** in general, **are** known to be **deficient in lysine and threonine,** but **contain high amount of methionine.**
- **Legumes and pulses,** on the other hand, **are good sources of lysine and threonine** but are **poor in methionine.**
- When proteins from these two sources are **taken together, excess of an amino acid present in pulses effectively supplement the limiting amino acid in the cereals,** and vice versa. As a result of it, the limiting amino acid from one source is compensated from the other.
- Thus, **proteins from two different sources when taken together, improve their biological value.**
- It provides a strong biochemical basis for the **traditional Indian dietary habit of taking rice or wheat bread with pulses.**

NITROGEN BALANCE

Nitrogen balance refers to the amount of nitrogen (N) retained by the body, i.e. the difference between N intake (dietary protein) and its excretion, which is the sum of all the sources of nitrogen excretion such as urine and faeces, skin and hair, and other body fluids (Fig. 8.4).

Nitrogen balance is calculated to assess protein status of the body. Determination of N balance, thus, requires a careful estimation of protein (nitrogen) intake (I) and its excretion (O) by all routes, namely urine, faeces and dermal losses, etc. Difference in N intake and its output may be zero (N equilibrium), positive (N retention) or negative (N loss).

- **Nitrogen equilibrium:** When the amount of nitrogen intake is equal to the amount of nitrogen excretion, an individual is said to be in nitrogen equilibrium (i.e. zero N balance). As a result

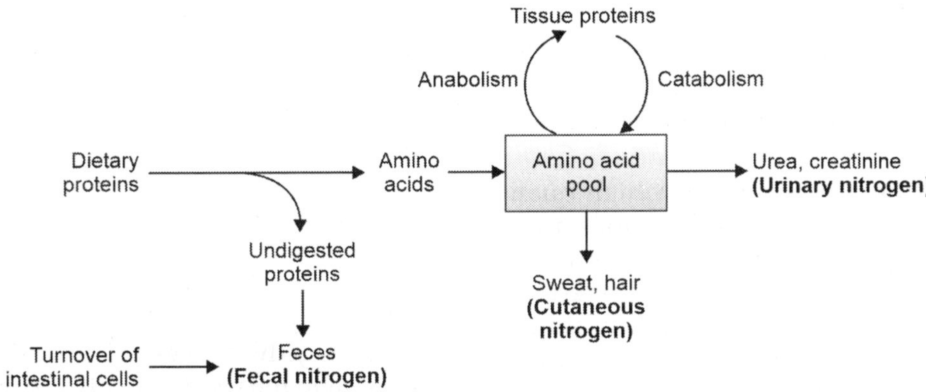

Fig. 8.4: Nitrogen balance

of it, there is no net gain or loss of nitrogen from the body. Ideally, a normal adult should be in a state of zero nitrogen balance.

- **Positive nitrogen balance:** When nitrogen intake is more than the nitrogen excretion, body is said to be in positive nitrogen balance, which means that proteins are being retained (deposited) in the body tissues. Positive nitrogen balance is essential during growth such as in growing children, pregnant women and people recovering from protein deficiency or illness.
- **Negative nitrogen balance:** When nitrogen excretion is more than the intake, body is said to be in a negative nitrogen balance. This means that body is losing protein. Conditions such as injury, chronic diseases (such as tuberculosis, rheumatoid arthritis, cancer), increased muscular activity, inadequate protein intake, lack of essential amino acids and increased metabolic stress lead to negative nitrogen balance (Table 8.5).

CALORIC VALUE OF PROTEIN

Caloric value of proteins is similar to the carbohydrates but is nearly half of fat. Accordingly, each gram of protein provides 4 kcal.

RECOMMENDED DAILY ALLOWANCES OF PROTEIN

Protein requirements vary with age, physiological state and stress. Accordingly, there is an extra requirement for growth in infants and children, and for pregnant and lactating women.

ICMR-NIN (2020) Expert Group has adopted the FAO/WHO/UNU (2007) approaches to define protein requirements for Indians of different age groups.

- As per its recommendations, **10–15% of the total energy requirement should be derived from proteins.**
- **RDA for maintenance in adults** has been suggested as **0.64 g/kg/d** while the **safe intake has been suggested as 0.83 g/kg/d.** However, for people consuming

Table 8.5: Type of nitrogen balance and examples of the prevailing conditions

Nitrogen balance	*Protein intake (I)/output (O)*	*Condition*
Equilibrium	I = O	Normal/healthy individuals
Positive	I > O	Growth, pregnancy, convalescence
Negative	I < O	↓ Protein intake, trauma, chronic illness (e.g. tuberculosis)

cereal-based diet with low quality protein such as **vegans,** the recommended protein intake is suggested as **1 g/kg per day.**

Accordingly, **total requirement** for protein has been suggested as **54 g/d for adult male moderate worker** and **46 g/d for adult female moderate worker.**

- **During pregnancy,** as we know, additional protein is necessary for the synthesis of foetal, placental and maternal body proteins. The Committee has suggested revised recommendations for protein during pregnancy, based on the gestational weight gain (GWG).

  Accordingly, it has been suggested that the pregnant woman, with pre-pregnant weight of about 55 kg and the GWG of 8–12 kg, should receive an additional 9.5 g of protein during the second trimester and 22.0 g during the third trimester, which should be available from high quality proteins. The requirement would further increase, if plant-based proteins are consumed.
- **During lactation:** It has been suggested that additional 16.9 g of protein should be added (to the total daily amount recommended for non-pregnant women) during the first six months and 13.2 g between 6 and 12 months of lactation.
- **For infants and children:** Adequate dietary protein is essential during growth when new tissue proteins are being synthesized. The estimates of daily protein requirements for infants have been defined as 1.40 g/kg **during the first six months of life,** and 1.23 g/kg between **6 and 12 months** of age.

  The requirement for children has been suggested as 0.97 g/kg between 1 and 3 year(s) of age.
- **In disease conditions:** In some disease conditions, protein intake must be controlled, e.g. in **acute liver failure** (the intake has to be restricted in order to avoid hepatic coma) and **uremia** (when the capacity of the kidneys to excrete nitrogenous end products is limited).

DIETARY SOURCES OF PROTEIN

Animal-based foods like milk, meat, fish and eggs, and **plant-based foods** such as pulses and legumes are rich sources of proteins (Fig. 8.5).

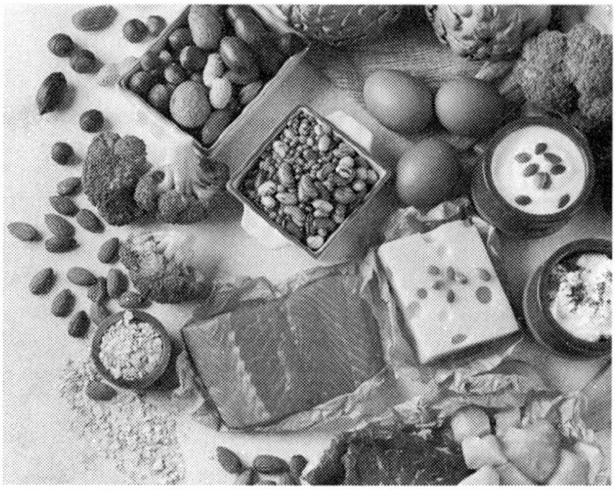

Fig. 8.5: Dietary sources of proteins

DIGESTION, ABSORPTION AND STORAGE OF PROTEINS

DIGESTION OF DIETARY PROTEIN

Digestion (enzymatic hydrolysis) of proteins **begins in the gastrointestinal tract** and is carried out **by proteases secreted by the stomach, the pancreas and the small intestine:**

- Digestion of proteins starts **in the stomach** by the action of proteolytic enzyme **pepsin,** at pH of the gastric juice. Pepsin is secreted by the cells of the gastric mucosa in the form of a zymogen (proenzyme) called **pepsinogen** which is activated by hydrogen ions of the gastric juice (HCl) and later autocatalytically by pepsin itself.
- **Proteolytic products of pepsin** pass on to **small intestine** where these **are hydrolyzed by** various other proteases **(trypsin, chymotrypsin and carboxypeptidases)** which are secreted by the pancreas.

- **Trypsin is secreted** in the zymogen form **as trypsinogen** which is **converted to trypsin by** another enzyme, called **enterokinase** (entero-peptidase). Once trypsin is formed, it acts on trypsinogen and converts it to trypsin, autocatalytically.
- **Chymotrypsin** is also synthesized and **secreted** as a zymogen designated as **chymotrypsinogen.** It is **activated by trypsin.**
- In addition, **procarboxypeptidase A** and **procarboxypeptidase B** are also **secreted as zymogens** and are **activated by trypsin.**
- **Carboxypeptidase A hydrolyzes the C-terminal** amino acid in peptides, particularly, of those where the terminal amino acid is an **aromatic or aliphatic amino acid.**
- **Carboxypeptidase B hydrolyzes the terminal** peptide bond of the **basic amino acid** (arginine or lysine).

- Pancreatic juice also secretes **collagenase** and **elastase,** which specifically act on collagen and elastin, respectively.
- The digestion of proteins, thereafter, is completed by the action of **amino-peptidases** and **dipeptidases,** which are secreted by the mucosa of the small intestine.
- Any part of the protein that is not hydrolyzed in the small intestine enters the large intestine and excreted in the feces.

ABSORPTION OF AMINO ACIDS

Amino acids are **absorbed from the small intestine** into the portal blood. It is a **Na^+-dependent active transport** which **requires ATP and specific transport proteins. Vitamin B_6 (pyridoxal-phosphate) is also required** for the absorption of amino acids.

There are several **transport systems for the uptake of different amino acids.** These include:

- A transport system for **neutral amino acids** with short or polar side **chains** such as Ala, Ser and Thr;
- For **neutral amino acids with an aromatic or hydrophobic side chain** such as Phe, Tyr, Met, Val, Leu, Ile;
- For **imino acids,** i.e. Pro and hydroxyproline (HO-Pro);
- For basic amino acids like **Lys, Arg and Cystine** (Cys-Cys);
- For **acidic amino acids,** i.e. Asp and Glu;
- For **β-amino acids,** e.g. β-Ala and taurine; and
- For **dipeptides,** e.g. peptide-1 (pep-1), glycyl-sarcosine, etc. These dipeptides are absorbed through the intestinal cells where these dipeptides are hydrolysed by dipeptidases to the constituent amino acids.
- Besides, the small intestine of the foetus and the neonate also absorbs intact proteins by endocytosis (pinocytosis).

METABOLISM OF AMINO ACIDS

Proteins differ from fat and carbohydrates in the way that proteins are **not stored in the body.** On the other hand, all the dietary proteins are digested and hydrolyzed into amino acids, which enter the bloodstream and forms amino acid pool.

In the liver, amino acids are utilised in different ways such as for protein synthesis and synthesis of various specialised products. Those in excess are **catabolized to release ammonia,** which is **converted to urea,** and the carbon skeletons, which are converted to **glucose.** Thus, proteins are also **used as a source of energy.** So,

- A part of the free amino acids, from the amino acid pool, is incorporated into **tissue proteins.**
- Some amino acids are also used for the synthesis of several **N-containing compounds** such as purine bases, creatine and epinephrine, etc.
- Excess of the free amino acids undergo **catabolic** degradation **(transamination** and **deamination)** and are used as a source of energy.

UTILIZATION OF PROTEINS FOR ENERGY

As discussed above, excess of the dietary **amino acids are** degraded to some metabolites which are **used as a source of energy (metabolic fuel).** According to the formation of the end product, i.e. glucose and/or ketone bodies, various amino acids are classified into three groups, as follows:

1. **Glucogenic amino acids:** These amino acids serve as precursors of glucose, which are used in gluconeogenesis, for glucose formation. For example, alanine, glutamate and valine form pyruvate, α-ketoglutarate and succinyl-CoA, respectively. As these are the intermediates of the citric acid cycle and can be converted to glucose by gluconeogenesis, these amino acids are called glucogenic amino acids. Glucogenic amino acids include **glycine, alanine, serine, aspartic acid, asparagine, glutamic acid, glutamine, proline, valine, methionine, cysteine, histidine and arginine.**
2. **Ketogenic amino acids:** These amino acids are degraded to form ketone bodies. These include **leucine and lysine.** End products of the catabolism of leucine are acetyl-CoA and aceto-acetyl-CoA, whereas the end product of the catabolism of lysine is aceto-acetyl-CoA.
3. **Both glucogenic and ketogenic amino acids:** Catabolic products of these amino acids are used in the formation of both ketone bodies and glucose. For example, catabolism of phenylalanine, in addition to fumarate, an intermediate of the citric acid cycle, also forms acetoacetyl-CoA, a precursor of ketone bodies. Therefore, these amino acids are referred to as glucogenic as well as ketogenic. These include **isoleucine, phenylalanine, tryptophan and tyrosine.**

Classification of amino acids based on metabolic fate, as a source of energy, is shown in Table 8.6.

PROTEIN ENERGY RATIO

Protein utilization and deposition are dependent on the intake of adequate energy. Adequate nonprotein energy from carbohydrates and fat is essential for dietary amino acids to be utilized for protein synthesis and for the other amino-acid related functions in the body. If adequate dietary energy is not available from carbohydrates and fat,

Table 8.6: Classification of amino acids based on metabolic fate

Metabolic fate of amino acids	*End products of their catabolism*
Glucogenic	
Gly, Ala, Ser, Cys, HO-Pro	Pyruvate
Glu, Gin, Pro, Arg, His	α-ketoglutarate
Val, Met	Succinyl-CoA
Asp, Asn	Oxaloacetate
Ketogenic	
Leu	Acetyl-CoA and acetoacetyl-CoA
Lys	Acetoacetyl-CoA
Glucogenic and ketogenic	
Ile	Succinyl-CoA and acetyl-CoA
Phe and Tyr	Fumarate and acetoacetyl-CoA
Trp	Pyruvate and acetoacetyl-CoA
Thr	Pyruvate and acetyl-CoA

dietary protein is used for energy, and is not available for other functions.

REMOVAL OF THE AMINO GROUP FROM AMINO ACIDS

There are two processes by which the α-amino group can be removed from amino acids. These are referred to as **transamination** and **deamination**.

TRANSAMINATION

Transamination is a process of the **transfer of the α-amino group from amino acid to keto acid.** As a result of it, the amino acid is converted to keto acid while the keto acid is converted to amino acid (Fig. 8.6).

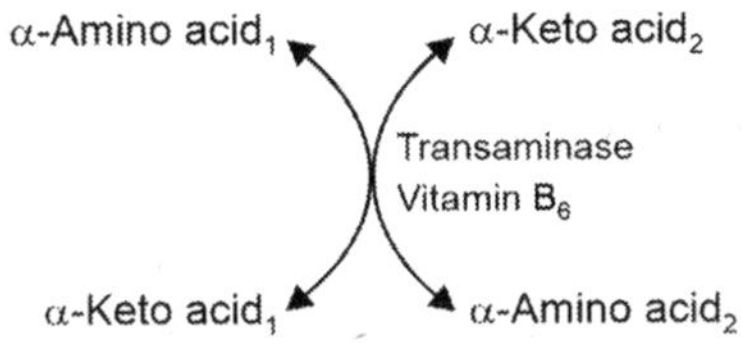

Fig. 8.6: Transamination reaction

Enzymes which catalyze transamination reactions are called transaminases or **aminotransferases.** Transaminases catalyzed reactions are shown in Fig. 8.7.

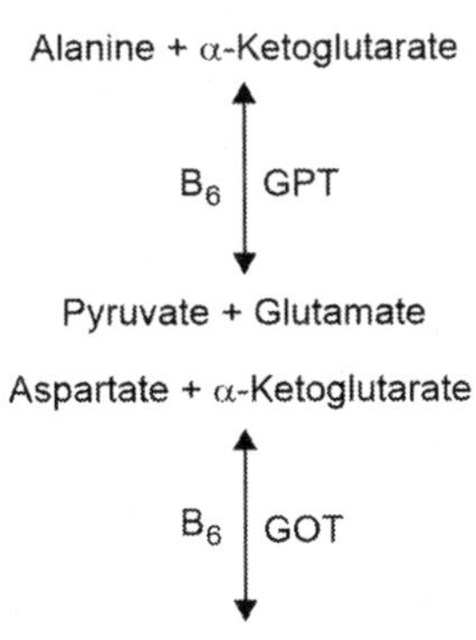

Fig. 8.7: GPT and GOT catalysed reactions

Diagnostic Significance of Transaminases

Liver contains several transaminases but most important of these are glutamate pyruvate transaminase (GPT, also called **alanine aminotransferase or ALT**) and glutamate oxaloacetate transaminase (GOT, also called **aspartate aminotransferase or** AST) which have diagnostic significance. These are present in large amounts in cardiac muscle and liver, respectively. Although, serum levels of both the enzymes are raised in heart as well as liver diseases, AST is markedly raised in myocardial infarction while ALT is more increased in liver disorders such as viral hepatitis or toxic liver necrosis (Table 8.7).

Table 8.7: Diagnostic significance of transaminases

Enzyme	*Comparatively more raised in*
SGOT	Cardiac disorders, e.g. myocardial infarction
SGPT	Liver disorders, e.g. viral hepatitis

Significance of Transamination Reactions

Besides the diagnostic significance of transaminases, transamination reactions are also important for the synthesis of nonessential amino acids and utilization of proteins as a source of glucose and thus, energy, in the body.

Synthesis of Nonessential Amino Acids

Except tyrosine, all the nonessential amino acids are synthesized from intermediates of the major metabolic pathways. As the carbon skeletons of the nonessential amino acids form α-ketoacids, by the reversal of the reactions, these α-ketoacid will form the corresponding nonessential amino acid. For example, the conversion of pyruvate to alanine, oxalo-acetate to aspartate or α-ketoglutarate to glutamate (Table 8.4).

Synthesis of Glucose

As discussed above, various glucogenic amino acids transfer their α-amino group by transamination and release carbon skeletons, which form intermediates of the citric acid cycle and are converted to glucose by the process of gluconeogenesis.

DEAMINATION

The process of the removal of α-amino group from the amino acids is referred to as deamination. Liver and kidney are the main organs which are responsible for deamination of amino acids. Deamination may take place either by oxidative or nonoxidative process.

Oxidative Deamination

Liver and kidney contain several enzymes which catalyze deamination of amino acids, such as amino acid oxidases. There are two types of amino acid oxidases, called L-amino acid oxidases and D-amino acid oxidases:

- **L-Amino Acid Oxidases:** L-amino acid oxidase is linked to FMN (the prosthetic group) and catalyzes the oxidation of L-amino acids, producing α-keto acids, ammonia and water as the final products (Fig. 8.8).

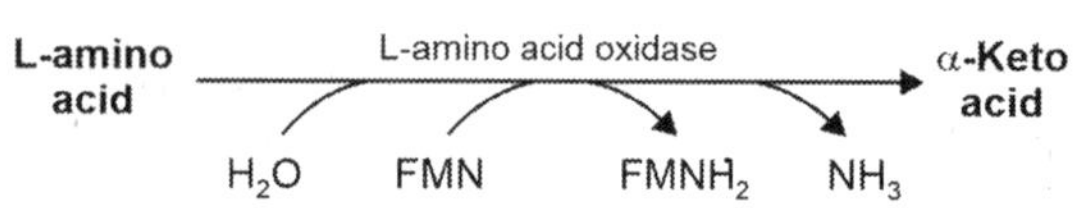

Fig. 8.8: L-amino acid oxidase reaction

- **D-Amino Acid Oxidases:** Some of the tissues also contain FAD-linked D-amino acid oxidases which catalyze oxidation of glycine and the D-amino acids.

Nonoxidative Deamination

Dehydratase, sulf-hydrase and histidase catalyze deamination of serine, cysteine and histidine, respectively. They catalyze dehydration followed by nonoxidative deamination of the amino acid, spontaneously (Fig. 8.9).

PROTEIN MALNUTRITION

Proteins are constantly broken down and used in the body. Hence, it is essential that the diet should provide enough protein, to replace what is being used, each day.

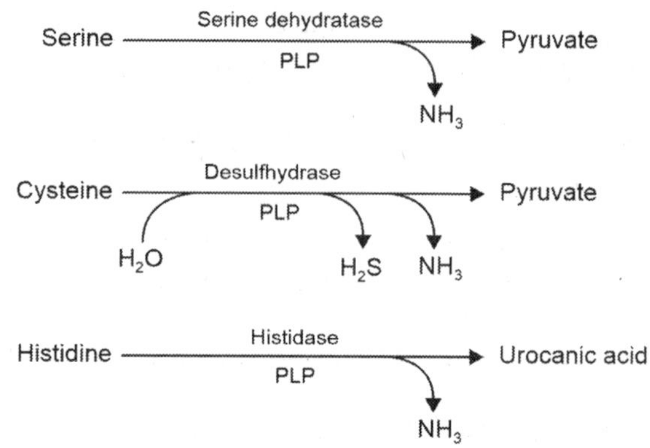

Fig. 8.9: Nonoxidative deamination reactions

Negative nitrogen balance may be a result of protein deficiency.

PROTEIN DEFICIENCY

Normally, it is difficult to separate protein intake and energy intake, since a diet, adequate in energy, usually, has adequate protein. Similarly, a diet which lacks energy, also inhibits the use of dietary protein for the synthesis of various proteins, required by the body. A deficiency of dietary protein and/or energy is called **protein–energy malnutrition** (Chapter 2).

PROTEIN OVERCONSUMPTION

High protein intake can cause several health problems.

- High protein intake can **alter kidney function,** since kidneys excrete urea, a product of protein catabolism.
- High protein intake also leads to increased excretion of calcium and thus, increases **risk of osteoporosis**.
- A diet high in proteins is also often high in fat thus, it contributes to **obesity**.
- High intake of animal proteins also increases the risk of heart diseases, since foods high in animal proteins are also high in saturated fat and cholesterol.
- Diets which have high content of animal proteins, have also been shown to be associated with increased risk of certain types of cancer such as that of colon, breast, pancreas and prostate.

SOME IMPORTANT QUESTIONS

1. **Define amino acid. How do you classify amino acids?**
2. **Describe sources, calorific value, recommended daily allowances and biological significance of proteins.**
3. **Differentiate between:**
   i. Essential and nonessential amino acids
   ii. Positive and negative nitrogen balance
   iii. Transamination and deamination
   iv. High quality and poor quality proteins
4. **Write notes on:**
   i. Nitrogen equilibrium
   ii. Semi-essential amino acids
   iii. Complementary action of proteins
   iv. Nutritional quality of proteins
   v. Biological value of proteins
5. **Briefly describe:**
   i. Protein deficiency
   ii. Nitrogen balance
   iii. Transamination and its significance
   iv. Digestion of proteins
   v. Absorption of amino acids

CHAPTER

9

Vitamins

Vitamins are the organic constituents of food, called protective accessory food factors. These are the micronutrients, which are essential for life and well-being. Vitamins, in general, cannot be synthesized by the body and have to be supplied in the diet.

CLASSIFICATION OF VITAMINS

Based on their solubility, vitamins are grouped into two categories, as **fat soluble** vitamins and **water soluble** vitamins.

WATER SOLUBLE VITAMINS

Water soluble vitamins include **B vitamins** (vitamin B complex) and **vitamin C.** As these are soluble in water, these are rapidly absorbed from the gastrointestinal lumen.

- Water soluble vitamins are **used as coenzymes** in various metabolic reactions.
- Due to their water solubility, most of the water-soluble vitamins are **not stored in the body.** Since, these cannot be stored, a dietary deficiency quickly becomes manifest.
- Typical deficiency symptoms, for most of the water-soluble vitamins, particularly, those of vitamin B complex, include **dermatitis, glossitis, cheilosis and diarrhea,** besides some of the neurological symptoms, such as peripheral neuropathy and malaise.
- Water soluble vitamins are susceptible to destruction by heat and alkalinity. Some cooking practices also destroy water soluble vitamins.

B-VITAMINS

The B-vitamins or **vitamin B complex** consists of various vitamins, which are generally referred by their names. These include:

- Thiamine (vitamin B_1)
- Riboflavin (vitamin B_2)
- Nicotinic acid (vitamin B_3)
- Pantothenic acid (vitamin B_5)
- Pyridoxine (vitamin B_6)
- Biotin (vitamin B_7)
- Folate (vitamin B_9)
- Cyanocobalamine (vitamin B_{12})

Most of the B-vitamins are synthesized in the GIT by the intestinal flora. As mentioned above, they, primarily, act as coenzymes, and help in catalyzing various metabolic reactions, particularly, energy producing reactions.

THIAMINE (VITAMIN B_1)

Thiamine is also referred to as **vitamin B_1** as it was the first water-soluble vitamin. It occurs in three forms, which are referred to as thiamine, thiamin monophosphate (TMP) and thiamine pyrophosphate (TPP).

Biochemical Functions

- The **coenzyme form** of thiamine is referred to as **TPP** (thiamin pyrophosphate).
- As a component of TPP, thiamine is **used** as a coenzyme **in** several **energy yielding metabolic pathways.**
- Accordingly, thiamine **requirement is related to the amount of energy consumed.**
- Thiamine is **also involved in** the normal functioning of the **nervous system** and other excitable tissues such as **skeletal muscle** and the **heart.**

Daily Requirement

RDA for thiamine has been suggested between **1.4–2.3 mg/day.**

Its **RDA** has been suggested as **1.8 mg/d for adult male moderate worker and 1.7 mg/d for adult female moderate worker.**

ICMR-NIN (2020) has recommended additional allowances of thiamine **depending upon** the additional **calories intake.**

Thiamine requirement is increased during fever, hyperthyroidism, and in alcoholics and pregnant women.

Sources

Rich sources of thiamine include **whole grain cereals, oilseeds, nuts, legumes, green-leafy vegetables, organ meats, liver, eggs, and milk and milk products.**

Deficiency Symptoms

Thiamine deficiency occurs with the consumption of raw fish, which contains thiaminase that destroys thiamine.

Thiamine deficiency manifest as **beriberi,** which may be:

- **Wet beriberi:** It **affects cardiovascular system** and results in edema, and dilated heart.
- **Dry beriberi:** It, normally **affects central nervous system** and causes peripheral neuropathy with myelin degeneration, leading to foot-drop and paralysis.

In alcoholics, particularly, in those consuming poor quality of diet with low thiamine content, thiamine deficiency may lead to a condition referred to as **Wernicke-Korsakoff syndrome (Wernicke's encephalopathy).**

Common deficiency symptoms include neuropathies and numbness, **nausea, vomiting, weakness and tenderness of the calf muscles.**

RIBOFLAVIN (VITAMIN B_2)

Riboflavin is also referred to as **vitamin B_2.** It is also called **lactoflavin,** due to its presence in milk. It is needed for the normal structure and functions of mucous membrane and skin.

Biochemical Functions

- Riboflavin is a component of the **coenzymes FMN** (flavin mononucleotide) and **FAD** (flavin adenine dinucleotide).
- As a component of FMN and FAD, riboflavin **acts as electron and hydrogen acceptor,** and **participates in** several **oxidation–reduction reactions** in the citric acid cycle, β-oxidation of fatty acids, and oxidative deamination.
- Thus, vitamin B_2 is required to release energy from proteins, carbohydrates and fat.

Daily Requirement

RDA for riboflavin has been suggested between **1.9–3.2 mg/day.**

Its RDA is suggested as **2.5 mg/d for adult male moderate worker and 2.4 mg/d for adult female moderate worker.**

ICMR-NIN (2020) has recommended additional allowances **depending upon** the additional **calories intake**.

Sources

Milk, liver, kidney, egg-white, green-leafy vegetables, mushrooms and almonds are rich sources of riboflavin.

Deficiency Symptoms

Riboflavin deficiency may be observed with malabsorption, prolonged fever, hyperthyroidism and pregnancy. Deficiency symptoms include chelosis (lesions at angles of the mouth), **glossitis,** and **angular stomatitis.** There may be reduced iron absorption and diminished visual activity, as well.

NIACIN (Vitamin B_3)

Niacin is also referred to as vitamin B_3. **Nicotinic acid** and **nicotinamide** (or **niacinamide**) refer to two similarly functioning compounds which **have niacin activity.** It is also known as **pellagra-preventive factor,** due to its role in the prevention of pellagra.

Biochemical Functions

- Niacin is a component of the **coenzymes NAD** (nicotinamide adenine dinucleotide) and **NADP** (nicotinamide adenine dinucleotide phosphate).
- Both, NAD and NADP **participate in oxidation–reduction reactions.**
- **NAD** accepts electrons and hydrogen, and **is reduced to NADH,** that **carries electrons to the electron transport chain.**
- **NADP is reduced to NADPH,** which is **used in the synthesis of fatty acids, cholesterol and steroid hormones.**
- Both, NAD and NADP are catabolized to yield nicotinamide, which can be deaminated into nicotinic acid or methylated to yield 1-methyl-nicotinamide.

Daily Requirement

ICMR-NIN (2020) has recommended the requirement of niacin based on **calories intake.**

RDA for niacin has been suggested between **11–23 mg/day.**

Its **RDA** is suggested as **18 mg/d for adult male moderate worker** and **14 mg/d for adult female moderate worker.**

Sources

Nuts and oilseeds are good sources of nicotinic acid, whereas nicotinamide is absorbed in the liver from animal foods.

Synthesis of Niacin

Niacin can also be synthesized in the liver in the form of NAD. Sixty mg of tryptophan gives one mg equivalent of niacin. This is called tryptophan–niacin conversion ratio, whose value has been given as 60:1.

Milk and milk products, though are not important sources of niacin, but have **high tryptophan** content. Thus, milk and milk products play an important role in niacin biosynthesis and prevention of pellagra.

Deficiency Symptoms

Niacin deficiency is **common in persons whose staple food is maize and jowar** (called millets). Such individuals develop pellagra-like symptoms, since maize and jowar are **deficient in tryptophan.** On the other hand, these millets are rich in **isoleucine.** Low tryptophan and high isoleucine results in amino acid imbalance, which reduces biosynthesis of niacin in the body.

Deficiency of niacin can lead to a disease called **pellagra** which is characterized by **3Ds,** i.e. dermatitis, diarrhea and dementia.

- **Dermatitis** results in pain, particularly, in those parts of the body which are exposed to sunlight such as face, neck, hands and feet. These parts become bronze, resembling sunburn, and get thickened.
- **Diarrhea** is accompanied with anorexia, abdominal discomforts and other symptoms of gastrointestinal tract.
- **Dementia** is due to impaired ability of the brain to utilize carbohydrates. Symptoms like depression, confusion and psychosis are commonly observed.
- Prolonged deficiency of niacin may result in 4th D, i.e. death.

PANTOTHENIC ACID (VITAMIN B_5)

Pantothenic acid is also referred to as vitamin B_5. It, **structurally,** is a combination of pantoic acid and **β-alanine.**

Biochemical Functions

- Pantothenic acid forms an **integral part of coenzyme A** (CoA) as well as **acyl carrier protein** (ACP).
- **CoA is** essentially **required in fatty acid metabolism.**
- CoA is also required in the **metabolism of proteins, carbohydrates and fat.**
- **ACP is used in fatty acid synthesis.**

Daily Requirement

RDA for pantothenic acid for normal adults has been suggested as **5 mg per day.**

Sources

Rich sources of pantothenic acid are **yeast, liver, eggs, potatoes, whole cereals and legumes.**

Deficiency Symptoms

- Pantothenic acid deficiency, in human beings, **affects nervous and digestive systems.**
- Its deficiency has also been shown to result in **adrenal insufficiency.**
- Deficiency symptoms include **headache, fatigue, impaired motor activity, muscle cramps and gastrointestinal disturbances.**
- Pantothenic acid is also **used in burning-feet syndrome** as well as **healing of ulcers and bedsores.**

PYRIDOXINE (VITAMIN B_6)

Pyridoxine, also called vitamin B_6, refers to three different compounds (vitamers), which include:

- Pyridoxine
- Pyridoxal, and
- Pyridoxamine.

Biochemical Functions

- The **coenzyme form** of vitamin B_6 is called pyridoxal-5-phosphate **(PLP).**
- **PLP is used as a coenzyme** with different enzymes which are involved in the **transfer of amino group** (NH_2), **carboxyl group** (–COOH) or **water** from one compound to another. Thus, PLP is also called cotransferase.
- PLP also plays a role in the **synthesis of non-essential amino acids.**
- PLP also **promotes gluconeogenesis** and facilitates glycogenolysis.
- **Vitamin B_6** also **helps in the production of several neurotransmitters,** such as serotonin, γ-aminobutyric acid, dopamine and norepinephrine.
- It also helps in the **conversion of tryptophan to niacin.**
- Vitamin B_6 is also important in the **synthesis of hemoglobin** and its binding with oxygen.
- Dietary vitamin B_6, along **with folate and vitamin B_{12}, lowers blood homocysteine levels,** which, in turn, is associated with the risk of cardiovascular disease.

Daily Requirement

RDA for vitamin B_6 has been suggested between **1.9–3.1 mg per day.**

Its RDA is suggested as **2.4 mg/d for adult male moderate worker** and **1.9 mg/d for adult female moderate worker.**

Sources

Rich sources of vitamin B_6 include **nuts and seeds, poultry, chicken and liver.**

Deficiency Symptoms

Deficiency symptoms include **cheilosis, glossitis and peripheral neuritis.**

- **In infants,** deficiency of B_6 affects central nervous system and results in **convulsions, demyelination** of the peripheral nerves and **degeneration of axons.** Its deficiency also associated with **hypochromic microcytic anemia.**

- Pyridoxine has also been shown to be **helpful in the treatment of nausea and vomiting during pregnancy, radiation therapy and muscular dystrophy.**

Vitamin B_6 Antagonists

Deficiency of vitamin B_6 has been shown to **occur in patients** with tuberculosis, who are **taking antitubercular drug INH** (isonicotin-hydrazide), since **INH acts as an antagonist to vitamin B_6** (Fig. 9.1).

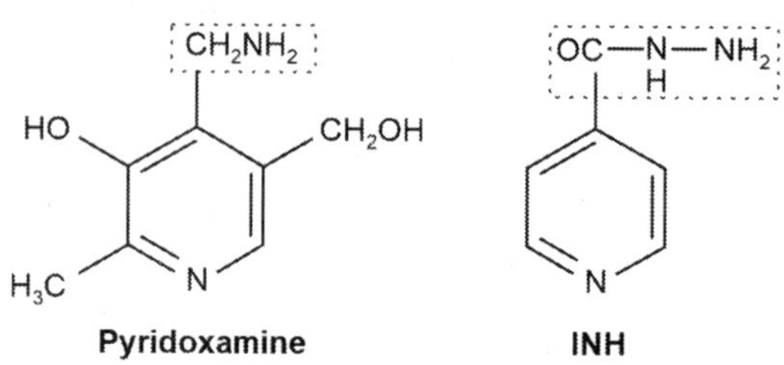

Fig. 9.1: Pyridoxamine and INH

BIOTIN (VITAMIN B_7)

Biotin is also referred to as vitamin B_7. It is involved in a wide range of metabolic processes, primarily, related to the utilization of fat, carbohydrates and amino acids.

Biochemical Functions

- Biotin forms **prosthetic group of the biotin-containing enzymes.**
- It is important in **carboxylation reactions,** where **carbon dioxide is added to the substrate,** e.g. in the conversion of pyruvate to oxaloacetate, propionyl-CoA to succinyl-CoA and acetyl-CoA to malonyl-CoA. Thus, it is also called as cocarboxylase.

Daily Requirement

RDA for biotin for normal adult has been suggested as **25 µg/day.**

Sources

Rice polish, whole cereals, milk, yeast and organ meat such as liver and kidney are good sources of biotin.

Deficiency Symptoms

Raw egg-white contains a heat labile **biotin-binding protein** called **avidin** which binds to biotin and **inhibits its absorption.** If raw egg-white is taken in large amounts, avidin acts as **antivitamin** for biotin and causes biotin deficiency.

Heating raw egg white denatures avidin and prevents its effect.

Deficiency of biotin **may cause mild dermatitis, nausea and loss of appetite, muscular pain and anemia.**

FOLATE (VITAMIN B_9)

Folate is also referred to as folic acid or vitamin B_9. It refers to a **group of derivatives of pteroylglutamic acid.** The synthetic form of folate, available commercially, is used as supplement in food fortification.

Biochemical Functions

- The **coenzyme form** of folate is referred to as tetrahydro-folate **(FH_4).**
- Tetrahydro-folate is **important in one-carbon metabolism.**
- It also plays an important role in **amino acid metabolism,** particularly, in the metabolism of serine and methionine, and in **purine synthesis.**
- With vitamin B_{12}, folate also helps in the **formation of red blood cells.**
- It is also required for normal **cell division,** structure of the nervous system, specifically, in the **development of the neural tube,** which develops into the spinal cord and skull, in the embryo.
- With vitamin B_6 and vitamin B_{12}, folate is also required for the **maintenance of blood homocysteine level.**

Daily Requirement

RDA for folate (dietary folate) has been suggested between **220 and 300 µg/day**.

Its RDA is recommended as **300 µg/d for adult men** and **220 µg/d for adult women.**

Sources

Green leafy vegetables such as spinach and cabbage, **yeast, liver and kidney** are good sources of folate.

Deficiency Symptoms

- Folate **deficiency may be seen in stressful conditions,** during pregnancy, intestinal malabsorption such as steatorrhea, and during antibiotic therapy.
- Its deficiency may result in macrocytic **(megaloblastic) anemia.**
- Combined deficiency of folate and vitamin B_{12} may result in **psychosis and mental retardation.**
- Folate deficiency in early pregnancy, has also been implicated in **neural tube defects.**

Folic Acid Antagonists

- Several compounds **interfere with the metabolic functions of folic acid.** These are referred to as folic acid antagonists. Most potent of these include **aminopterin and amethopterin.**
- **Amethopterin** (N10-methylfolic acid or **methotrexate**) **inhibits folic acid reductase,** thus, affects the conversion of folic acid to FH_4.
- **Aminopterin** (4-aminofolic acid) inhibits the conversion of folic acid to folinic acid and, thus, **inhibits biosynthesis of nucleic acids.**
- Both of these act as competitive inhibitors of dihydrofolate reductase, and, thus, are **used as anticancer agents,** particularly, in the treatment of childhood leukemias.

CYANOCOBALAMIN (VITAMIN B_{12})

Vitamin B_{12}, also called **cyanocobalamin,** refers to a family of cobalamin-containing compounds, which include **cyanocobalamin** and **hydroxy-cobalamin.**

Biochemical Functions

- **Coenzyme forms** of vitamin B_{12} include **deoxyadenosyl-cobalamin** and **methyl-cobalamin.**
- Vitamin B_{12} is also important for the **metabolism of folate.**
- With folate, **deoxyadenosyl-cobalamin** plays a key **role in one-carbon metabolism.**
- **Methyl-cobalamin** is **essential in amino acid metabolism, DNA synthesis and cell multiplication.**
- It is also **required in propionate metabolism** (in the conversion of methyl-malonyl-CoA to succinyl-CoA).
- Vitamin B_{12} also helps to maintain **myelin sheath.**
- It is also important for the nervous system and formation of red blood cells.

Daily Requirement

RDA for vitamin B_{12} for normal adults has been suggested as **2.2 µg/day.**

Sources

Liver, kidney, eggs, fish and milk are the good sources of vitamin B_{12}.

Deficiency Symptoms

- Vitamin B_{12} deficiency **can be seen in geriatric persons,** particularly, in those who are **strict vegetarians.**
- Its deficiency may also occur on **prolonged reduced intake, intestinal malabsorption, atrophy of the gastric mucosa,** or due to deficiency of the intrinsic factor such as in **pernicious anemia.**
- Vitamin B_{12} deficiency can result in **methylmalonic aciduria.**
- Measurement of the **urinary excretion of methylmalonic acid** is used to **confirm deficiency of this vitamin.**

VITAMIN C

Vitamin C is also called **ascorbic acid.** Due to its role in the prevention of scurvy, vitamin C is also called **anti-scurvy factor.**

- Majority of the animals can synthesize vitamin C from glucuronate, but men, primates, and guinea pigs **cannot synthesize it.**
- Vitamin C is **destroyed by heat.**

Biochemical Functions

Ascorbic acid performs several functions in the body. These include:

- **Collagen synthesis:** Ascorbic acid plays an important role in hydroxylation reactions. **Hydroxylation of proline** by the enzyme prolyl-hydroxylase converts it to hydroxyproline which is an important constituent of collagen.
- **Antioxidant activity:** Ascorbic acid acts as an antioxidant and **prevents damage caused by free radicals.** This, in turn, reduces the risk of certain chronic diseases such as heart disease, cancer and cataract.
- Ascorbic acid also helps in **recycling of** the oxidized form of **vitamin E** for its reuse within the cells.
- Vitamin C also **stabilizes** the reduced form of **folate.**
- **Absorption of iron:** As a reducing agent, vitamin C also enhances the absorption of non-heme iron from plant foods.
- **Synthesis of vital compounds:** Ascorbic acid also helps in the synthesis of various vital compounds such as **carnitine, norepinephrine, epinephrine, serotonin, thyroxine, bile acids, steroid hormones and purines.**
- **Immune functions:** Vitamin C also enables lymphocytes and other cells of the immune system to function properly. Accordingly, high doses of vitamin C may reduce severity and duration of cold-related symptoms.

Daily Requirement

RDA for vitamin C has been suggested between **65 and 80 mg/day.**

Its RDA has been suggested as **80 mg/d for adult males** and **65 mg/d for females.**

Women need more vitamin C during pregnancy and lactation. Smokers also need more vitamin C, as smoke increases metabolic turnover of the vitamin.

Sources

Amla is the richest source of vitamin **C. Citrus fruits, green chilies, guava and tomatoes** are also good sources of vitamin C.

Deficiency Symptoms

Prolonged deficiency of vitamin C causes **scurvy.**

- Early symptoms of the disease include **swollen, spongy and bleeding gums; loosening of teeth; and pain in joints.** In severe cases there may be **multiple hemorrhages** including bleeding from nose, gastrointestinal tract and genitourinary tract.

  Prolong deficiency of vitamin C inhibits prolyl-hydroxylase, as a result of which hydroxyproline cannot be synthesized, thereby resulting in defective collagen synthesis and bleeding of gums. Thus, **low levels of vitamin C in blood increase the risk of gum bleeding** (one of the symptoms of scurvy), which can be resolved by increased intake of vitamin C.
- **Infants may lose appetite and body weight** with **painful tenderness of the extremities, bleeding from gums** and **mucous membrane, and cessation of osteogenesis of long bones.**
- Because of its role in the absorption, transport and storage of iron, vitamin C deficiency may also cause **anemia.**

Vitamin C toxicity: Vitamin C is not normally toxic but large doses may result in a**bdominal pain, diarrhea, and nausea.** More than 3 g/day may lead to **urolithiasis** (formation of oxalate stones).

Water soluble vitamins, their coenzyme forms, major **biochemical functions, principal deficiency diseases and daily requirements** are shown in Table 9.1.

FAT SOLUBLE VITAMINS

Fat soluble vitamins include vitamin A, vitamin D, vitamin E and vitamin K. These are absorbed from the gastrointestinal lumen, in the presence of dietary fat (triacylglycerols) and bile salts.

VITAMIN A

Vitamin A refers to a group of compounds, collectively, called retinoids. These include **retinol** (vitamin A alcohol), **retinal** (vitamin A aldehyde or retinaldehyde) and **retinoic acid** (vitamin A acid).

Provitamin A

Plants contain a group of compounds called **carotenoids.** Carotenoids are referred to as **provitamin A** (precursors of vitamin A), because these are converted to retinoids (vitamin A), when metabolized in the body.

Physiological Functions

Vitamin A is essential to the normal structure and functions of the skin and mucous membrane in eyes, lungs and digestive system. It is, therefore, vital for vision, embryonic development, growth and cellular differentiation, and immune system. Besides,

- **Retinal** is essential for **night and color vision.**
- **Retinol** is required in **reproduction and bone health.**

Table 9.1: Water soluble vitamins, their coenzyme forms, biochemical role, deficiency diseases and daily requirements for adults

Vitamin	*Coenzyme*	*Major biochemical role*	*Deficiency diseases*	*Daily requirement*
Vitamin B complex				
Thiamin (B_1)	TPP	Oxidative decarboxylation	Beriberi	1.4–2.3 mg
Riboflavin (B_2)	FMN, FAD	Oxidation–reduction with flavo-proteins	Lesions on lips, cheilosis	1.9–3.2 mg
Niacin	NAD^+, $NADP^+$	Hydrogen acceptor for dehydrogenases	Pellagra	11–23 mg
Pyridoxine (B_6)	Pyridoxal-5-PO_4	Transamination, decarboxylation	Peripheral neuritis	1.9–3.1 mg
Pantothenic acid	Coenzyme A	Formation of CoA, component of the acyl carrier protein	Muscle cramps, burning feet	5 mg
Biotin	Carboxybiocytin	Cocarboxylase	Anemia, dermatitis	25 μg
Folate	FH_4	Carrier of one-C moiety	Megaloblastic macrocytic anemia	220–300 μg
Cobalamin (B_{12})	Cobamides	Transmethylation with FH_4	Pernicious anemia	2.2 μg
Vitamin C (Ascorbic acid)	L-Ascorbate	Hydroxylation	Scurvy	65–80 mg

- **Retinoic acid** is important for **cell growth and differentiation.**
- **Provitamin A** (carotenoids) functions as a potent **antioxidant** and **prevents damaging effects of free radicals.** Thus, carotenoids help to prevent damage from chemical carcinogens and lower the risk of certain types of cancer.

Role of Vitamin A in Visual Process

Retinal (vitamin A aldehyde), as mentioned above, is essential for vision, both in rods as well as cones:

- **In rods:** Rod cells contain a conjugated transmembrane protein called **rhodopsin,** which consists of an apoprotein **opsin** and a nonprotein prosthetic group called **11-cis-retinal** (11-cis-retinene).

  Rhodopsin is essential for vision in dim light.
  - **When light falls on retina, rhodopsin** is bleached and **generates all-trans-retinal,** which cannot form a complex with opsin.
  - All-trans-retinal is **reduced to all-trans-retinol by** the enzyme **all-trans-retinol dehydrogenase** (retinene reductase).
  - It is then **transported to the liver and stored** there.
  - In the liver, it is **isomerized to 11-cis-retinol by an isomerase.**
  - After its delivery to the retina, 11-cis-retinol is **changed to 11-cis-retinal,** which again **conjugates with opsin** and **reforms rhodopsin, in dark.**
  - This is called vision cycle (Fig. 9.2).
- **In cones:** Similar to rhodopsin, which is present in rods for the black and white vision, **cones contain** 3 different pigments which are sensitive to three primary colors, i.e. **porphyropsin (for red), iodopsin (for green)** and **cyanopsin (for blue).** Prosthetic group in these pigments is the same, i.e. **11-cis-retinal.**

Daily Requirement

Vitamin A requirement is expressed in terms of retinol equivalents **(RE). One RE** represents one **μg of retinal** or **12 μg of α-carotene.** Accordingly, the general **conversion ratio of 6:1 for β-carotene** and **12:1 for α-carotene has been suggested.**

RDA for **vitamin A** has been suggested between **840 and 1000 μg/day.**

Its RDA has been suggested as **1000 μg/d for adult males** and **840 μg/d for adult females.**

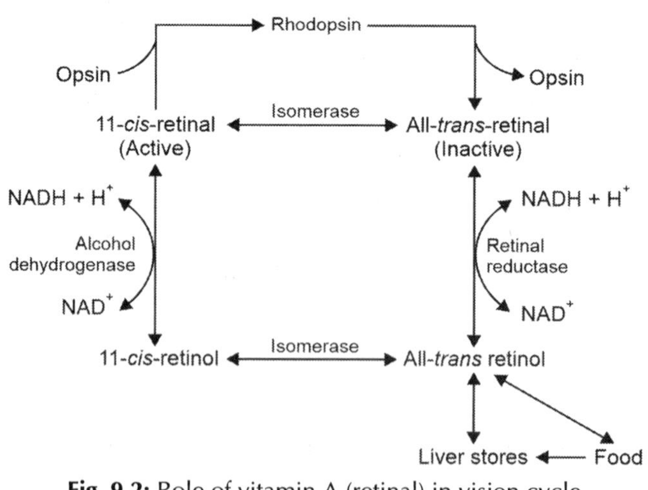

Fig. 9.2: Role of vitamin A (retinal) in vision cycle

Its requirement is **increased by about 10% during pregnancy and 20% during lactation.**

Sources

Liver oil, fish-liver oil, eggs, milk and milk products are good sources of **vitamin A.**

On the other hand, **papaya, carrots, sweet potatoes, and green leafy vegetables** are good sources of **β-carotene.**

Deficiency Symptoms

Vitamin A deficiency is observed, primarily, due to its low intake. Its deficiency is aggravated by infections, which reduces its absorption and utilization. Vitamin A deficiency affects many tissues:

- It is most detrimental for eyes. Deficiency of vitamin A may result in **xerophthalmia,** which is characterized by **drying of conjunctiva and cornea, followed by destruction of cornea, leading to blindness.** Manifestations of xerophthalmia are shown in Fig. 9.3.
- Vitamin A deficiency also affects osteoblastic activity and results in **defective resorption of bone,** affecting growth.
- Deficiency of vitamin A also results in xerosis and keratinization of the mucous membrane, resulting in **dry and rough skin.** Keratinization of the mucous membrane increases its susceptibility to infections.

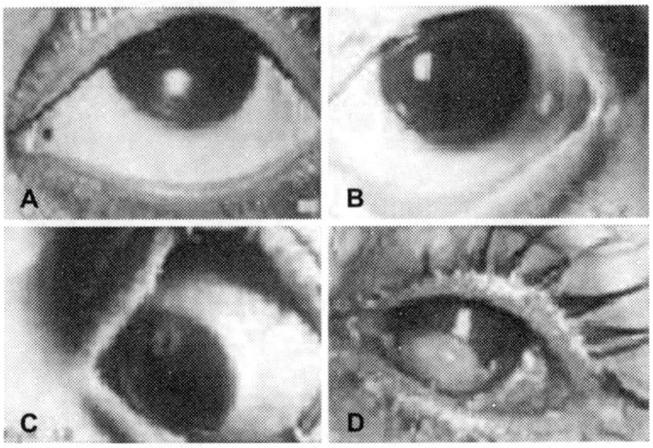

Fig. 9.3: Manifestations of xerophthalmia. (A) Bitot's spot; (B) Corneal xerosis; (C) Keratomalacia; and (D) Corneal scar

- Keratinization of the urinary tract may lead to **urolithiasis.**
- Vitamin A deficiency also results in certain abnormalities of the reproductive system, such as **degeneration of testes, abortions** and production of the **malformed-offsprings.**
- Keratinization of epithelium of the seminiferous tubules may also lead to **infertility.**

Hypervitaminosis A

If taken in large quantities for a longer period, vitamin A is toxic, since it is a fat-soluble vitamin and stored in the liver.

Toxicity symptoms include skin abnormalities such as **dry and rough skin, scaly dermatitis, headache, nausea, vomiting** and **loss of appetite, hepatomegaly, painful joints** and several bone abnormalities.

VITAMIN D

Vitamin D is a **sterol (steroid alcohol),** also called **sunshine vitamin.** Although several forms of vitamin D have been shown to exhibit antirachitic properties, most important of these are:

- Vitamin **D_2 (ergocalciferol)** found in **plant foods, and**
- Vitamin **D_3 (cholecalciferol)** found in **animal foods.** It is also **synthesized in the skin.**

Vitamin D is, classically, a **prohormone.** It acts as a **precursor to** the hormone calcitriol (1,25-dihydroxycholecalciferol).

Provitamin D

A derivative of cholesterol, called **7-dehydrocholesterol,** is a precursor of vitamin D_3 in animals. It is also called provitamin D. It is synthesized in the human beings from cholesterol and is **converted to vitamin D_3 by UV light, in the skin.** This process is referred to as **photo-biogenesis.**

Active Vitamin D

Vitamin D is activated by two sequential hydroxylation reactions:

- The first step takes place **in the liver,** where it is hydroxylated by cytochrome P450-dependent 25-hydroxylase to **25-hydroxycholecalciferol** [25(OH).D_3].
- From liver, 25-hydroxycholecalciferol is **transported to kidney,** where it is further hydroxylated at position-1, by the mitochondrial enzyme 1-α-hydroxylase, forming **1,25-dihydroxycholecalciferol** [1,25$(OH)_2$.D_3], also called **calcitriol.**

Calcitriol is the physiologically **active form of the vitamin,** which **functions as a hormone** and is **essential for calcium homeostasis.**

Physiological Functions of Vitamin D

- Primary role of vitamin D, in the form of **calcitriol,** is to **regulate blood calcium** level, through its action on **bone, kidneys** and **small intestine.**
- Receptors for calcitriol are also found in a variety of other tissues, hence, vitamin D has also been shown to **inhibit cell proliferation** and **enhance cell differentiation.**

Role of vitamin D in calcium metabolism—Calcitriol **induces synthesis of calcium-binding protein, Ca^{2+}-dependent ATPase and alkaline phosphatase,** which are essential for the regulation of serum calcium and phosphorus.

Net result is achieved through its action in the intestine, bone and kidney:

- **In the intestine,** due to stimulation of synthesis of the calcium-binding protein, 1,25$(OH)_2$.D_3 **increases intestinal absorption of calcium** as well as phosphorus.
- **In the bone,** calcitriol **stimulates synthesis of osteocalcin,** which, in turn, mobilizes calcium from bone, i.e. it **causes demineralization of bone.**
- **In the kidney,** active vitamin D **increases tubular reabsorption of calcium** and **excretion of phosphorus.**

Overall effect of the three processes, thus, is to **increase serum calcium level towards normal.**

Daily Requirement

ICMR-NIN (2020) has emphasized the importance of outdoor activities for achieving adequate vitamin D status in tropical countries like India.

RDA for vitamin D for normal adult has been suggested as **600 IU** (15 μg) **per day.**

Sources

As vitamin D can be synthesized in the body by the action of the ultraviolet light on the skin, hence, **sunshine** is the best source of vitamin D.

Besides sunshine, rich sources of vitamin D are **milk, butter, egg yolk, fish oil and liver oil.**

Deficiency Symptoms

Deficiency of vitamin D, generally, does not occur, as it can be synthesized in the body. Deficiency, however, may occur due to lack of sunshine.

Vitamin D deficiency leads to **rickets in children and osteomalacia in adults** (Fig. 9.4).

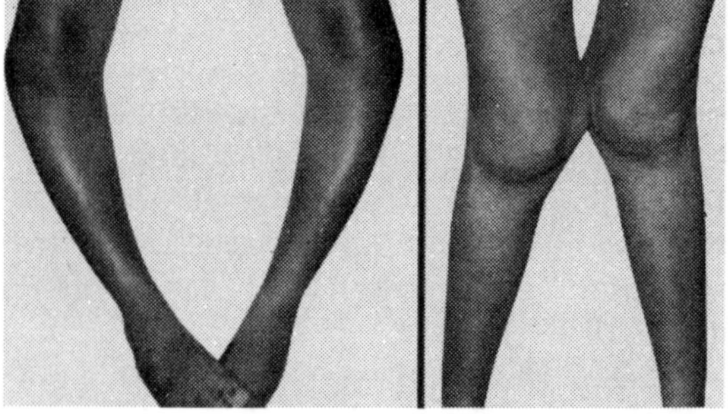

Fig. 9.4: Rickets (bowed-legs and knock-knees)

Hypervitaminosis D

Extremely large doses of vitamin D, over a long period, may lead to **hypercalcemia, hyperphosphatemia, anorexia, nausea, vomiting** and **diarrhea,** besides **bone pain** and metastatic **calcification of the soft tissues** including kidney, myocardium, pancreas and uterus.

VITAMIN E

Several compounds belonging to the group of tocopherols, such as **α, β, γ and δ tocopherols, exhibit vitamin E activity.**

- The α-tocopherol has highest biological activity as well as widest distribution. It is an alcohol with a **phytol** and **trimethylhydroquinone.**
- Commercially, vitamin E is available, both, as a natural substance as well as a synthetic compound.
- **Natural** vitamin E is **d-α-tocopherol** and is a single stereoisomer.
- **Synthetic** vitamin E **is dl-α-tocopherol,** which is **produced commercially.**

Physiological Functions of Vitamin E

Vitamin E performs several functions:

- Vitamin E acts as an **antioxidant.**
- It stabilizes cell membrane and **defends cells against oxidative damage** from free radicals. Since cells damaged by free radicals, are prone to mutations, thus, vitamin E **helps to prevent cancer.**
- Vitamin E also maintains antioxidant status of **α-carotene.**

Daily Requirement

ICMR-NIN (2020) has suggested that requirement of vitamin E varies depending upon the level and nature of physical activity, diet, psychological stress, exposure to pollutants and intake of polyunsaturated fatty acids.

It is recommended that, normally, **0.8 mg of vitamin E** is required **per g of PUFA.**

Its RDA for normal adult has been suggested as **8–10 mg/day.**

Sources

Tocopherols are present in small quantities in **green leafy vegetables** such as spinach and lettuce, **milk and milk products,** and **egg yolk.**

Oils, such as **corn oil, cottonseed oil and sunflower oil** are also rich sources of vitamin E.

Deficiency Symptoms

Vitamin E deficiency results in a range of **degenerative diseases.**

- Its **deficiency is seen in patients with abetalipoproteinemia,** who cannot form chylomicrons and VLDL. As a result of abetalipoproteinemia, vitamin E can neither be absorbed nor distributed.
- Deficiency of vitamin E is **also seen in children with fat malabsorption,** where it results in **severe progressive neuropathy and retinopathy.**
- **Hepatic necrosis, muscular dystrophy, defects in vascular system** and certain **reproductive defects** are also known to occur due to deficiency of vitamin E in various animal species.

VITAMIN K

Vitamin K refers to a family of compounds known as **naphthoquinones.** These include:

- Vitamin K_1 (**phylloquinone,** obtained from plant sources). It is the most biologically active form.
- Vitamin K_2 (**menaquinone,** obtained from animal sources and synthesized by intestinal bacteria) and
- Vitamin K_3 (**menadione,** the water-soluble form, available commercially).

Physiological Functions of Vitamin K

- Vitamin K plays a key role in the formation of **blood clot.** It is required for many reactions in the blood-clotting cascade, which involves the **production of** a series of proteins such as **prothrombin, factor VII, factor IX and factor X, and fibrin.**
- It also helps in **bone formation,** where it is required in the **carboxylation of osteocalcin,** which is required for mineralization and maturation of bone.

Role of Vitamin K in Gamma Carboxylation

Vitamin K is essential for maintenance of the normal levels of various blood clotting factors such as prothrombin, factor VII, factor IX and factor X. These proteins are synthesized in the liver in their inactive forms and get **converted to their biologically active forms by γ-carboxylation,** with the help of vitamin K (Fig. 9.5).

> ***Note:*** Reduced synthesis of blood clotting factors forms the basis of internal bleeding arising due to vitamin K deficiency.

Daily Requirement

RDA for vitamin K for normal adults has been suggested as **55 μg/day.**

Further, it is advised to administer a **single prophylactic dose of 1 mg of vitamin K_1 to a newborn on the first day of life.**

Sources

Green leafy vegetables such as spinach, lettuce and cabbage, are the rich sources of vitamin K. **Fish, liver and skeletal muscle** are also good sources of this vitamin.

Deficiency Symptoms

Deficiency of vitamin K is seen **in newborns,** due to their sterile intestine, particularly, in **premature infants,** who show **reduced levels of vitamin K, prothrombin and Christmas factor.** This also forms the basis of internal bleeding arising due to vitamin K deficiency.

Common deficiency symptoms include **cutaneous and intramuscular hemorrhages** with **bluish-red discoloration in different** parts of the body.

Vitamin K Antagonists

Anticoagulants such as **dicumarol and warfarin,** due to their **structural similarities** with vitamin K_1, act as antagonists **(anti-vitamins)** of vitamin K.

These compounds act as **competitive inhibitors for the enzymes,** which are concerned with the **activation of** prothrombin and other **coagulation factors,** and require vitamin K for their activation.

Table 9.2 lists various **fat soluble vitamins,** their **physiological functions, deficiency diseases, sources and daily requirements** for adults.

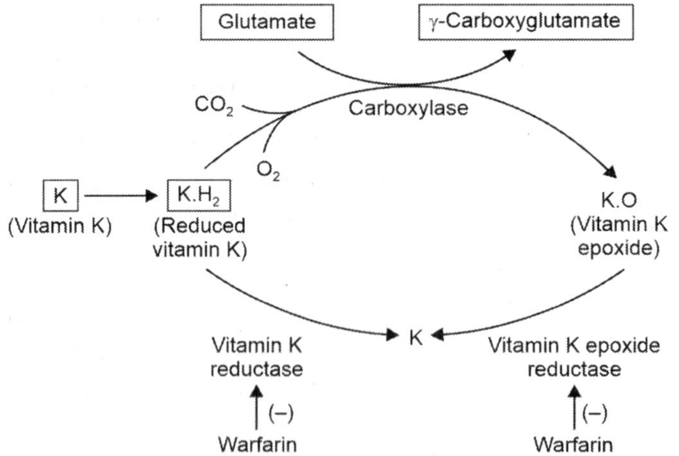

Fig. 9.5: Role of vitamin K in carboxylation of blood clotting factors

Table 9.2: Fat soluble vitamins, their biological functions, deficiency diseases, sources and daily requirements for adults

Vitamin	*Provitamin*	*Biological functions*	*Deficiency diseases*	*Sources*	*Daily requirement*
Vitamin A (Retinol)	β-Carotene (Carotenoids)	In vision cycle, growth and maintenance of epithelium	Night blindness; disorders of mucous membrane, bone, nerves and reproduction	Liver oil, fish oil and vegetable oils	840–1000 μg
Vitamin D (Calciferol)	7-Dehydrocholesterol	Regulation of serum calcium and phosphorus	Rickets and osteomalacia	Fish oil	600 IU
Vitamin E (Tocopherols)	—	As antioxidant	Hemolytic anemia (in infants) and muscular dystrophy	Plant seed oils	8–10 mg
Vitamin K	—	In blood coagulation	Blood clotting failure	Plant seed oils	55 μg

SOME IMPORTANT QUESTIONS

1. **Name fat soluble vitamins. Mention their dietary sources, physiological functions and deficiency symptoms.**
2. **Describe physiological functions and deficiency symptoms of vitamin A.**
3. **How is vitamin D activated? Describe its role in calcium metabolism.**
4. **Describe dietary sources, biochemical functions and deficiency symptoms of folate and vitamin B_{12}.**
5. **Give an account of dietary sources, biochemical functions and deficiency symptoms of vitamin C.**
6. **Describe coenzyme forms and biochemical roles of:**
   i. Riboflavin
   ii. Pantothenic acid
   iii. Biotin
   iv. Vitamin B_6
   v. Thiamin
   vi. Niacin
7. **Discuss briefly:**
   i. Role of pyridoxal-5-phosphate in amino acid metabolism
   ii. Physiological functions of vitamin D
   iii. Role of vitamin A in vision

8. Write notes on:

i. Pellagra
ii. Beriberi
iii. Scurvy
iv. Calcitriol
v. Role of vitamin D in calcium metabolism
vi. Role of vitamin K in γ-carboxylation
vii. Pyridoxine
viii. Wernicke's encephalopathy
ix. Provitamin A
x. Xerophthalmia
xi. Provitamin D
xii. Active vitamin D
xiii. Rickets
xiv. Vitamin K antagonists
xv. Hypervitaminosis A

CHAPTER

10

Minerals

Minerals are the inorganic substances and represent about 4 to 5% of body weight. These are required by the body in small amounts and perform a variety of functions such as for the formation of bones and teeth, are essential constituents of body fluids and tissues, components of several enzymes and are required for normal nerve functions.

CALCIUM

Calcium (Ca) is the most abundant mineral, found in highest concentration in the body and is needed by all the cells. **Adult human body contains,** nearly, **1.0–1.5 kg of calcium,** out of which about **99% is found in bones and teeth,** and 1% in the extracellular fluid. Calcium level in the blood is regulated by balancing calcium absorption from the gut, excretion via kidneys, and mobilization and deposition in the bone. These sites are **regulated by** feedback mechanisms, which are controlled by several hormones, **including parathyroid hormone (PTH) and active vitamin D.**

Recommended Daily Allowance

RDA for calcium has been suggested between **1000 and 1200 mg/day.**

Its RDA **for adult men and women** has been suggested as **1000 mg/day.**

RDA of calcium **for the postmenopausal women** has been recommended as **1200 mg/day.**

Dietary Sources

Milk, cheese and other dairy products are rich sources of calcium. **Eggs, dry fruits, legumes, green-leafy vegetables** (such as broccoli and cabbage), **fortified soya products and fish** eaten with the bones (such as tinned salmon and whitebait) **are also good sources of calcium.**

Uptake and Excretion of Calcium

- Only about **10–30%** of the dietary calcium is normally **absorbed,** mostly in the duodenum.
- Absorption of calcium **depends upon** several factors:
  - In **vitamin D** deficiency, calcium absorption is impaired.
  - Excess of **phosphate** lowers calcium absorption.
  - **Phytic acid** and related substances present in unrefined cereals interfere with the absorption of calcium.
  - Excessive amounts of **fat, fiber and oxalate** in the diet reduce calcium absorption, due to the formation of insoluble salts.
  - Higher amounts of dietary **protein, lactose** and acidic **pH** promote calcium absorption.

- Calcium is excreted in the feces, urine and sweat:
  - Dietary calcium, which is not absorbed in the intestine, is excreted in the feces.
  - Amount of calcium excreted in the urine varies from 50 to 200 mg/day.
  - Urinary **excretion is increased** (hypercalciuria) **by ingestion of the excessive** amount of **protein** in the diet, in **acidosis, thyrotoxicosis, hypo-parathyroidism** and **restricted physical activity.**
  - **In tropical climate,** calcium **excretion is increased in sweat.**

Physiological Functions

Calcium performs several functions in the body:

- **Formation of bones and teeth:** Bones are the reservoir of Ca in the body.
- **Mediates muscle contraction:** Ca mediates excitation and contraction of muscle fibers.
- **Helps in nerve conduction:** Transmission of nerve impulses from pre-synaptic to post-synaptic region.
- **Mediates secretion of hormones:** Calcium mediates secretion of **insulin, PTH, calcitonin and vasopressin.**
- **Acts as second messenger:** Ca and cAMP act as second messengers of different hormones, such as glucagon.
- **Membrane integrity and permeability:** Calcium influences transport of several substances across the membranous barrier.
- **Role in blood coagulation:** Calcium is essential for factor IV in blood coagulation cascade and in the conversion of prothrombin to thrombin.
- **Action on heart:** Ca prolongs systole. High Ca concentration also **increases myocardial contractility.**
- **Activation of enzymes:** Calmodulin (Ca-binding regulatory protein) **binds with 4 Ca ions** and leads to activation of several enzymes.

Regulation of Serum Calcium (Calcium Homeostasis)

Maintenance of serum calcium level, within the normal limit, is called **calcium homeostasis.** Serum Ca^{2+} level is **regulated** in a complex manner **by** parathyroid hormone **(PTH), vitamin D and calcitonin** (Fig. 10.1).

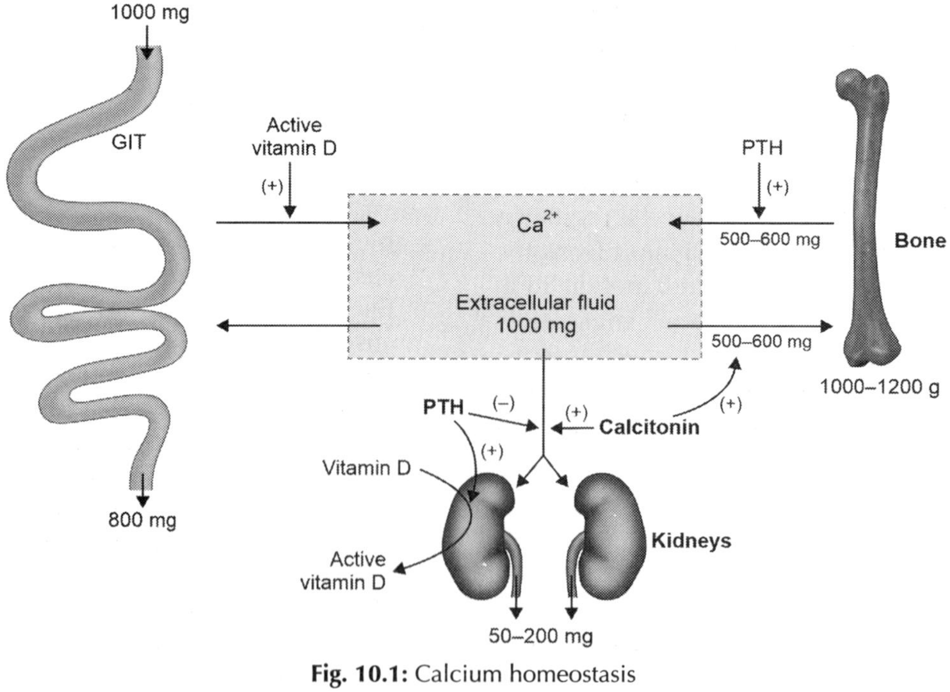

Fig. 10.1: Calcium homeostasis

Parathyroid hormone: If serum Ca^{2+} concentration falls, secretion of PTH is increased:

- **PTH acts** directly **on osteoclasts** and increases dissolution of **bone mineral.** This process is called bone resorption.
- It also increases the **reabsorption of Ca^{2+} from the kidney tubules.**
- PTH also stimulates 1-α-hydroxylase activity in the kidney which, in turn, **activates vitamin D.**
  - **Active vitamin D:** It increases serum Ca^{2+} concentration by promoting intestinal absorption as well as renal tubular reabsorption of Ca^{2+}.
  - **Calcitonin:** It is secreted when serum Ca^{2+} level rises. Its action is to lower serum Ca^{2+} level by promoting deposition of calcium by the osteoblasts. It also promotes renal Ca^{2+} excretion. Thus, PTH and calcitonin act in opposite directions in regulating serum calcium.

Deficiency Disorders

- Inadequate intake of calcium, in addition to an inadequate intake of vitamin D, has been demonstrated to contribute to **rickets** in children, and **osteomalacia** in adults.
- Hypocalcemia may also lead to **osteoporosis, which is characterized by loss of bone matrix and progressive demineralization. Decreased calcium intake, particularly, during menopause, leads to increased fragility of bones, mainly, of the extremities and pelvis.**
- **Hypocalcemia may also result in** tetany **of skeletal muscles. It is characterized by muscle twitching, spasms and, eventually, convulsions.**

Toxicity

- Very high intake of calcium (2000 mg or more per day) may lead to excessive **calcification of soft tissues,** especially, the kidneys.
- Long-term high intake of calcium may lead to **increased bone fractures in the elderly,** perhaps, due to high bone remodeling that leads to exhaustion of osteoblasts.
- High intakes of calcium may also **interfere with the absorption of other divalent cations,** such as iron, zinc and manganese.
- Another potential adverse effect of excessive calcium intake is **constipation.**

PHOSPHORUS

A normal **adult body contains** nearly **600–800 g of phosphorus.** About **85%** of it **is present in the skeleton and teeth,** as calcium phosphate crystals. It is **essential for the structure of cell membranes,** as phospholipids. Phosphorus, in the cells also contributes to a number of processes associated with **energy metabolism.**

Recommended Daily Allowance

ICMR-NIN (2020) recommendation for **phosphorus is similar to that of calcium,** i.e. in the 1:1 ratio for all age groups except for infants whose requirement is recommended as 1.5 times of the calcium.

RDA for phosphorus for normal adults has been suggested between **1000 and 1200 mg/day.**

Dietary Sources

Phosphorus is found in foods containing phosphoproteins, nucleoproteins, phospholipids and glycerophosphates, as well as in the form of inorganic phosphates (chiefly of Ca and Na).

Phosphorus is abundant in **red meat, dairy products, fish, poultry, bread, rice and oats,** and is, usually, found in foods that also contain calcium.

Uptake and Excretion

- Depending upon the presence of other constituents, **about 10–40% of the dietary**

phosphorus is absorbed as inorganic phosphate in the small intestine.
- Organic phosphate is hydrolyzed in the intestinal lumen and released as inorganic phosphate, through the action of pancreatic/intestinal phosphatases, e.g. alkaline phosphatase.
- **Absorption** of phosphorus also **depends upon the dietary content of phosphorus** (absorption of phosphorus is increased when its intake is low), as well as **calcium and vitamin D.**
- An increase in dietary magnesium also results in reduction in phosphate absorption.
- About **two-thirds** of the dietary phosphorus is **excreted in the urine,** while the remaining **one-third** is excreted in feces.
- PTH increases excretion of phosphate by inhibiting its tubular reabsorption.

Physiological Functions

- As **phosphates,** phosphorus participates in numerous essential functions of the body, e.g. **as a component of DNA and RNA, ATP and other high energy phosphate compounds,** such as creatine phosphate, glucose-6-phosphate, phosphoenolpyruvate, etc.
- **Phosphate with calcium forms hydroxyapatite,** the major inorganic molecule in teeth and bones.
- As part of the phospholipids, phosphorus is present in every cell membrane in the body. Numerous **phospholipid molecules also act as secondary messengers,** within the cytosol.
- As a part of **phosphate buffer,** it is important in intracellular fluid and kidney tubules, where phosphate functions in the **excretion of hydrogen ions.**

Serum Phosphorus Regulation

Absorbed phosphate exists in plasma in two forms, i.e. as phospholipids (organic form) and in the inorganic form. The inorganic form, like calcium, can be either protein bound or free. In normal adult human beings, **serum phosphorus** (as inorganic phosphorus) varies from **2.5 to 4.5 mg/100 mL.** Circulating phosphates are in equilibrium with the skeletal and cellular inorganic phosphates, as well as the organic phosphates. **PTH and serum calcium regulate** the **level of phosphorus in the serum** as well as its reabsorption by the renal tubules.

Deficiency Disorders

- Phosphate deficiency may **result from** long-term administration of glucose, or total parenteral nutrition (TPN) without sufficient phosphate, **excessive use of phosphate-binding antacids, hyperparathyroidism,** during treatment of diabetic acidosis, and in those who are **alcoholics.**
- Phosphate deficiency may lead to **neural, muscular, skeletal, hematological, renal and other abnormalities.**

Toxicity

Persistently high PTH, because of the chronic consumption of low calcium and high phosphorus, may contribute to **increased bone turnover** that, potentially, can result in a reduction of bone mass and density. If this condition is chronic, it could contribute to **fragility fractures** because of excessive resorption and **thinning of trabecular plates at bone sites** throughout the skeleton.

MAGNESIUM

Adult human body contains nearly **20–25 g of magnesium** (Mg). About **75% of it is present in bones,** in combination with calcium and phosphorous. Remaining of it is present in soft tissues such as muscle and nervous tissue and in body fluids. Most of the **magnesium in blood is intracellular.**

Recommended Daily Allowance

RDA for magnesium has been suggested between **370–440 mg/day.**

Its RDA has been suggested as **440 mg/ day for adult males** and **370 mg/day for adult females.**

Dietary Sources

Whole **grains cereals, potato and seafoods** are good sources of magnesium. Beverages such as **coffee, tea and cocoa are also rich in magnesium.**

Physiological Functions

1. Magnesium is a **component of the bone structure.**
2. It also plays an important role in **nerve impulse transmission.**
3. Magnesium ions (Mg^{2+}) also act as **activator for several enzymes,** particularly those requiring ATP, such as glucokinase, hexokinase, acyl CoA synthetase, alkaline phosphatase, and DNA and RNA polymerases, etc.
4. Mg^{2+} is also required in the synthesis of cAMP and, thus, **mediates the effects of numerous hormones.**
5. Mg^{2+} also **participates in electron transfer** and stabilizes the arrangement of redox centers in cytochrome C oxidase.
6. Mg^{2+} also helps in **contraction of the cardiac and smooth muscles.**

Deficiency Symptoms

Magnesium **deficiency is often observed in alcoholics** and in **patients taking certain types of diuretics,** and those with metabolic acidosis.

Magnesium deficiency may also be observed **in uremics** and children suffering from **kwashiorkor.**

Low serum magnesium levels are also observed **during pregnancy,** particularly during **toxemia of pregnancy, rickets, diarrhea and vomiting.**

Deficiency symptoms include **tremors, depression, hyperirritability, cardiac arrhythmia, muscular weakness** and convulsions.

Low levels of serum magnesium may also result in **tetany.**

Toxicity

Magnesium toxicity may be observed due to increased use of magnesium-containing laxatives and antacids. Chief symptoms include **drowsiness, lethargy and weakness.**

IRON

Total quantity of iron (Fe), in normal adult human body is about 4 g. Iron may be incorporated in the protoporphyrin ring, both in the Fe^{2+} and Fe^{3+} forms. **Fe^{2+}-protoporphyrin complex** is called **heme,** while **Fe^{3+}-protoporphyrin complex** is designated as **hematin.**

- **Heme-containing proteins** include **hemoglobin, myoglobin** and several enzymes, such as **catalase and peroxidases.**
- **Nonheme proteins** include **ferritin, transferrin, cytochromes and iron-sulfur proteins.**

Recommended Daily Allowance

Requirement for iron during the reproductive age has been recommended taking into account the menstrual losses. It is further suggested that at least 20 mg/1000 kcal of vitamin C should be consumed daily for the better absorption of iron.

RDA for iron has been suggested between **19–29 mg/d.**

Its RDA has been suggested as **19 mg/day for normal adult males and 29 mg/day** (due to loss during menstruation) for normal adult females.

During pregnancy RDA is **27 mg** while during lactation it is **23 mg.**

Dietary Sources

Dietary iron is found in two forms, i.e. as **heme iron** (from **animal sources**) and **nonheme iron** (from **plant sources**).

- Food cooked in **iron cookware** is the best source of iron.
- Animal foods such as **meat, fish and egg,** are good sources of **heme iron.** It is the most bioavailable form of iron.
- **Green-leafy vegetables, cereals, legumes, pulses and beans (whole grains), nuts and fruits,** are good sources of **nonheme iron,** the predominant form of iron found in plant foods.

Uptake and Transport

Absorption of iron, mainly, occurs **in the stomach, duodenum and upper part of the small intestine.** Normally, only about 10% of the dietary iron is absorbed. Efficiency of absorption is increased up to 30% during severe iron deficiency.

Heme iron is **absorbed across the brush border** (mucosa) of the intestinal absorbing cells **(enterocytes)** after it is obtained from the animal sources. After the heme enters cytosol, its **ferrous iron** is enzymatically removed from the ferroporphyrin complex and **combines with apoferritin** to **form ferritin,** similar to free non-heme iron. Ferritin carries it from brush border to the basolateral membrane of the absorbing cells. Brush border iron transporter, called divalent metal transporter 1 (DMT 1), transports ferrous iron.

Ferric iron is reduced by the brush border enzyme **ferric reductase,** for its absorption.

Nonheme iron is transported by transferrin, from intestinal absorbing cells to various tissues.

Unabsorbed iron is **excreted in the feces.**

Physiological Functions

Iron forms a component of several **heme** and **nonheme** proteins:

- **Hemoproteins:**
  - **Hemoglobin** is required for the **transport of O_2** and CO_2.
  - **Myoglobin** is an **oxygen-storage** protein in muscles.
  - **Cytochromes** are required in the **electron transport chain** and **oxidative phosphorylation.**
  - **Cytochrome P450 system** is responsible for many **biotransformation reactions.**
  - Several enzymes contain heme iron, as a part of their prosthetic group, e.g. **catalase, peroxidase, tryptophan pyrrolase, nitric oxide synthases, prostaglandin synthase,** etc.
  - As a component of the lysosomal enzyme myeloperoxidase, iron is required for **phagocytosis** and, thus, killing of bacteria by the neutrophils.
- **Nonheme proteins: Transferrin, ferritin and iron-sulfur proteins** (ferridoxins).
  - **Ferridoxins:** These are nonheme iron proteins called **iron–sulfur centers** or **iron-sulfur proteins.**
  - Due to the presence of iron, Fe–S centers **occur in the oxidized as well as the reduced state.**
  - These are **involved in** various enzymatic oxidation processes, such as in the **mitochondrial electron transport chain.** For example, complex I which passes electrons from NADH to CoQ, contains one molecule of FMN and 6 to 7 Fe–S clusters, that participate in the electron transport.
- **Ferritin:** Ferritin is an iron containing protein **involved in the storage of iron.**
  - The protein component is called **apoferritin,** which consists of 24 sub-units of the H chains and the L chains, that are arranged spherically.
  - **Apoferritin,** also called mucosal iron-receptor protein in the upper small intestine, thus, **controls absorption of iron** as it has a very rapid turnover.
  - **Intake of iron regulates the rate of synthesis of apoferritin** so that more protein is available for iron binding when the intake is high.
  - Ferritin, therefore, **acts,** both, **as a sink for iron during its excess intake** as well as **its source during iron deprivation.**

- **Transferrin:** Transferrin is a non-heme iron-**containing serum glycoprotein** (β_1-globulin) synthesized in the liver.
  - Transferrin **transports iron to the sites where it is required,** such as in the bone marrow.
  - The apoprotein part of transferrin is designated as **apotransferrin.** There are two iron-binding sites in an apotransferrin molecule.
  - In a normal healthy adult, nearly one-third of the iron-binding sites are occupied. Thus, total iron-binding capacity **(TIBC) of the serum is directly related to its transferrin concentration.**
  - **In iron overload,** serum **transferrin may be fully saturated.**

Deficiency Disorders

The commonest disorder is iron deficiency **anemia.** It is the commonest disorder of iron metabolism and the commonest form of nutritional anemia.

Causes of anemia: Anemia may be due to several causes, which may include:

- **Inadequate intake:** Malnutrition, pregnancy (increased fetal demand), etc.
- **Poor absorption:** Prolonged gastroenteritis, complete/partial gastrectomy, etc.
- **Increased losses:** Excessive blood loss during menstruation, gastrointestinal hemorrhage, hookworm infections, etc.

Types of anemia: Anemia is a condition, which is characterized by the reduced number of circulating erythrocytes or reduced amount of hemoglobin in them, or both. Based on the RBC size and the hemoglobin content, anemia is of three types:

- **Microcytic hypochromic anemia:** The **erythrocytes are much smaller in size** and **have reduced hemoglobin content.** Their number may also be reduced but to a smaller extent. It is **caused by iron deficiency** (Fig. 10.2).

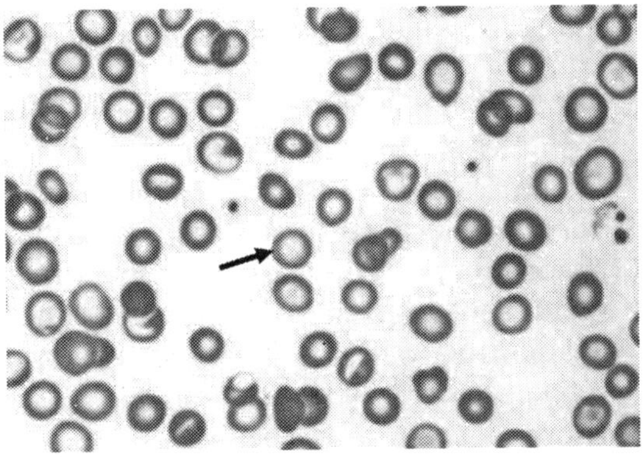

Fig. 10.2: Iron deficiency anemia morphologically characterized by variable degrees of microcytosis and hypochromia which results in widening of the central pallor accounting for greater than one-third of the total RBC diameter (arrow)

- **Macrocytic hyperchromic/normochromic anemia:** The **size of the erythrocytes is increased** while their **number is reduced,** presenting the characteristic blood picture of megaloblastic anemia including pernicious anemia. It is **caused by the deficiency of vitamin B_{12} and/or folate.**
- **Normocytic normochromic anemia:** The **size as well as the hemoglobin content of the erythrocytes remains normal** but **number of the circulating erythrocytes is reduced.** It is, usually, a **result of internal or external hemorrhage.**

Symptoms: Anemia is a common feature in children, adolescent girls and females of the childbearing age, particularly, in the developing countries.

- **Children become dull, inactive, lose appetite and have poor growth.**
- Deficiency of iron in **females reduces their work capacity.** On exertion, such women get **breathless** and remain **fatigued.**
- Iron deficiency is also associated with **decreased immunocompetence and susceptibility to infections.**

Toxicity

Major **cause** of iron overload is **hereditary hemochromatosis.** Frequent blood transfusions and long-term ingestion of large amount of iron can also lead to abnormal accumulation of iron in the liver.

- Consumption of, abnormally, large amount of iron, or in those with a genetic defect resulting in excessive iron absorption, can develop an iron storage condition called **hemosiderosis.** When associated with tissue damage, it is referred to as **hemochromatosis.**
- Increased dietary intake of iron by adult men and postmenopausal women, may contribute to enriched oxidative environment in the body and favors **oxidation of LDL cholesterol, arterial vessel damage and other adverse effects, involving the cardiovascular system.**
- Excess iron also **generates excessive amounts of free radicals** that attack cellular molecules, thereby, increasing the number of potentially carcinogenic molecules within cells.

IODINE

Nearly 20–30 mg of iodine is present in adult human body.

Recommended Daily Allowance

RDA for iodine has been suggested as **140 µg/day.**

Dietary Sources

Iodine requirement is, mostly, fulfilled from **drinking water.** Adequate supply of iodine can also be met from **iodized salt.** Besides, **seafoods, fruits, vegetables, cereals and meat** are good sources of iodine.

Physiological Functions

Important function of iodine is the **synthesis of the thyroid hormones** (T_3 and T_4). These hormones perform several functions, which include:

- **Regulation of basal metabolic rate**
- **Growth and development in children.**
- **Synthesis of the thyroid hormones**
  - **In the thyroid gland,** thyroid hormones are synthesized, as a result of **iodination of the tyrosyl residues of** the glycoprotein **thyroglobulin** (Fig. 10.3).

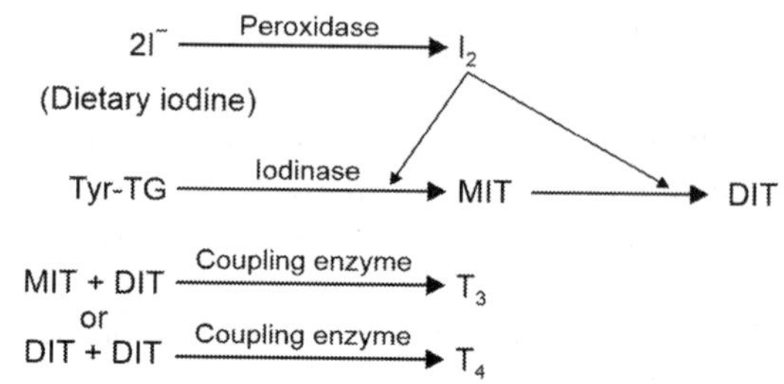

Fig. 10.3: Role of iodine in the synthesis of thyroid hormones (T_3 and T_4); (Tyr–TG = Tyrosine amino acids (tyrosyl-residues) in a thyroglobulin molecule)

  - For iodination with the tyrosyl residues of thyroglobulin, iodine is first activated by the enzyme peroxidase.
  - Subsequently, iodinase catalyzes iodination of the tyrosyl residues in thyroglobulin, and converts the tyrosine to mono-iodotyrosine (MIT) and di-iodotyrosine (DIT).
  - Thereafter, coupling of either a molecule of MIT with DIT or two molecules of DIT, forms tri-iodothyronine (T_3), or tetra-iodothyronine (called thyroxine or T_4), respectively. This is an intra-molecular process and these hormones are synthesized within the protein chain (thyroglobulin).

Thyroid Hormones (T_3 and T_4) Perform Various Functions

- **Development of the central nervous system:** Thyroid hormones **stimulate growth of the nerve cell bodies, branching of dendrites and rate of myelination of axons.**
- **Regulation of normal body growth:** Thyroid hormones **promote general growth and calcification of bones.**
- **Regulation of basal energy economy:** Thyroid hormones stimulate **synthesis**

of various cytochromes, cytochrome oxidase and Na^+/K^+-ATPase enzymes, uncoupling protein-1 (UCP-1, in brown adipose tissue) as well as other uncoupling proteins (UCP-2 and UCP-3) in many tissues, and, thus, **regulate** basal metabolic rate **(BMR).** This is also called **thermogenic action of thyroid hormones.**

- **Regulation of fuel metabolism:** In addition to their ability to regulate BMR, thyroid hormones also **promote** a **positive nitrogen balance** and **synthesis of structural proteins.** The effects of these hormones on carbohydrate metabolism are opposite to that of insulin, hence, thyroid hormones tend to **increase blood glucose levels.** They also upregulate hepatic LDL receptors, and increase **uptake of LDL-cholesterol.**

Deficiency Disorders

Iodine deficiency causes **abnormal enlargement of the thyroid gland,** which is situated in the neck region. In childhood, iodine deficiency causes reduced thyroid functioning, which results in retarded physical and mental growth. It may result in **goiter** (also called endemic goiter) as well as **cretinism,** which result in developmental delays and other health problems.

Iodine deficiency is associated with the development of **endemic goiter,** enlargement of the thyroid gland, **commonly observed in mountainous areas and in regions of high goitrogens intake** (Fig. 10.4).

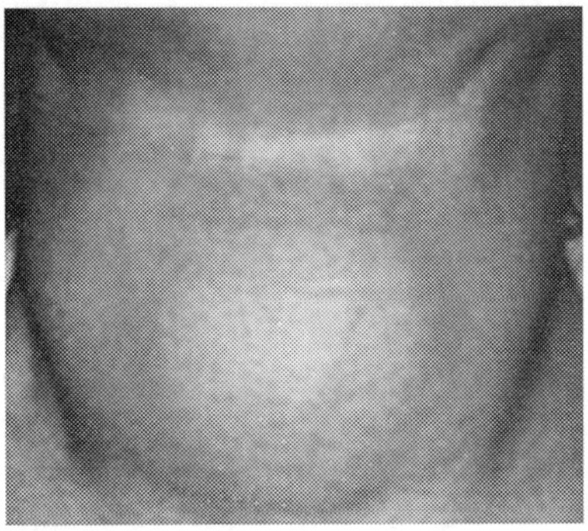

Fig. 10.4: Endemic goiter

Goitrogens are the substances that **exist, naturally, in foods.** These can cause goiter by blocking uptake of iodine, from blood, by the thyroid cells. Foods, containing goitrogens, include **cabbage, turnips, rapeseeds, peanuts, cassava, sweet potatoes and soybeans.** Goitrogens can be inactivated by heating or cooking.

Severe iodine deficiency during gestation and early postnatal growth, results in cretinism in infants, a syndrome **characterized by mental deficiency, spastic diplegia or quadriplegia, deaf mutism, dysarthria, a characteristic shuffling gait, short stature and hypothyroidism** (Fig. 10.5).

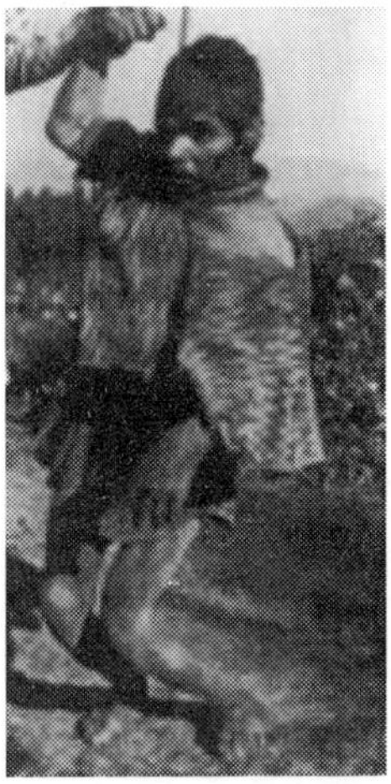

Fig. 10.5: Cretinism

Toxicity

Long-term iodine intake, much higher than the physiologic requirement, may result in **hypothyroidism,** goiter formation or **hyperthyroidism.**

FLUORIDE

Fluoride is present in traces, in several tissues, mainly, bone, teeth, thyroid gland and skin.

Recommended Daily Allowance

RDA for fluoride has been suggested between **2 and 3 mg/day.**

Dietary Sources

Drinking water is an important source of fluoride, in a human diet. Besides, fluoride can also be obtained from **tea and fish.**

Functions of Fluoride

- The main function of fluoride is in the **mineralization of bone and teeth.**
- Fluoride also acts as an **antibacterial agent,** in the oral cavity and **protects teeth from dental caries.**

Deficiency Disorders

Deficiency of fluoride promotes development of **dental caries** in children, and osteoporosis in adults, particularly, in the postmenopausal women.

Dental caries: Dental caries is characterized by destruction of the tooth enamel due to the action of microorganisms (which are normally present in the oral cavity) on carbohydrates, particularly, during the formation of teeth. Breakdown of the enamel, in turn, exposes the dentine and leads to the development of caries (Fig. 10.6).

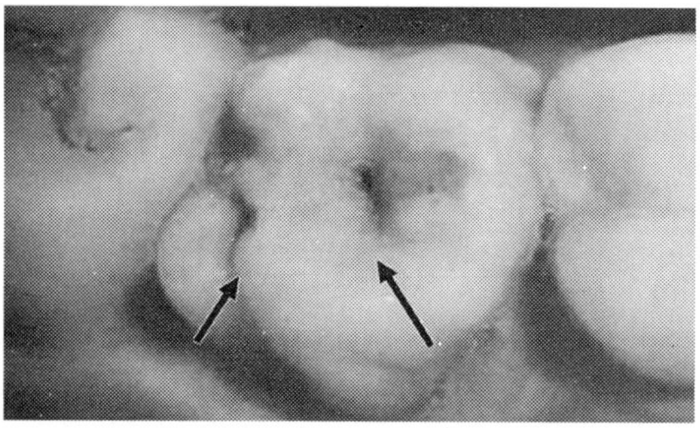

Fig. 10.6: Dental caries (formation of cavities)

Toxicity

Large doses of fluoride may be toxic. It may lead to **fluorosis,** which is an important public health problem in many parts of the world. It is due to the reason that high content of fluoride in rocks results in increased level of fluoride in the groundwater. Fluoride toxicity may manifest in two major forms, i.e. as **dental fluorosis and skeletal fluorosis,** which **together** constitute **endemic fluorosis:**

- **Dental fluorosis:** It occurs, mainly, in children, who are exposed to high fluoride intake, before the completion of mineralization of the tooth enamel. Their teeth exhibit mottled enamel. **Mottling** is confined to the permanent teeth and is **characterized by multiple, minute white flecks and yellow/brown spots,** which are **scattered irregularly over the tooth surface** (Fig. 10.7).

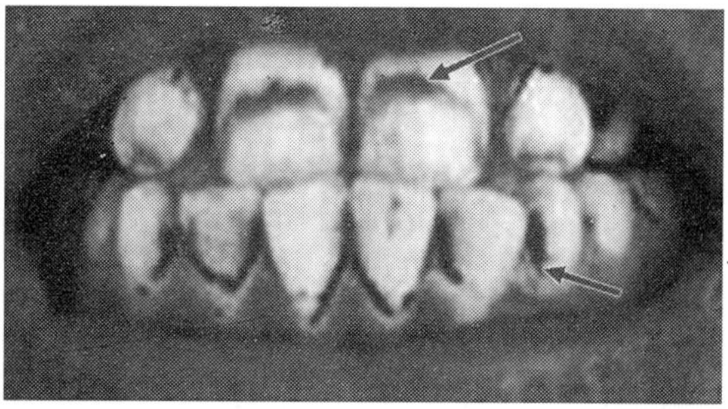

Fig. 10.7: Dental fluorosis. The teeth of the upper jaw (the two central incisors) show mottling and discoloration (red arrow) horizontally aligned on the enamel surface, away from the gums. It cannot be cleaned by a dentist. However, the teeth of the lower jaw show discoloration along the gums (blue arrow) due to dirty teeth (not fluorosis), which can be cleaned by a dentist

- **Skeletal fluorosis:** Its clinical features include **pain, inflammation and restricted movement of the joints** and **stiffness of the spine.** Further, significantly higher intake of fluoride (more than 3 mg/L, in drinking water) results in a variant of severe form of the skeletal fluorosis called **genu valgum** (Fig. 10.8).

COPPER

Adult human body contains 100–150 mg of copper, out of which, nearly, 50% is found in muscles and 25% in bones.

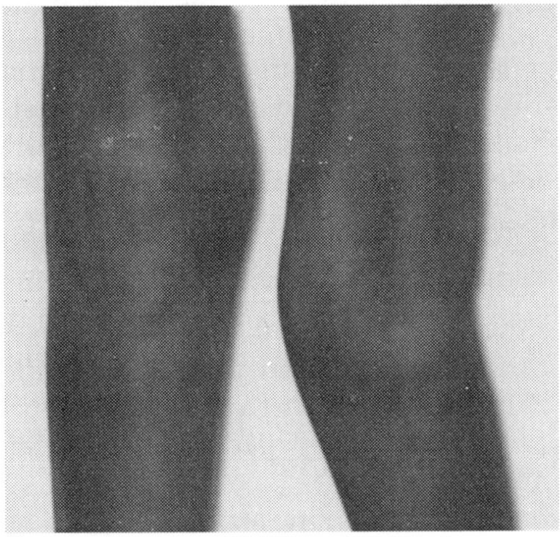

Fig. 10.8: Skeletal fluorosis. Deformed but mobile joints

Recommended Daily Allowance

RDA for copper has been suggested as **1.5–1.7 mg/day.**

Dietary Sources

Nuts, leafy vegetables, dried legumes, egg yolk, and fish and liver meat, are good sources of copper.

Physiological Functions

- Copper is a **component of many enzymes,** particularly, those which require vitamin C, such as **cytochrome oxidase, ferroxidase (ceruloplasmin), tyrosinase, ascorbic acid oxidase, superoxide dismutase,** etc.
- It is also a constituent of α-aminolevulinate synthase and ferroxidase I, and thus, **helps in the metabolism of iron and biosynthesis of hemoglobin.**
- Copper is also an important **constituent of** several other proteins, such as **erythrocuprein, cerebrocuprein and hepatocuprein,** which are present in the bone marrow, brain and liver, respectively.
- It also helps in the **formation of bone and elastin fibers,** and **maintenance of myelin sheath.**
- Copper is also important for **infant growth, brain development, immune system and strong bones.**

Deficiency Disorders

- Some of the symptoms of copper deficiency include **hypercholesterolemia, demineralization of bones, leukopenia, demyelination of the neural tissue and alopecia** (loss of hair).
- There is also **microcytic normochromic anemia,** which cannot be cured by iron supplementation alone, since copper (as ferroxidase) is essential for the intestinal absorption of iron and its metabolism.
- Copper deficiency in infants has been found to be associated with a condition described as **Menkes disease.**

Menkes disease is an X-linked hereditary disease due to **failure of copper absorption** across the serosal membrane of intestinal mucosal cells. This, in turn, leads to **low concentration of copper** in the plasma and the liver. It also results in **deficiency of various copper-containing oxidases** (tyrosinase, lysyl oxidase, etc.), leading to various systemic manifestations such as **skeletal malformation, mental retardation, defective thermoregulation and immunodeficiency.** Menkes disease is also called **kinky hair syndrome,** due to the failure to keratinize **hair which becomes kinky and steel grey** (Fig. 10.9).

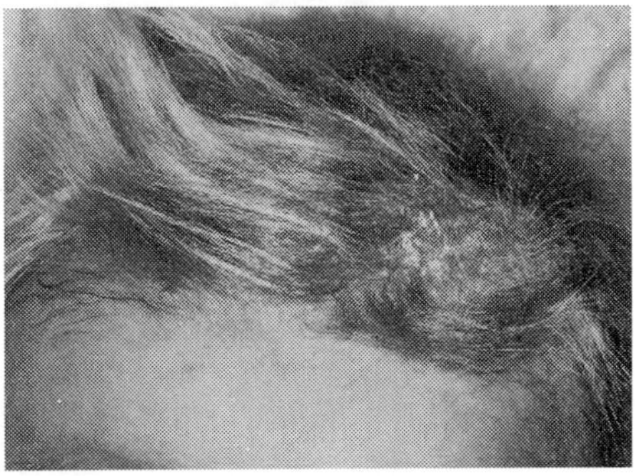

Fig. 10.9: Copper deficiency results in defective keratinization: Menkes kinky hair which feels like steel wool (steely hair syndrome)

Copper Toxicity

Copper toxicity may manifest as **diarrhea, blue-green discoloration of the saliva, hemolysis, proteinuria and renal failure.** Increased amount of copper is deposited in the liver and brain in Wilson's disease.

Wilson's disease (also known as hepatolenticular degeneration) is an **autosomal recessive inherited disorder** in which there is a **positive copper balance** due to **deficient synthesis of ceruloplasmin in the liver.** The net result is the **accumulation of Cu^{2+}** to highly toxic levels, mainly, in the liver and the basal nuclei of the brain. This, in turn, promotes the **generation of free radicals** leading to **extensive cell damage.** There may be **liver failure, neurological disturbances and characteristic Kayser-Fleischer rings in the cornea** (Fig. 10.10).

ZINC

Total **body content** of zinc in an adult man **is about 2.0 g.** Choroid of the eye, liver, prostate gland and prostate fluid contain high concentration of zinc.

Recommended Daily Allowance

RDA for zinc has been suggested between **13–17 mg/day.**

Its RDA has been suggested as **17 mg/day for adult males and 13 mg/day for adult females.**

Dietary Sources

Zinc is present in many foods, but is most readily absorbed from **meat. Colostrum** is a rich source of zinc. It is also present in **milk, cheese, eggs, shellfish, wholegrain cereals, nuts and pulses.**

Physiological Functions

- Zinc, primarily, an intracellular ion, **functions with more than 300 enzymes.** It **participates in the metabolism of carbohydrates, lipids, proteins and nucleic acids.**
- In the nucleus, zinc **stabilizes RNA and DNA structure,** and is required for the activity of **RNA polymerases.**
- Zinc also functions in **chromatin proteins, involved in transcription and replication.**
- It is also involved in the **integrity of subcellular organelles, in transport processes, immune functions and expression of genetic information.**

Deficiency Disorders

Since body stores of zinc are small, dietary deficiency can therefore produce symptoms promptly, particularly, when the soil content is low.

- Severe zinc deficiency is **seen in alcoholics, chronic renal disease, severe gastroenteritis and malabsorption, and protein-energy malnutrition.**

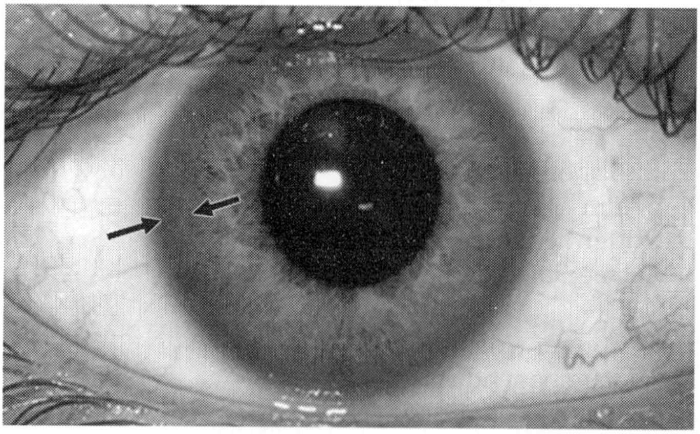

Fig. 10.10: Wilson's disease (Kayser-Fleischer ring)

- There is **poor wound healing, loss of appetite, poor growth and alopecia** (loss of hair).
- **Impairment of sexual development in children.**
- **Impairment in brain functions.**
- Certain **fetal abnormalities during pregnancy** besides hypogonadism, dwarfism (stunted growth) and gross skin lesions with severe acrodermatitis.
- **Delayed recovery from diarrhea.**

Zinc Toxicity

- Zinc, when consumed in excessive amounts, produces toxic effects, such as **acute gastrointestinal irritation, gastric ulcers, nausea and vomiting.**
- It also interferes with the utilization and functions of copper, and may cause anemia.

MANGANESE

Total body manganese (Mn) content of an adult man is about 10–12 mg. It is mainly concentrated in the bone, liver, and kidney.

Recommended Daily Allowance

RDA for manganese **for normal adult** is suggested as **4.0 mg.**

Dietary Sources

Nuts, whole grain cereals, legumes and leafy vegetables are good sources of manganese. Tea is also a rich source of manganese.

Functions

Manganese is required for bone formation and energy metabolism. It is also a constituent of an antioxidant enzyme, and helps prevent free radical mediated damage to cells.

1. Manganese is a component of many enzymes, including glutamine synthetase, pyruvate carboxylase and mitochondrial superoxide dismutase.
2. Manganese is also associated with the formation of connective and skeletal tissues, growth and reproduction, and carbohydrate and lipid metabolism.

Absorption, Metabolism, Storage and Excretion

- Manganese is absorbed throughout the small intestine.
- It is transported bound to a macroglobin, tansferrin and transmanganin.
- Excretion of manganese occurs, mainly, in the feces, after secretion into intestine via bile.

Deficiency Diseases

Due to its role in reproduction, manganese deficiency results in sterility, in both the sexes. Striking skeletal abnormalities and ataxia characterize the offspring of mothers, who are manganese deficient.

Toxicity

Manganese toxicity is developed in mine workers, as a result of its absorption through respiratory tract. Its accumulation in the liver and central nervous system produces Parkinson-like symptoms.

Toxicity symptoms include headache, dizziness and hepatic dysfunctions.

CHROMIUM

Total body chromium (Cr) content of adult men varies between **5 and 10 mg. Trivalent form of chromium (Cr^{3+}) is biologically active.** An organic compound of chromium, termed **glucose tolerance factor,** potentiates the effects of insulin, may be by facilitating its binding to the cell-receptor sites. Thus, it is **important in the removal of ingested glucose.**

Recommended Daily Allowances

RDA for chromium for normal adult is suggested as **50 µg/day.**

Dietary Sources

Sources of chromium include meat, nuts, cereal grains, Brewer's yeast and molasses. Besides, mushroom, black pepper, meat (liver), and cheese are also good sources of chromium.

Functions

1. Chromium potentiates insulin action and, as such, influences carbohydrate, lipid and protein metabolism.
2. As a glucose tolerance factor (GTF), chromium regulates the synthesis of a molecule that potentiates insulin action.
3. It is also required in the regulation of gene expression.

Absorption, Metabolism, Storage and Excretion

- Organic and inorganic forms of chromium are absorbed differently.
- Organic chromium is readily absorbed but quickly passes out of the body. Less than 2% of the trivalent chromium consumed is absorbed. Chromium absorption is increased by oxalate and is higher in iron-deficient animals than in animals with adequate iron, suggesting it shares some similarities with the iron absorption pathway.
- Chromium and iron are carried by transferrin.
- Primarily, the kidneys excrete inorganic chromium with small amounts being excreted through hair, sweat and bile.
- Organic chromium is excreted through bile.

Deficiency

Chromium deficiency results in impaired glucose tolerance, insulin resistance and lipid profile abnormalities.

Toxicity

Chromium toxicity may be observed on occupational exposure to chromium dust in industrial workers, or in athletes and power lifters, who take chromium picolinate, as a supplement, in high doses.

Its toxicity may result in some adverse effects, primarily skin lesions. Excessive exposure to chromium dust may induce lung cancer.

SELENIUM

Selenium is **present in high amounts in renal cortex, pancreas, pituitary, and liver.**

Recommended Daily Allowances

Recommended intake of selenium **for adults** is **40 µg/day.**

Dietary Sources

Selenium is found in a variety of foods, especially, Brazil nuts, bread, fish, meat and eggs. The selenium content of cereals is directly proportional to the selenium content in the soil. Thus, plant foods, cereals, fish and meat are rich in selenium.

Functions

The main function of selenium is as a component of some of the important antioxidant enzymes (e.g. glutathione peroxidase; GSH-Px), and therefore to protect the body against oxidative damage.

1. It is also necessary for the use of iodine in thyroid hormone production, for immune system and reproductive functions.
2. Selenium, as seleno-methionine or selenocysteine, exists in several proteins that are widely distributed in the body.
3. Antioxidant effects of selenium and vitamin E may reinforce each other, by the overlap of their protective actions against oxidative damage. Whereas, GSH-Px acts in the cytosol and mitochondrial matrix, vitamin E exerts its action within cell membranes

Absorption, metabolism, storage and excretion:

- Absorption of selenium, which occurs in the upper segment of the small intestine, is more efficient under conditions of deficiency.

- Selenium is transported bound to albumin initially and subsequently to α_2-globulin.
- Increased intake frequently results in increased excretion of selenium in the urine.

Deficiency Diseases

Selenium deficiency has been reported in malnourished patients, particularly, in those receiving long-term total parenteral nutrition (TPN).

The best characterized selenium deficiency condition is referred to as **Keshan disease,** a heart condition that affects children and women of child bearing age. It occurs in some parts of the world, where soil is deficient in selenium.

Toxicity

Selenium toxicity, referred to as **selenosis,** is observed in workers in the paint, glass and ceramic industries. Symptoms include brittle nails and hairs, skin lesions, tooth decay, and nonspecific gastrointestinal and neurologic abnormalities.

MOLYBDENUM

Adult human body contains, nearly, **5 mg of molybdenum (Mo). Liver and kidney** contain large amount of it.

Recommended Daily Allowances

Daily requirement is about **100–200 µg.**

Dietary Sources

Pulses, cereals, green leafy vegetables, and meat are good sources of molybdenum.

Functions

Molybdenum is a prosthetic group for several enzymes, such as xanthine oxidase, aldehyde oxidase and sulfite oxidase, which catalyze oxidation–reduction reactions. Sulfite oxidase is also important in the degradation of cysteine and methionine, and catalyzes formation of sulfate from sulfite.

Absorption, Metabolism, Storage and Excretion

- Molybdenum, which is found in minute amounts in the body, is readily absorbed from the stomach and small intestine, with the rate of absorption being higher in the proximal small intestine than in the distal small intestine. As with other minerals, molybdenum is absorbed by two mechanisms, i.e. carrier-mediated and passive diffusion.
- Molybdenum is excreted primarily in the urine. Some molybdenum is also excreted in the bile.

Deficiency Diseases

Symptoms of molybdenum deficiency include mental changes, and abnormalities of sulfur and purine metabolism.

Toxicity

An excessive molybdenum intake of 10 to 15 mg/day is associated with a gout-like syndrome. Molybdenum toxicity may cause weight loss, anorexia, anemia, severe diarrhea and skeletal deformities.

COBALT

Adult human body contains **2–3 mg of cobalt.** It is, mainly, present in the **liver and kidneys.**

Recommended Daily Allowances

Requirement of cobalt is **1–2 µg/day.**

Dietary Sources

Liver meat is a rich source of cobalt.

Functions

Cobalt is a component of vitamin B_{12} (cobalamin), which is essential for the

Table 10.1: Recommended daily allowances for adults, dietary sources, physiological functions and deficiency disorders of some of the minearls

Minerals	*Recommended daily allowances**	*Dietary sources*	*Physiological functions*	*Deficiency disorders*
Sodium	2000 mg	Common salt	Water and electrolyte balance	
Potassium	3500 mg	Fruits, vegetables and dairy products	Acid–base balance	Cardiac arrhythmia
Calcium	1000–1200 mg	Milk and milk products, eggs, dry fruits, legumes, cabbage and cauliflower	Calcification of bones and teeth, blood coagulation, cofactor for adenylate cyclase, Ca^{2+}-ATPase, and protein kinases	Rickets in children and osteomalacia in adults
Phosphorus	1000–1200 mg	Milk and milk products, eggs, meat, legumes and cereals	Calcification of bones and teeth, component of nucleic acids, regulation of blood pH and activator for enzymes involved in phosphorylation/dephosphorylation	Neural, muscular, skeletal, hematological and renal abnormalities
Magnesium	370–440 mg	Whole grain cereals, potatoes and seafoods	Cofactor for various ATP-dependent enzymes required in the synthesis of fatty acids and proteins, phosphorylation of glucose and its derivatives in the glycolytic pathway and transketolase reaction	Tremors, muscle spasms, personality changes, anorexia, nausea and vomiting, tetany, convulsions and coma
Iron	19–29 mg	Meat, fish, eggs, green leafy vegetables, cereals and legumes	Component of heme and nonheme proteins, such as hemoglobin, catalase and cytochromes	Iron deficiency anemia, reduced work capacity and immunocompetence
Zinc	13–17 mg	Meat, seafoods, eggs legumes and milk	Cofactor for various enzymes that participate in reactions involving either synthesis or degradation of carbohydrates, lipids, proteins and nucleic acids	Short stature, hypogonadism, mild anemia and reduced immune functions
Copper	1.5–1.7 mg	Nuts, leafy vegetables, dried legumes, egg-yolk, fish and liver meat	Component of several enzymes, such as cytochrome oxidase, ferroxidase (ceruloplasmin), tyrosinase, ascorbic acid oxidase and superoxide dismutase	Anemia, neutropenia, skeletal abnormalities and Menkes syndrome
Iodine	140 µg	Drinking water, iodized salt, seafoods, fruits, vegetables, cereals and meat	Synthesis of iodine-containing hormones (T3 and T4), regulation of BMR in adults, growth and development in children	Endemic goiter and cretinism
Fluoride	2–3 mg	Drinking water and tea	Development of tooth enamel and as antibacterial agent	Dental caries and osteoporosis
Selenium	40 µg	Plant-foods, cereals, fish and meat	Component of selenoproteins, such as glutathione peroxidase and selenoprotein-P	Liver necrosis

Contd...

Table 10.1: Recommended daily allowances for adults, dietary sources, physiological functions and deficiency disorders of some of the minearls (*Contd...*)

Minerals	*Recommended daily allowances**	*Dietary sources*	*Physiological functions*	*Deficiency disorders*
Manganese	4 mg	Nuts, whole grain cereals, legumes and leafy vegetables	Component of many enzymes, such as glutamine synthetase, pyruvate carboxylase and superoxide dismutase	Sterility, skeletal abnormalities and ataxia in off-springs
Chromium	50 μg	Brewer's yeast, mushroom, black pepper, liver, whole grains, nuts and cheese	Potentiates insulin action and influences carbohydrate, lipid and protein metabolism	Insulin resistance and lipid profile abnormalities
Molybdenum	100–200 μg	Pulses, cereals, green leafy vegetables and meat	Component of enzymes, such as xanthine oxidase, aldehyde oxidase and sulfite oxidase	Mental changes, abnormalities of sulfur and purine metabolism
Cobalt	1–2 μg	Food from the animal origin	Component of vitamin B_{12}	Macrocytic anemia and pernicious anemia

* ICMR-NIN (2020)

maturation of red blood cells and the normal functioning of all cells.

Absorption, Metabolism, Storage and Excretion

- Cobalt may share at least part of the same intestinal transport mechanism as iron.
- Absorption is higher in patients with deficient iron intake, portal cirrhosis with iron overload and idiopathic hemochromatosis.
- The major route of cobalt excretion is the urine. Small amounts are also excreted via feces, sweat and hair.

Deficiency Diseases

Cobalt deficiency results in vitamin B_{12} deficiency, which, in turn, causes **macrocytic anemia.**

Toxicity

High intake of inorganic cobalt (existing freely from cobalamin) in animal diets produces **polycythemia** (an overproduction of red blood cells), hyperplasia of bone marrow, reticulocytosis and increased blood volume.

Physiological role, sources, daily requirement, deficiency disorders and toxicity symptoms of the various minerals are described in Table 10.1.

SOME IMPORTANT QUESTIONS

1. **Describe dietary sources, daily requirement and physiological functions of calcium.**
2. **Describe role of parathyroid hormone, vitamin D and calcitonin in calcium metabolism.**
3. **Name iron-containing proteins found in the body and describe their functions. Describe disorders related to iron metabolism.**

4. Describe:

i. Regulation of calcium metabolism
ii. Fluoride as a nutrient
iii. Role of copper in iron metabolism
iv. Significance of zinc for the body
v. Factors affecting absorption of iron
vi. Physiological functions of phosphorus
vii. Physiological functions of chromium

5. Write notes on:

i. Copper
ii. Wilson's disease
iii. Physiological functions of calcium
iv. Ferritin
v. Transferrin
vi. Anemia
vii. Menkes disease
viii. Kinky-hair syndrome

6. Discuss:

i. Hepatolenticular degeneration
ii. Endemic goiter
iii. Factors affecting absorption of calcium

CHAPTER

11

Water and Electrolytes

Water is a very special kind of nutrient, since it is consumed at more frequent intervals and in large quantity, as compared to other nutrients.

- It is the **most abundant substance presents in the body.**
- It is **more important than food,** as if one is given water but no food, the individual may survive for several weeks, in spite of the loss of most of the body fat and 50% of the tissue proteins. On the other hand, only about 10% loss of the body water may cause illness and a loss of 20% of body water may even cause death.
- Increased fluid intake is very **beneficial for the individuals with renal calculi, urinary tract infections and chronic obstructive respiratory diseases.**

DISTRIBUTION OF BODY WATER

Human body consists of about 50–70% of its weight as water. Water content of the body, expressed as per cent of body weight, falls with age.

- **At birth, about 75% of the total body mass is water.**
- Water content is **reduced to nearly 60% in an average adult male** and the value further falls to about 50%, thereafter.
- Due to relatively high fat content, **females have nearly 5% less water.**
- **Most tissues,** except bone and adipose tissue, **contain more than 70% water.**
- Proportion of **water in a tissue depends upon its fat content.**

Human body consists of about 50–70% of its weight as water. Most tissues contain more than 70% of water, though bone and adipose tissue contain relatively lesser amounts. This is due to the reason that the proportion of water in a tissue depends upon the proportion of fat in the tissue (Table 11.1).

Table 11.1: Average water content of different tissues

Tissue	*Water content (% of total body weight)*
Whole body	60–70
Muscles	75–80
Nervous tissue	70–85
RBCs	60
Bones	25
Adipose tissue	20

BIOLOGICAL FUNCTIONS OF WATER

Water is needed for various physicochemical processes in the body:

- It is a **common solvent** in which most of the chemical reactions of the body occur.
- It **participates in various metabolic processes** within the cell.

- It **transports vital substances** via blood, lymph and other body fluids.
- It is also essential for the **elimination of waste products** from the body.
- Water intake helps to **maintain water content of the feces** and, thus, promotes regular bowel movement.
- Increased water intake **prevents urinary tract infections and kidney stones** by increasing the flow of urine.
- It helps to provide **lubrication in various strategic locations** of the body, e.g. synovial fluid between the joints, mucus in the respiratory passage, etc.
- As the latent heat of evaporation of water is high, it assists in the **regulation of body temperature**.

Sources of Body Water

Drinking water and beverages (milk, tea, fruit juices, coconut water, cold drinks and butter milk, etc.) and **food** are the sources of water for the body.

The amount of water available to the body as a result of metabolic degradation of food for energy (oxidation of nutrients), however, depends upon the type of the nutrient used in the body, e.g. 100 g of fat produces 107 ml of water, while 100 g of carbohydrates produces 56 ml and 100 g of proteins produces 41 ml of water. On an average, the amount of endogenous water produced by an individual is nearly 300 ml per day.

Daily Requirement

Daily requirement for water **varies** widely, **with** variations in **body surface area, amount of body fat, metabolic rate, physical activity and environmental factors, such as temperature, humidity, altitude, clothing,** etc. During very hot weather and while undertaking vigorous physical activity, this requirement increases, as a considerable amount of water is lost through sweat.

ICMR-NIN (2020) Expert Group has suggested daily water requirement based on the energy requirement (estimated average ratio) and the WHO guidelines of **1.5 ml per calorie ingested.**

Accordingly, **total water requirement for sedentary elderly** persons is suggested as **2800 ml/day for males and 2550 ml/day for females.**

Infants need more water because of limited capacity of their kidneys to handle renal solute load, higher percentage of body water and large surface area per unit body weight.

Lactating woman's need for water increases to 2850 mL/day because of the large amount required for milk production.

DISTRIBUTION OF BODY WATER

Total body water is distributed in two compartments, referred to as the intracellular fluid (ICF) and the extracellular fluid (ECF) as shown in Fig. 11.1.

- **Intracellular fluid:** ICF is composed of the **fluid within the** trillions of **cells** in our body. It **accounts for two-thirds of total body water.**
- **Extracellular fluid:** ECF is commonly estimated to **account for one-third of the total body water** (or 20% of the body weight), and includes the water in plasma, interstitial fluid, lymph, spinal fluid and various secretions.

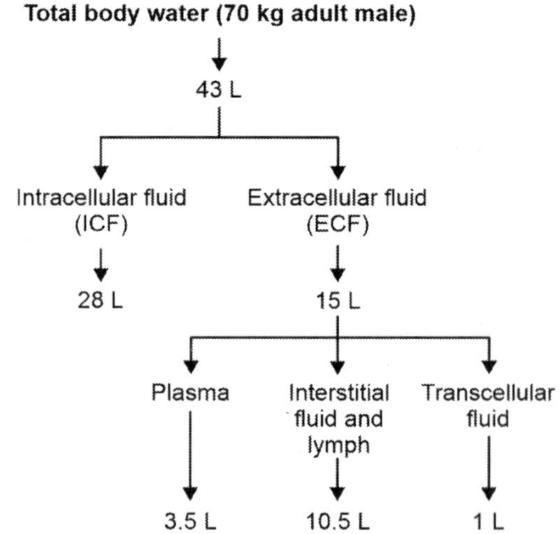

Fig. 11.1: Distribution of body water in different compartments

In humans, the normal **glucose concentration of the ECF is approximately 5 mmol/L.** Its **pH is** tightly regulated by buffers and is maintained **around 7.4.** Total **volume of ECF** is around **15 L** (of which 12 L is interstitial fluid and 3 L is plasma).

ECF contains, both cations and anions, which are important for water transport throughout the body. **Cations include sodium** (Na^+ = 136–145 mEq/L), potassium (K^+ = 3.5–5.5 mEq/L) and calcium (Ca^{2+} = 8.4–10.5 mEq/L). Anions include chloride (Cl^- = 96–106 mEq/L) and bicarbonate (HCO_3^- = 22–26 mmol).

- **Plasma:** Plasma is the ECF **found within the vascular system.** It is the **fluid portion of the blood in which blood** cells are suspended. The plasma water **compromises about 3.5 L** for an average 70 kg man.

  Plasma makes up **about 55% of total blood volume.** It is **mostly water** (93% by volume) and **contains dissolved proteins** (fibrinogens, globulins and albumins), **glucose, clotting factors, mineral ions** (Na^+, Ca^{2+}, Mg^{2+}, HCO_3^-, Cl^-, etc.), **hormones and carbon dioxide.** These dissolved substances are important for various physiological processes such as exchange of gases, immune functions and drug delivery throughout the body.
- **Interstitial fluid and lymph:** These are **considered together,** because these cannot be separated easily. Both are the **ultrafiltrates of plasma.** The **interstitial fluid directly bathes most body cells** while the **lymph is the fluid within lymphatic vessels.**

  On an average, a person has **about 11 L of interstitial fluid and lymph.** It is important to provide nutrients to the cells and for the removal of waste products. The interstitial matrix comprises mainly **connective tissues** and **proteins** (such as collagen) which are important in blood clotting and wound healing.

  Transcellular fluid: Transcellular fluid is the portion of total body water contained within the epithelial-lined spaces. It is the smallest component of extracellular fluid, i.e. **about 2.5% of the total body water.** It includes **cerebrospinal fluid (CSF), ocular fluid, joint fluid** and **pleural fluid,** which is only found in their respective epithelium-lined spaces. The function of transcellular fluid is mainly lubrication of these cavities and sometimes electrolyte transport. Some of the **electrolytes present in the transcellular fluid are sodium ions, chloride ions** and **bicarbonate ions.**

  Cerebrospinal fluid is similar in composition to blood plasma, but lacks most proteins, such as albumins, because these are too large to pass through the blood–brain barrier.

  Ocular fluid contains high concentration of proteins, including antibodies.

REGULATION OF BODY WATER

In a normal adult, the quantity of **water intake is balanced by** that what is eliminated from the body **(output)** every day, thus, maintaining a state of equilibrium (water homeostasis).

Water Intake

Volume of the fluid ingested is, primarily, regulated by thirst which is under the control of the thirst center. Besides several other factors, which include obligatory losses, disease conditions and diet, also play some role.

- **Thirst:** Thirst is the basic instinct or urge that drives us to ingest water. It is an important component of blood volume regulation. Thirst is a **sensation created by the hypothalamus** (the thirst center of the human body) and the **renin-angiotensin system.**
  - **Hypothalamus**: When osmolarity of the blood changes, water diffusion into and out of the osmoreceptor cells alters. After these **osmoreceptors** detect high plasma osmolarity (often a sign of a low blood volume), they **send signals to the hypothalamus,** which

creates biological sensation of thirst. Osmoreceptors **also stimulate ADH secretion,** which starts the events that will reduce plasma osmolarity to normal.

  - **Renin–angiotensin system:** Thirst is **induced through angiotensin II,** one of the hormones involved in the renin-angiotensin system. Stimulation of the sympathetic nervous system and low blood pressure in the kidneys (decreased GFR) stimulates renin–angiotensin system and causes an increase in thirst.
- **Obligatory losses:** There is an obligatory but variable loss of water in **insensible perspiration, breath** and **feces.** Sweating can greatly increase fluid loss and, thus, its demand.
- **Disease conditions:** Fluid intake is also associated with physical condition and injury, e.g. **fluid loss increases due to watery diarrhea** or **blood loss,** etc.
- **Dietary factors:**
  - **Sodium:** As sodium tends to hold water, so extra sodium (salt) intake may increase water content of the body.
  - **Carbohydrate:** Carbohydrate content of the diet affects both sodium and water balance. Increased amount of carbohydrate in the diet increases water retention while a low carbohydrate intake results in a loss of body fluid.
  - **Protein:** Serum proteins influence water balance by their osmotic effect since proteins draw water from the interstitial fluid into the blood. If a low protein diet is consumed for a longer duration, serum albumin levels fall to such an extent that fluid accumulates between the cells and thus total body water is increased.

Water Output

Water is removed from the body in the form of urine, feces, perspiration and expiration by lungs.

- **Urine:** It is an important medium for the elimination of water present in the body in excess of its requirement. Normally, about **1.2 to 1.5 L** of water is excreted in the form of urine, daily. This is **regulated by** antidiuretic hormone **(ADH),** which promotes reabsorption of water from the distal renal tubules. In the absence of ADH (such as in diabetes insipidus), the urine is not concentrated and its output is highly increased and may reach up to 15 L/day.
- **Feces:** Normally, about **80–150 ml** of water is excreted in the feces of an adult, daily. The value may increase considerably on a high vegetable diet, particularly in the presence of diarrhea.
- **Perspiration:** Normally, from an adult human being about **300–700 ml** of water is eliminated by this route, daily. The amount of water lost in the perspiration, however, varies enormously. When the environmental temperature or humidity increases, sweat glands become active and, thus, **in summer excessive water is lost** via perspiration. It includes:
  - **Insensible perspiration** is the process whereby the **body loses water** continuously from the skin surface and lungs.
  - **Visible perspiration removes hypotonic solution.**
- **Expiration:** Nearly, 500 ml of water is lost daily in the exhaled air.

ELECTROLYTES

An electrolyte is **a substance that ionizes, when dissolved in suitable ionizing solvents** such as water. This includes most soluble salts, acids and bases. Chemically, electrolytes are substances that become ions in solution and acquire the capacity to conduct electricity. Electrolytes are present in the human body and the **balance of the electrolytes in our body is essential for normal function of cells and organs.**

These are involved in many essential processes in our body and play important role in conducting nervous impulses, contracting muscles, keeping us hydrated and regulate pH level of our body.

Common electrolytes that are **routinely measured** in blood **include sodium and potassium.**

Biological functions of sodium and potassium are described in Table 11.2.

SODIUM

An **adult human body contains nearly 90–100 g of sodium** as sodium ions (Na^+). It is essential for normal functioning of the cell and is the **major cation present in the** ECF (extracellular fluid) in our body.

Biological Functions and Metabolism

Sodium plays an important role in the **maintenance of plasma volume, acid–base homeostasis** (acid–base balance) and **transmission of nerve impulse.**

- Sodium **exists in the body in association with several anions,** such as chloride, bicarbonate, phosphate, lactate and proteinate.
- **Normal plasma sodium concentration** is in the range of **136–145 mmol/L** (mEq/L).
- **Sodium–potassium gradient across the cell membrane (high concentration of Na^+** along with the low concentration of K^+ **in the ECF) is maintained by** Na^+/K^+-ATPase **(Na^+/K^+ pump).**
- It is **completely absorbed by the gastrointestinal tract.**
- Sodium is **freely filtered by the glomerulus.** About **70%** of the filtered sodium is **reabsorbed by the proximal tubules,** 15% by the loop of Henle, 5% by the distal convoluted tubules and about 10% by the collecting ducts.
- **Active reabsorption of Na^+** in the **proximal tubule results in the passive reabsorption of Cl^- and HCO_3^-** along **with water.** This helps to **maintain electrical neutrality of the** ECF while **reabsorption of water ensures normal osmotic pressure.** Thus, kidney is the major organ which helps to regulate sodium concentration in the body.
- Sodium is, mainly, **excreted by the kidneys.**
- Only, **less than 2% of the ingested sodium is eliminated in the feces.**
- Under normal physiological conditions, its **daily urinary excretion is equal to its intake.**
- **Sodium homeostasis is influenced by** several general factors, including **aldosterone, renin-angiotensin system and natriuretic factor** (ANF).

Table 11.2: Biological functions of sodium and potassium in the body

Sodium	*Potassium*
1. Regulation of osmotic pressure of extracellular fluid	1. Regulation of intracellular osmotic pressure
2. Regulation of acid–base balance of extracellular fluid	2. Regulation of intracellular acid–base balance
3. GI and renal absorption of monosaccharides and amino acids	3. GI secretions
4. Maintenance of neuromuscular irritability and excitability	4. Maintenance of neuromuscular irritability and excitability
5. Maintenance of blood viscosity	5. Storage of proteins and glycogen
6. Cofactor for Na^+/K^+-ATPase	6. Cofactor for enzymes, e.g. Na^+/K^+-ATPase, pyruvate kinase, etc.

Sources of Sodium

Most important source of sodium is the **common table salt,** i.e. sodium chloride. Besides, **meat, seafoods, milk, cheese** and **bread** are also good sources of sodium. **Processed foods** and **pickles** are also good sources of sodium. Plant sources are, usually, low in sodium.

RDA of Sodium

ICMR-NIN (2020) has recommended daily intake of sodium as **2000 mg/day.**

Deficiency

Abnormally reduced level of plasma sodium is referred to as **hyponatremia.** It may be a result of some **kidney or liver disease, adrenal insufficiency, chronic diarrhea or excessive intake of water.**

Sodium deficiency may result in **nausea and vomiting, muscle weakness, state of confusion, seizures and coma.**

Sodium Toxicity

Increased plasma concentration of sodium is referred to as **hypernatremia.** It may be a result of **low intake of fluid** and **some kidney disorder.**

It has been well studied that there is a direct relationship between high salt (sodium) intake and **hypertension.**

POTASSIUM

Potassium is the **chief cation in the ICF** (intracellular fluid) in the body. A large part of it is present in **skeletal muscles.** Along with the sodium, potassium is also important for cell functions.

Biological Functions and Metabolism

- Potassium plays an important role in the regulation of plasma volume, acid–base balance, and water and electrolyte homeostasis.
- Potassium is also essentially required for various enzymes of glycolysis and oxidative phosphorylation.
- Normal plasma potassium concentration is maintained in the range of 3.5–5.0 mmol/L.
- Potassium is completely **absorbed from the gastrointestinal tract through diffusion.**
- It is freely **filtered at the glomerulus** and is **excreted,** almost, entirely **by the kidneys in the urine.**

Sources of Potassium

Potassium is **widely distributed in plants as well as animals,** as the chloride, phosphate and carbonate salts of inorganic acids, organic acids and proteins.

Coffee, cocoa, dried beans, wheat bran, most of the vegetables (potato and tomato), **dairy products, fish, eggs, meat and fruits** (banana, peach and oranges) are good sources of potassium. **Coconut water is a rich source of potassium.**

RDA for Potassium

ICMR-NIN (2020) has recommended daily intake of potassium as **3500 mg/day.**

Deficiency

Low plasma potassium level is referred to as **hypokalemia.** It may be a result of **excessive sweating and diarrhea, chronic kidney disease** and by **use of diuretics.**

Deficiency symptoms include **nausea and bloating, constipation, muscle cramps and depression.**

Toxicity

Increased plasma potassium concentration is referred to as **hyperkalemia.**

It may be a **result of dehydration, excessive bleeding, some kidney disease or uncontrolled diabetes.**

MAINTENANCE OF FLUID AND ELECTROLYTE BALANCE

The kidneys are essential for the regulation of volume and composition of bodily fluids, and prevent our body against all possible disturbances in the volume and osmolarity of the bodily fluids such as dehydration and over-hydration.

- As discussed above, water balance is achieved in the body by ensuring that the **amount of water consumed** in food and drink (and generated by metabolism) **equals the amount of water excreted.**
- Its consumption is regulated by the **behavioural mechanisms,** including **thirst** and **salt cravings.** While almost a liter of water per day is lost through the skin, lungs, and feces, the **kidneys are the major site of excretion of water.**
- **Either the kidneys can conserve water by producing urine that is concentrated** relative to plasma, or they can rid the body of excess water by producing urine **that is dilute** relative to plasma.
- Direct control of water excretion by the kidneys is exercised by **anti-diuretic hormone** (**ADH** or vasopressin), a peptide hormone secreted by the hypothalamus.
- ADH causes the insertion of water channels into the membranes of cells lining the collecting ducts, allowing **water reabsorption** to occur.
- In **ADH** deficiency very little of water is reabsorbed resulting in **dilute urine.**
- ADH secretion is influenced by several factors, which include:
  - **Receptors in the hypothalamus** that are sensitive to increasing plasma osmolarity and **stimulate ADH secretion.**
  - **Stretch receptors in the atria of the heart** which are activated by a larger than normal volume of blood returning to the heart from the veins. They **inhibit ADH secretion.**
  - **Stretch receptors in the aorta and carotid arteries** which are stimulated when blood pressure falls. They **stimulate ADH secretion.**
- Regulation of osmolarity is achieved by balancing the intake and excretion of sodium with that of water.
- To prevent osmolarity from decreasing below normal, kidneys also have a regulated mechanism for reabsorbing sodium in the distal nephron, which is controlled by **aldosterone** (hormone of the adrenal cortex).
- Aldosterone secretion is controlled as follows:
  - **When the osmolarity increases aldosterone secretion is inhibited.**
  - The **juxtaglomerular cells** in the afferent and efferent arterioles **produce renin** (a peptide hormone) that produces **angiotensin II.** Angiotensin II **stimulates the adrenal cortex to produce aldosterone.**
  - Lack of aldosterone **causes less sodium to be reabsorbed in the distal tubule.** The net effect on urine excretion is a decrease in the amount of urine excreted, with an increase in the osmolarity of the urine.
- The kidneys also sense low blood pressure, which triggers a complex response to raise blood pressure and conserve volume.

OVERHYDRATION

Overhydration or **hyperhydration** may be a result of the excessive intake of water. It may also be due to **reduced excretion** or **increased retention** of water that may be a result of some **kidney or liver disease, congestive heart failure or hormonal disturbances.**

Overhydration, in turn, may result in **hyponatremia, muscle cramps** and **generalized weakness.** This, in turn, can lead to water intoxication.

DEHYDRATION

Dehydration is defined as **excessive loss of body fluid.** It is a state of negative fluid balance caused by **decreased intake, increased loss or fluid shift.**

Several conditions, such as **excessive perspiration, diarrhea, uncontrolled diabetes mellitus** and **diabetes insipidus** may lead to dehydration.

It can result in **high electrolyte concentrations in cells** and tissues. Most commonly seen type of dehydration is isotonic. Symptoms include **headache, decreased blood pressure and dizziness.**

WATER AND ELECTROLYTES IMBALANCE

In some circumstances, **electrolyte levels in the blood can become too high or low,** causing an imbalance. Disturbances in electrolytes can have a harmful effect on our health and can even be fatal.

- Electrolyte imbalances often occur **due to dehydration caused by excess heat, vomiting or diarrhea.**
- Some illnesses, including **kidney disease, eating disorders** and **injuries, like severe burns,** can also cause electrolyte imbalances.
- Severe imbalances can cause **symptoms like fatigue, fast or irregular heartbeat, numbness and tingling, confusion, muscle weakness and cramping, headache and convulsions.**
- **Long periods of exercise** or activity, particularly, in the heat, can cause significant electrolyte loss.
- **When we sweat,** we lose both, water and electrolytes, especially, sodium and chloride. Accordingly, **we must take normal amount of sodium from foods and drinking water** to remain hydrated.
- **Endurance athletes,** who are exercising for more than two hours or those who exercise in extreme heat, **should drink electrolyte-enriched sports drinks** to replace their losses.
- In some circumstances, such as **during bouts of vomiting and diarrhea,** where electrolyte losses are excessive, **supplementing with a rehydration solution** that contains electrolytes should be given.

SOME IMPORTANT QUESTIONS

1. **Describe sources, recommended daily allowances and deficiency symptoms of water.**
2. **Describe:**
   i. Regulation of water metabolism
   ii. Distribution of body water
   iii. Composition of body fluids
   iv. Maintenance of fluid and electrolyte balance
3. **Write notes on:**
   i. Electrolytes
   ii. Over-hydration
   iii. Dehydration
   iv. Electrolyte imbalances

CHAPTER

12

Storage of Food and Preservation of Nutrients

Food, as discussed in Chapter 1, refers to any substance or stuff which is used by the human beings, animals or any other organism for their survival and nutrition support.

Man acquires food for his/her own consumption, consumption of the family and their animal(s) **to meet immediate needs.** We also acquire different foodstuffs **for our future consumption** and for that purpose it has to be properly stored.

Government agencies procure and store food grains for distribution to the public till the next harvest. **Businessmen also procure foods** during postharvest season **and store it for sale in the market** throughout the year.

SIGNIFICANCE OF FOOD STORAGE

1. Food, particularly the **foodgrains, is procured during the harvesting season, when it costs less, for use for the remaining part of the year when its cost is high.** Thus, **food storage saves cost.**
2. Foodstuff is procured during the postharvest season and is **stored to be made available during the period of shortage,** such as during flood, war or famine. Recently, every one of us has realized the significance of food storage during Covid.

CLASSIFICATION OF FOOD ACCORDING TO STORAGE

Various foods may be stored in room, freeze, refrigerator or cold room. This, however, depends upon the type of food and the storage conditions. Accordingly, various foods are classified into three groups:

1. **Nonperishable foods:** Foodstuffs **which can be stored** under normal appropriate conditions **for a longer period** (may be for **months or years**) are referred to as nonperishable foods such as **cereal grains, pulses, nuts and sugar,** etc.
2. **Semi-perishable foods:** This group includes the class of foods **which can be stored** under certain desired storage conditions **for comparatively a short period** (may be **for a few days or weeks** only). These foods are referred to as semi-perishable foods, e.g. **fruits, vegetables and poultry,** etc.
3. **Perishable foods:** Perishable foods are those foodstuffs **which cannot be stored for more than a few hours.** These **get spoiled very soon** and do not remain fit for human consumption, if not stored under the desired conditions and left unattended even for one day, e.g. **dairy, fish and meat,** etc.

STORAGE OF FOOD GRAINS

Food grains, like **cereals** (wheat and rice), **millets** (maize, bajra, jowar or sorghum), **grams** (Bengal gram or chana and garbanzo beans or chickpeas, i.e. *chole*), **legumes, pulses, beans** and **oilseeds,** etc. are the most common food items which are stored throughout the world for personal consumption as well as for distribution to the public.

FOR DOMESTIC USE

Several studies have reported that in most of the countries including India, nearly half of the crop is **stored by** the farmers, particularly **the small farmers, for household consumption in the traditional indigenous storage structures.** These storage spaces are, generally, **made of locally available materials** such as grass, wood, mud, etc. without any scientific design, which does not guarantee protection of the stored grains against pests for a long time.

Depending upon the geographical region, climate, type and quantity of the food grain to be stored, these methods include:

- **Earthen bins: Small farmers and consumers,** mainly in the rural areas, **store food grains for their family consumption in the indigenous storage structures prepared from the locally available material** (mud, grasses, etc.), that may be located indoor or outdoor. Depending upon the personal requirement, these structures may be of different sizes, shapes, designs and capacities.
- **Silo:** Silo (Greek-Siros, means **pit for holding grains**) refers to a **long cone like structure** which is used to store grains. It can be **made of mud, concrete, plastic or metal** with varying capacities. A silo, generally, is resistant to insects and pests, and has a long life.
- **Drums:** Drums **made of plastic or metal** are, generally, used for the storage of food grains in the urban set-up. It is, however, recommended that after storage of the grains, these drum **should be sealed air tight,** not only in the beginning but after every time, whenever it is opened to remove the desired quantity of the grain.
- **Bags:** Common practice to store food grains required in large quantities, is the use of **jute** or **polyethylene** bags of different capacities, varying from 25 to 100 kg. These bags can be easily handled, transported and stored in a room.

FOR COMMERCIAL USE

Large rooms and warehouses (godowns) are the structures with walls (made of bricks) with doors, windows and roof (generally made of metal or cement sheets) are used to store large number of bags of food grains.

These structures are mostly built and maintained by various Government agencies like State Warehouse Corporations and Food Corporation of India. Some of the big business houses and millers (flour mills, rice mills, dal mills, etc.) also own and maintain these structures.

Precautions During Storage of Food Grains

Before storage, it is, however, essential to take a few precautions to avoid wastage and spoilage of the food grains, such as:

- **Drying of the food grains:** The process of drying the food grains in sun, also referred to as **solarization,** is an **old age practice** that, in turn, **helps to kill insects,** naturally. Time of drying food grains under sun, however, depends upon the type of food grain, its moisture content and the intensity of sun.

  For the storage of food grains, the postharvest crop should be air dried in the sun. For this purpose, the postharvest **crop is spread in thin layers on jute bags, sheets, polythene, tarpaulin** (*tirpaal*, a heavy-duty waterproof cloth), **or directly on the ground** may be on the rooftop, floor in the open field or even on the road (such as the practice in local markets, *anaj mandies*, etc.), for any length of time depending upon the moisture content in it.

- **Clean and dry place:** After drying, grains should be **stored in a clean and dry place, away from direct moisture and air.** This, in turn, will not only help to **keep the food grains safe** for longer duration but will also **reduce the risk of its spoilage.** It will also prevent grains from coming in contact with moisture, insects and rodents.
- **Use of insecticides:** Some insecticide or any other natural material such as neem leaves, etc. may also be used to keep food grains safe from the attack of insects. Plant-based chemicals and products are also quite useful in food grain storage. Being biodegradable, these products are environmentally friendly and are comparatively safe for human health, as well. In this relation, several studies have reported that the leaves as well as oil extract from the leaves of *Chenopodium ambrosioides L.* useful and prevents the food grains from the attack of insects.
- **Fumigation:** Large storehouses should be fumigated periodically, may be by the use of chemicals such as methyl-bromide or phosphine, etc.

STORAGE OF OTHER FOODSTUFFS

Besides food grains, every house stores various other foodstuffs such as fruits and vegetables, milk and milk products, spices, etc., depending upon their use, for a few days to a month. These include:

- **Vegetables and fruits:** Most of the fruits and vegetables require different storage conditions.
  - **Fruits:** Commercially, fruits such as **apples can be stored for 5–6 months,** without spoilage, **in a cold storage.** For this purpose, only the riped apple fruits should be picked from the plants, these should be immediately transported and stored in the cold storage.

Bananas should be stored at room temperature but in a cool dry place away from direct sunlight and heat. Moreover, bananas **should not be stored with other fruits,** because during ripening, bananas also ripen other fruits.

Oranges and other citrus fruits can be stored in any house at room temperature for one week and in refrigerator for more than that.

  - **Vegetables:** As we know that all the **vegetables** are not alike, which means that there is no single way to store them **altogether.** For example, tomatoes contain a lot of water, and accordingly, cold temperatures destroy their flavor.

Green leafy vegetables such as palak (spinach), fenugreek (methi) or mustard leaves, etc. should be stored at low refrigerator such as in refrigerator, after these are wrapped in some paper (newspaper or paper, etc.) to soak any extra water from these vegetables, which otherwise will spoil these leafy vegetables.

Dry vegetables such as potatoes, onions and garlic, etc. can be stored in a cool and dry place for a week or more but away from heat which will cause some of these to sprout.

Other vegetables which have hard skin such as sweet potatoes, pumpkin, etc. can be stored in warm and dry atmosphere.

- **Dairy:** According to the Academy of Nutrition and Dietetics, dairy (milk and milk products) **should not be stored in the refrigerator door** but towards the back. Since the refrigerator door is frequently opened and thus, has an easy access to the warm air.

- **Fats and cooking oils:** Fats and cooking oils **should be stored in dark place** and **in dark-colored glass or metal containers.** It is due to the reason that fats and cooking oils contain polyunsaturated fatty acids (PUFA), as a result of which, their exposure to oxygen, light and heat make them rancid.
- **Spices:** Spices like **coriander, cumin, turmeric,** etc. contain oil which slowly gets evaporated with time and thus, lose their flavor. Thus, spices should be stored in glass, metal or plastic containers but for a limited time of use only.

PRESERVATION OF NUTRIENTS

Food storage facility should be such that it not only keeps the food safe from spoilage but also preserves its various nutrients. For this purpose, various storage methods are in practice. These include:

Washing

All the fruits and vegetables should be washed before storage. Washing removes most of the microbes, and thus, saves fruits and vegetables from spoilage. This, in turn, will also help to preserve their nutrients.

Curing

The earliest form of curing was dehydration or drying. Thereafter, smoking and salting improved the drying process. This, in turn, also includes addition of antimicrobial agents which further aid in preservation of food, e.g. during **smoking** of food there is also deposit of a number of compounds on food such as phenols and catechol, etc.

Cooling

Refrigeration preserves food by **slowing down the growth and reproduction of microorganisms,** and the **action of enzymes that cause food to degrade.** To preserve nutrients in food, particularly the **perishable items,** should be kept in refrigerator.

Some of the foods are also **stored in freezer, at temperature below −10°C,** to preserve their nutrients for a longer period. Chilling for longer duration, however, may affect color, texture, flavor and nutritive value of food.

Freezing is also used, commercially, for the transport of the perishable foods. These foods, however, should be **properly thawed and cooked immediately.**

Freezing and Dehydration

Freeze-dried food had been in use since the space age to provide food to the astronauts. Freeze-dried food is not only compact but also light in weight.

Freezing and dehydration of the food not only quickly removes moisture but also protects it from microbial growth as well as preserves all the nutrients, enzymes and taste. It is the best choice for long-term storage of food.

Heating and Boiling

Heating is a simple and common method of preserving food, particularly the leftover food. Heating destroys/inactivates most of the pathogens and thus, prevents spoilage of food.

Boiling liquid foods, such as milk, kills most of the existing microorganisms.

Use of Natural Compounds

Natural compounds such as **neem leaves, camphor** or **cloves** are used to store small quantities of a variety of food grains like pulses and legumes.

Chemical Preservatives

Various chemicals such as sucrose (sugar), ascorbic acid (vitamin C), benzoic acid, sodium nitrite, etc. which inhibit microbial growth and retard enzymatic degradation of food, are used as preservatives for the storage of various types of foods like the cut fruits and vegetables, candies, pickles, jam, jellies and syrups. At the concentration used as preservative, these chemicals are hazardous for the microorganisms but not to the human being.

Artificial food additives such as sodium nitrite, sulfur dioxide, sodium bisulfite, potassium hydrogen sulfite, etc., act as antimicrobials, whereas vitamin C, BHA (butylated hydroxyanisole) and BHT (butylated hydroxytoluene) act as antioxidants (which inhibit oxidation of the food constituents), and **prevent chemical reactions which cause oxidation of food that results in its spoilage**.

External Application of Compounds

A layer of wax or vinegar, etc. is applied on the external surface of some of the fruits such as apple, pomegranate, etc. to extend their shelf life and preserve their nutrients.

For preserving certain vegetables such as cauliflower, radish, green chilies, ginger, etc. a solution of (1–4%) acetic acid is, generally, used.

This, in turn, prevents spoilage of fruits and vegetables for a longer period and is, particularly, important for transportation of these foods for longer distances.

Change in Osmotic Conditions

Change in osmotic conditions of some of the foods by the addition of salt or sugar also prevent their nutrient contents as well as improve their shelf-life. For example, use of salt in the preparation of pickles or sugar in the process of the formation of jams, jellies and syrups, etc. This is also the principle of canning of foods.

- **Addition of sugar:** Use of sugar as a preservative is one of the earliest techniques that was in common practice to store fruits in honey. Sugar removes water thereby causing dehydration of the microbial cell and thus, kill the microbes.

  Sugar is commonly used to preserve fruits (such as apples, pears, peaches, apricots and plums, etc.). Sugar is either used in form of syrup with fruits or in the crystallized form wherein the preserved material is cooked in sugar to the point of crystallization and thereafter, the resultant product is stored dry. Sugar is also used in the production of jam and jelly.
- **Addition of salt:** Salt is also used as a preservative. Addition of some of condiments and spices along with the large quantity of salt is a common practice for the storage of various fruits and vegetables such as mangoes, lime and gooseberry (amla), etc. in the form of pickles. Pickling inhibits growth as well as kills bacteria and other microorganisms. Besides salt, vinegar and some of the vegetable oils are also used for this purpose.

Canning

Canning refers to the process of heating the food, which, in turn, kills bacteria and, thereafter, it is packed in a metallic or glass container which is sealed airtight, in the way there is no entry of oxygen or moisture. Sometimes, a preservative such as common salt, or a solution of sodium chloride, may also be added to prolong shelf life of the food. Nowadays, a variety of canned foods like **beans, lentils, semi-cooked vegetables,** etc. are available in the market.

Canning is a very old process of food preservation. Various studies have reported that after canning foods can be stored for longer duration, may be up to one year or more. Some of the researchers have also suggested that canned foods are equally good as the fresh foods, since it not only **increases shelf life of the food** but also **preserves some of the nutrients.** Further, it has also been reported that canning solubilizes dietary fiber and make it more useful for human consumption.

Canned food, however, **may contain more salt,** thus, the canned food should be consumed only after removing excess of water from the container.

Pasteurization

According to WHO, pasteurization is defined as the process of heating milk to about 70°C for 15–30 minutes and thereafter, cooling it quickly to 10°C. After pasteurization, the milk is stored in sterilized bottles or pouches, which are transported and stored in cold places. Pasteurization, in turn, kills most of the pathogens present in milk while causing minimal change in its composition, flavor and nutritive value. This technique was invented by Louis Pasteur, in 1862.

Vacuum Packing

It refers to the process of storage of food in high density polythene or aluminum packings in a vacuum environment, i.e. after packing all the air is sucked. This, in turn, prevents metabolic oxidation of food by the atmospheric air as well as stops microbial growth, as a result of which the nutrients present in food remains preserved.

Vacuum packing is commonly used for storing nuts to prevent oxidation and loss of flavour.

Vacuum drying, the form of preservation where food is packed in large containers and thereafter, the air is removed. It is also being practiced these days.

Airtight storage (sealed storage), also referred to as **hermetic storage,** is one of the common and popular methods of storage for a variety of cereals, pulses, flour, tea and coffee, etc. in several countries, due to the reason that it is very effective storage method to preserve nutrients without the use of chemicals. In this method, waterproof bags are used and sealed under high carbon dioxide concentration atmosphere. Several studies have shown that in this method of storage, due to high concentration of carbon dioxide, aflatoxin production ability of *Aspergillus flavus* is also significantly inhibited.

Irradiation

Irradiation refers to the exposure of food to ionizing radiation. Multiple types of ionizing radiation can be used, including beta-particles (high-energy electrons) and gamma rays (emitted from radioactive sources such as cobalt^{60} or cesium^{137}). Irradiation can kill bacteria, molds and insect and pests, and reduces ripening and spoilage of fruits. Different doses of rays are used for different types of foods.

Bio-preservation

Bio-preservation or **biological preservation** involves the use of natural or controlled microbes, or antimicrobials, as a way of preserving food and extending its shelf-life. In this process, enzymatic action involves alcoholic or acidic fermentation, wherein beneficial bacteria, or the fermentation products produced by these bacteria, are used to control spoilage and render pathogens inactive in food. These microbes not only increase shelf life of the food, but also its palatability and nutritive value. For example, bread, wine, tea, coffee and alcoholic drinks are prepared and preserved by this technique.

Microbial culture such as Lactobacillus from curd is used to convert milk into curd. Though in a different form, this, in turn, increases shelf life of milk. Curdling also preserves all the nutrients of milk and is more beneficial for human health, particularly, for those who have lactose intolerance. Fermentation of milk is also used in the formation of probiotics.

Accordingly, these methods not only prevent milk from spoilage and but also preserve nutrients and improve nutritional value of milk.

Storage in Gases

Some of the foods, particularly the highly perishable items, which are to be transported to very long distances are packed under gases such as nitrogen or carbon dioxide.

Food Circulation

Food circulation **(rotation)** refers to the **periodical removal of a part** of the **foodstuffs** from pantry **and replacement** of the quantity **with the fresh stock for its use later,** after the previous one has been exhausted.

Depending upon the family consumption, different foods can be procured for a definite period of use such as for a weak, month, quarter or year, and can be replaced accordingly. This, in turn, will help in the preservation of its nutrients.

Food Transportation

Dry foodstuffs, which does not require refrigeration, can be easily transported by transportation mode such as by road or rail to longer distances without much fear of spoilage.

Advances in transportation technologies and associated infrastructure have also reduced transport time of food, particularly the semi-perishable and perishable items such as some fruits and vegetables, dairy, fresh seafood and meat, etc. which spoil so rapidly, in turn, improves food storage and preserve their nutrients.

PREVENTION OF LOSS OF VITAMINS

Food is an ideal mix of vitamins, minerals and other nutrients, but certain nutrients, particularly, the vitamins, begin to deteriorate early and continues to decrease until the food is consumed. It is due to the reason that vitamins are susceptible to destruction by atmospheric air, light, water, acid, alkali, heat and the action of enzymes (that are present in food), with time. Further, some of the water-soluble vitamins, especially, thiamin, folic acid and vitamin C, get destroyed during improper storage and cooking (Table 12.1).

Table 12.1: Effect of heat, air, water or fat on loss of vitamins

Vitamin	*Factors causing loss of nutrient*
Vitamin A	Heat and cooking oils
Vitamin D	Cooking oils
Vitamin E	Heat, air and cooking oils
Vitamin C	Heat, air and water
Thiamin	Heat and water
Riboflavin	Water
Vitamin B_6	Heat, air and water
Folate	Heat and air
Vitamin B_{12}	Heat and water
Biotin	Water
Pantothenic acid	Heat

To prevent this loss of vitamins following points should be carefully observed:

- **Vitamins A, E and D:** To reduce the loss of vitamins A and E, cook with very little oil, e.g. bake or broil vitamin A rich liver or vitamin D rich fish, oil-free instead of frying it.
- **B-Vitamins:** B-Vitamins leak out into cooking liquid or drippings. So, use the cooking liquid in soup or sauce. Do not over wash grains (rice) before cooking. Each washing removes, nearly, 25 percent of thiamin. Toast or bake cakes and bread only until the crust is light brown to preserve heat-sensitive B vitamins.
- **Vitamin C:** To reduce the loss of vitamin C which is water soluble and oxygen sensitive, cook fruits and vegetables in the least possible amount of water. Serve cooked vegetables quickly. After 24 hours in the fridge, vegetables lose, nearly, one-fourth of their vitamin C content. Root vegetables such as carrots, potatoes and sweet potatoes, etc. should be baked or boiled whole with the skin, this, in turn, will retain about most of its vitamin C.

SOME IMPORTANT QUESTIONS

1. Define food preservation. Describe various methods of food preservation.

2. Describe various methods of prevention of loss of vitamins from foods.

3. Write notes on:

i. Food storage
ii. Food preservation
iii. Classification of foods according to preservation
iv. Curing
v. Pasteurization
vi. Prevention of loss of vitamins
vii. Vacuum packing
viii. Bio-preservation
ix. Canning

CHAPTER

13

Food Toxicity and Safe Food Handling

Toxicity refers to harmful effects of a substance, or a mixture of substances, on some organism, e.g. animals, bacteria, plants or cells/organs (such as liver).

Food toxicity, in everyday usage more or less synonymous to **food poisoning,** is illness that results due to the consumption of food or drink which is contaminated with pathogenic bacteria, viruses, parasites, toxins or chemicals. Natural enzymes present in food also lead to its deterioration. Besides, insects, rodents, adulterants, natural toxins and various chemical residues beyond permissible levels make the food unfit for consumption. In addition to moisture and environmental conditions like temperature and storage time also influence the quality of the food. The contamination of food can occur at any point beginning from food production (growing, processing and shipping) to consumption.

CAUSES OF FOOD TOXICITY

Food borne illness are, usually, infectious or toxic in nature and can be caused by bacteria, viruses, parasites or chemical substances that may entering the body through contaminated food or water, or arise from improper handling, preparation or storage of food. Thus, sources of food toxicity are diverse, which include, both **biological** as well as **environmental** in nature. Besides, natural toxins are also found in some foods of plants as well as animal origin.

Biological Sources

Major biological sources of food toxicity are:
- Bacteria, such as:
  - *Campilobacter jejuni*
  - *Clostridium perfringens*
  - *Salmonella species*
  - *Escherichia coli*
- Viruses, e.g. norovirus
- Parasites (Toxoplasmosis)
  - **Fresh produce** is, generally, more vulnerable to microbial infestation during post-harvest storage, while grains, dairy and meat products can harbor pathogens and toxic chemicals, both at the pre- and post-storage as well as during processing suggesting that not only storage but also processing conditions play an important role in food toxicity.
  - Consumption of **meat and dairy** products not properly processed is often associated with the risk of hemorrhagic colitis and diarrhea, which could be avoided by appr-opriated methods of processing and proper cooking.
  - Use of **contaminated water** for irrigation of vegetables, fruits and crops, and

during processing of fresh produce is also considered as a source of food toxicity.

The application of emerging technologies, such as gamma irradiation and cold atmosphere packaging techniques, have been widely recognized as safe alternatives to chemical preservatives for food preservation and processing, which have been helpful in reducing microbial infestation and decay of food products (Chapter 12).

Environmental Sources

Major environmental sources of food toxicity include:

- **BPA:** BPA (bisphenol-A) is a chemical **found in the plastic containers** of many common foods and beverages. BPA can leech of these containers into the food or beverage. Food sources, such as **bottled water, packaged foods and canned items** (like fish, chicken, beans and vegetables) make the biggest contribution to BPA levels in the body, which can be determined by measuring BPA in urine.

  BPA, in turn, has been reported to **mimic estrogen,** by binding to the receptor sites meant for the hormone. Thus, BPA exposure leads to several problems related to reproduction and also increases the **risk of breast and prostate cancer.** Increased BPA levels have also been shown to be associated with **infertility, insulin resistance, type 2 diabetes and obesity, altered thyroid hormones production** as well as their **functions.**

  BPA exposure can be reduced by the use of BPA-free bottles and containers as well as by eating whole unprocessed foods.
- **Trans fat:** Trans-fat is the unhealthiest fat, we eat. It is formed by pumping hydrogen into unsaturated oils, in order to turn them into solid fats. Our body does not recognize or process trans fats, as the naturally occurring fats. Eating trans fats can lead to a number of serious health problems, e.g. trans fat consumption **causes inflammation** and negative effects on heart health. In addition, chronic inflammation is at the root of many other serious conditions, such as **insulin resistance, type 2 diabetes and obesity.**
- **Polycyclic aromatic hydrocarbons:** Polycyclic aromatic hydrocarbons (PAHs) are released from red meat when it is grilled or smoked at high temperature. Incomplete burning of charcoal also causes the formation of PAHs. PAHs **are toxic and have been linked to an increased risk of breast and prostate cancer, kidney cancer and cancer of the digestive tract,** especially, **colon cancer.**
- **Heavy metals: Seafood consumption** is the largest contributor of heavy metals, such as **mercury,** in humans. Plants that grow in mercury contaminated waters are consumed by small fish, which are then consumed by larger fish. Over a period of time, mercury accumulates in the fish, which are eventually eaten by humans. Mercury is a **neurotoxin,** meaning that it can **damage the brain and nerves.** Pregnant women are, particularly, at high risk, since mercury **affects developing brain** and **nervous system of the foetus.**
- **Insecticides:** There are many types of poisons found in insecticides but the most dangerous types are the **organophosphates** which **generate nerve gas** for insects.
- **Other causes** There are many other causes of food poisoning. These include **wild nuts, leaves, flowers and berries under ripe tubers, botulism, cadmium from containers, lead or arsenic from fertilizers, and acids and lead from pottery,** etc.

Toxins that Occur Naturally in Foods

Natural toxins, inherently, found in foods of plant and animal origins can also be harmful, when consumed in large quantities.

Commonly found natural toxins, that can pose a risk to our health, include:

- **Cyanogenic glycosides:** Cyanogenic glycosides are phytotoxins, toxic chemicals produced by plants, of which a number of species are used as food in some areas of the World. Cassava, sorghum, stone fruits, almonds and bamboo shoots are, especially, important foods that contain cyanogenic glycosides (Fig. 13.1).

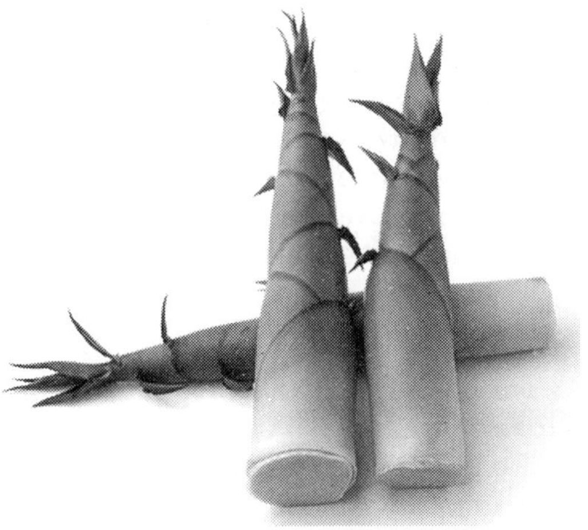

Fig. 13.1: Bamboo shoots

The potential toxicity of a cyanogenic plant depends upon the concentration of the cyanide produced, as a result of consumption of the toxin. In humans, the clinical signs of acute cyanide intoxication include rapid respiration, drop in blood pressure, dizziness, headache, stomach pains, vomiting, diarrhea, mental confusion, cyanosis with twitching and convulsions, followed by terminal coma and death.

- **Furocoumarins:** Furocoumarins are stress toxins that are released in response to stress, such as physical damage, in many plants like parsnips (closely related to carrots and parsley), celery roots, citrus plants (lemon, lime and grapefruit) and some medicinal plants. Some of these toxins cause gastrointestinal problems, particularly, in susceptible people. Furocoumarins are also phototoxic and can cause severe skin reactions under sunlight (UVA exposure).
- **Lectins:** Lectins are the toxins found in many types of beans, especially, red kidney beans. Consumption of a few types of raw beans can cause severe stomachache, vomiting and diarrhea. Lectins can be destroyed, when the dried beans are soaked for at least 12 hours, and then boiled, vigorously, for at least 10 minutes in water.
- **Mycotoxins:** Mycotoxins are naturally occurring toxic compounds produced by certain types of moulds, which grow on numerous foodstuffs, such as cereals, dried fruits, nuts and spices. Mould growth can occur before or after harvest, during storage, on/in the food itself, often under warm, damp and humid conditions. Most mycotoxins are chemically stable and survive food processing. Effects of food-borne mycotoxins can be acute, with symptoms of severe illness and even death appearing quickly after consumption of highly contaminated food products. Long-term effects on health of chronic mycotoxin exposure include the induction of cancers and immune deficiency.
- **Solanines and chaconine:** Most of the solanacea plants (tomatoes, potatoes and eggplants, etc.) contain natural toxins called solanines and chaconine, which are glycoalkaloids. Their higher concentrations are found in potato sprouts, and bitter-tasting peel and green parts, as well as in green tomatoes (Fig. 13.2).

Plants produce these toxins in response to stress, like bruising, UV light, microorganisms, and attacks from insect pests and herbivores. To reduce the production of solanines and chaconine, it is important to store potatoes in a dark, cool and dry place, and not to eat the green or sprouting parts.

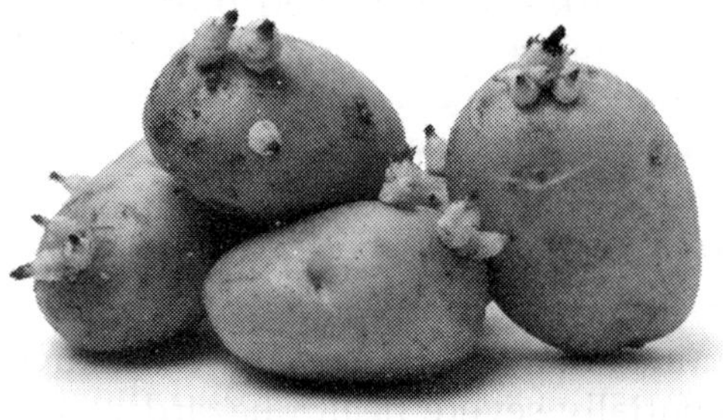

Fig. 13.2: Sprouted potatoes

- **Poisonous mushrooms:** Wild mushrooms may contain several toxins, such as muscimol and muscarine, which can cause vomiting, diarrhea, confusion, visual disturbances, salivation, and hallucinations. Onset of symptoms occurs between 6 and 24 hours, or more, after ingestion of these mushrooms. Fatal poisoning is, usually, associated with delayed onset of symptoms, which are very severe, with toxic effects on the liver, kidney and nervous system. Cooking or peeling does not inactivate the toxin. It is recommended to avoid any wild mushrooms, unless definitively identified as non-poisonous.
- **Pyrrolizidine alkaloids:** Pyrrolizidine alkaloids are toxins produced by several plant species. The main plant sources are the families Boraginaceae, Asteraceae and Fabaceae. Many of these are weeds that can grow in fields and contaminate food crops. They can be acutely toxic and cause a variety of adverse health effects. Some have the DNA-damaging potential, leading to cancer. They are stable during processing, and have been detected in herbal teas, honey, herbs and spices, and other food products, such as cereals and cereal products.

COMMITTEE ON FOOD TOXICITY

For a healthier life and better world, food safety is a must focused agenda for food producers, traders, policy makers and consumers, which can be attained collectively, by employing hygienic practices, integrated safety measures and by the use of safe food processing technologies.

Committee on Toxicity of Chemicals in Food, Consumer Products and the Environment

The Committee on Toxicity of Chemicals in Food, Consumer Products and the Environment **(COT)** is a UK independent scientific committee that provides advice to the Food Standards Agency, the Department of Health and other Government Departments and Agencies on matters concerning the toxicity of chemicals. The Committee started work in 1978 and replaced the toxicology sub-committee of the Committee on Medical Aspects of Chemicals in Food and the Environment.

SAFE FOOD HANDLING

As we know, food remains fit for human consumption only if stored properly and for the period till it is not spoiled.

Food spoilage refers to any **change in texture, flavor or taste of the food.**

CAUSES OF FOOD SPOILAGE

Several causative factors such as contamination of food by the microorganisms (bacteria, molds or fungi), its deterioration (fermentation or metabolic degradation) by the endogenous enzymes present in food and infestation by the insects and the rodents are responsible for the spoilage of food. These factors not only make food unfit for human consumption but also reduces germination of food grains.

- **Contamination by microorganisms:** Microorganisms, particularly the pathogens (disease-causing microorganisms) such as **bacteria, molds** and **fungi,** etc. contaminate our food at various stages. These microbes grow rapidly and multiply fast, which, in turn, spoil the food and make it unfit for human consumption.

Besides, a large amount (25–40%) of the cereal grains, especially **maize, peanuts,** etc. has also been reported worldwide, to be **contaminated by mycotoxins** during their storage. This, in turn, also makes these foods unsuitable for human consumption.

- **Endogenous enzymes:** Various environmental factors such as **atmospheric air and moisture** also **activate various endogenous enzymes** which are **present in food.** This, in turn, will **stimulate metabolic degradation and fermentation** of food.
- **Insects and rodents:** Smell and flavor of the foodstuff (food grains, dry fruits, etc.) attracts **insects and rodents,** which, in turn, **destroys food.** It has been reported from various countries that every year a large quantity of food grains is spoiled by insects and rodents.

GENERAL PRECAUTIONS TO PREVENT FOODBORNE ILLNESSES

- **Use of fresh ingredients** and **personal hygiene** are the most important concepts of safe food. Food turns harmful, when dirty hands are used to serve cooked food.
- Use of rotten and unwashed vegetables makes food unsafe. As physical and biological contaminants are the major hazards, **raw foods should be thoroughly washed/cleaned,** to make them free from physical contaminants and suitable for consumption.
- **Cooked food,** particularly, purchased from restaurants, eateries, take away, etc. is also considered to be unsafe, since one cannot be sure of the quality of ingredients, used in it. Moreover, since it is prepared in large quantity, it may not be possible to take full care during its preparation.
- **Packed foods** may be considered safer than the one that is kept in open and sold in eateries, since packets protect it from exposure to flies, insects and dust, etc. However, one cannot be certain about the ingredients used in it.

PRACTICES OF SAFE FOOD HANDLING

Safe food handling includes a number of routines that should be followed to avoid potentially severe health hazards, since a significant proportion of the food borne illnesses arise from practices in the kitchen.

In developed countries, there are intricate standards for food preparation, whereas in lesser developed countries the main issue is the availability of adequate safe water, which is usually a critical item. Besides the use of safe water for drinking and cooking, several other precautions are required to be taken for safe food handling. These include **general precautions** and specific steps at different stages such as **during shopping, storage in the house, freeze or refrigerator;** before, during and after **preparation for cooking;** and **storage of the leftover food,** to prevent food borne illnesses.

During Shopping

Selection of the right food is the first step to ensure safe and good quality diet. For this purpose:

- Food items should be purchased from reliable sources, having a high turnover ensure their freshness.
- We should purchase foods that carry certification mark, assuring good quality, e.g. AGMARK for honey and ghee; FPO (Fruit Products Order) for fruit and vegetable products, such as jams, squashes; and ISI (Bureau of Indian Standards) for food colours and essences, etc.
- While purchasing packaged food always look for its date of packaging, such as best before or date of expiry, such as:
  - **Best before:** This term is appropriate for most foods. It relates to the quality of food and is an indication of the

period for which a food can reasonably be expected to retain its optimal condition.
- **Use by:** This term is appropriate for perishable foods. These foods present a microbiological risk to the consumer, if sold after the indicated date. It is an offence for shops to sell food that is after the use by date.
- **Sell by:** Products may be labeled with sell by and display until dates, but these are not required by law and are used mainly for stock control premises.

- Food grains purchased should be **free from infestation and foreign matter,** such as rodent excreta or insect remains, etc. Further, they should be of uniform size and should not be shrivelled, shrunken or mouldy.
- Foodstuffs should be **free from artificial colors.**
- **Fats/oils should not be purchased loose,** from unsealed containers, to avoid the risk of adulteration.
- One must buy **pasteurized milk** in sachets from a reputed dairy, or from a reliable vendor, to avoid the risk of adulteration and contamination. Milk products, such as butter, ghee and khoa should also be purchased from reliable sources.
- **Whole spices** should be preferred, which should be uniform in color, size and shape. Since powdered spices are more likely to be adulterated. Also, always buy certified products.
- **Fruits and vegetables** that show patches, physical damage with bruises or wilted and decayed with visible evidence of insects and moulds, should be avoided.
- **Eggs** should be fresh and free from cracks.
- **Meat or poultry** must be examined for characteristic color, odor and texture, and should be purchased fresh or frozen.
- Freshness of fresh-water **fish** is indicated by a stiff body, bright, clear and bulging eyes, reddish gills, tight scales and absence of stale odor or discoloration. Fresh fish will not show any pitting on finger pressure.

During Storage

- **Always refrigerate perishable food** within 2 hours (1 hour when the atmospheric temperature is above 32°C). Check the temperature of refrigerator and freezer with a thermometer. The refrigerator should be between 0 and 4°C while the freezer below –10°C (Chapter 12).
- Perishable foods such as meat and poultry should be wrapped securely, to maintain quality and to prevent meat juices from getting onto other foods.
- Always **keep eggs in the refrigerator.**
- **High-acid canned foods** such as tomatoes, grapefruit and pineapple, **can be stored on the shelf** for up to 12 months. **Low-acid canned foods** such as meat, poultry, fish and most vegetables **can be stored for even more time,** if the can remains in good condition and has been stored in a cool, clean and dry place. Discard cans that are dented, leaking, bulging or rusted.

Before Cooking

- Always **wash hands** with warm water and soap for 20 seconds before and after handling food, using the bathroom, changing diapers, or handling pets.
- Since **kitchen towels and clothes** can harbor bacteria, so **wash** them regularly. Also, replace sponge after every few weeks.
- **Do not cross contaminate food.** Keep raw meat, poultry, fish and their juices away from other foods.
- After every use **wash cutting board, utensils and countertops** with hot and soapy water, or sanitize by using a solution of 1 tablespoon of unscented, liquid chlorine bleach (in 4 liters of water).

- **Thaw frozen food** in the microwave or refrigerator. Do not thaw the items on kitchen counter, since it will allow bacteria to grow in the outer layer of the food, before the inside thaws. For faster thawing, place food in a leakproof plastic bag. Submerge in cold tap water and change the water every 30 minutes.
- Cook food immediately after thawing.

During Cooking

- Preferably, **use fresh vegetables** and **wash them** thoroughly by dipping in a container of water.
- Cook the food thorough, since cooking kills harmful bacteria. Raw or partially cooked meat, poultry, fish or eggs may result in exposure to bacteria that can affect health. Some of the bacteria such as Salmonella, that causes food poisoning, can grow inside fresh unbroken eggs. This is, particularly, important for children, pregnant women, the elderly and for those whose immune system is compromised.
- If food has been cooked ahead of time, divide large portions into small shallow containers and refrigerate the same. This ensures rapid and safe cooling.
- Though the microwave oven is time saver, but it has food safety disadvantage. It, sometimes, leaves cold spots in the food where bacteria may grow. Hence, be sure to cover food with a lid or plastic wrap. Leave a small section uncovered so that steam can escape.
- Stir and rotate food for even cooking. If there is no turntable in the oven, rotate the dish by hand once or twice during cooking.

After Cooking

- Keep cold food on ice or refrigerated until the time to replenish platters. If serving hot maintain it at 60°C or divide into small serving platters which can be refrigerated until time to warm them up for serving.
- Always use clean dishes and utensils to serve food and not those which were used to prepare food. If the food is being grilled, serve it on a clean plate, not on the one that held the raw meat, poultry or fish.
- When serving food at a buffet, keep food hot with slow cookers or warming trays.
- Perishable food should not be left out for more than 2 hours at room temperature (1 hour when the temperature is above 32°C). Bacteria, that can cause food poisoning, grow quickly at warm temperature.
- Pack lunch in an insulated carrier with a cold pack. Be sure not to leave lunch in direct sunlight or on warm radiator.
- Carry picnic food in a cool pack carrier (cooler) with a cold pack. Do not open the lid any more than it is necessary.

Leftover Food

- Discard any food left out at room temperature for more than 2 hours (1 hour, if the temperature is above 32°C).
- Also, discard any food with a strange color, or odor, immediately.
- Divide large amounts of leftover food into small shallow containers for quick cooling in the refrigerator.
- With poultry or other stuffed meats remove stuffing and refrigerate it in a separate container.
- Bring sauces, soups and gravy to a boil. Heat other leftover food thoroughly to above 70°C.
- Microwave the leftover food using a lid or vented plastic wrap to ensure thorough heating.
- Use cooked leftover within 4 days.
- Discard any thawed food that has risen to room temperature and remained there for 2 hours or more.

SOME IMPORTANT QUESTIONS

1. What is food toxicity? Describe various causes of food toxicity.

2. Briefly describe:

i. Biological sources of food toxicity
ii. Environment sources of food toxicity
iii. Symptoms and prevention of food toxicity
iv. Natural toxins inherently found in foods
v. Safe food handling

3. Write notes on:

i. Committee on Toxicity of Chemicals in Food, Consumer Products and the Environment
ii. Polycyclic aromatic hydrocarbons
iii. Food toxicity

CHAPTER

14

Food Standards

Food standard is a **set of criteria that a food must meet,** if it is to be suitable for human consumption, such as source, composition, appearance, freshness, permissible additives and maximum bacterial content.

Food standards are the body of rules directly governing foodstuffs, whether they are issued by official, semiofficial or factory authority. Food standards, such as those that specify the maximum allowable level of contaminants in food or the amount of food additives permitted, are important for the assurance of food safety.

Significance of Food Standards

Food **standards** aim to lower the incidence of food-borne illness.

- **Food quality must meet the expectations of the consumer.**
- It must be as described, and **not presented, in a way that misleads the consumer,** and
- **Nothing may be added or removed from food that would make it harmful to the consumer.**

Food standards are adopted and used as models **by many countries** in their domestic **food legislation** and **regulations.**

- **WHO** and **FAO,** in 1963, published the **Codex Alimentarius,** which serves as a **guideline to food safety.**
- In **Australia, food safety standards** place obligations on Australian food businesses, to produce food that is safe and suitable to eat, and also place health and hygiene obligations on food handlers.
- In **United Kingdom,** the **Food Standards Agency** is a non-ministerial Government Department, of the Government of the United Kingdom. It is responsible for protecting public health in relation to food in England, Wales and Northern Ireland. It is led by a board appointed to act in the public interest with its headquarter in London.
- In **India,** the **Food Safety and Standards Authority of India** (FSSAI) has been created for laying down science-based standards for articles of food and to regulate their manufacture, storage, distribution, sale and import, to ensure availability of safe and wholesome food for human consumption.

FOOD SAFETY AND STANDARDS AUTHORITY OF INDIA

Food Safety and Standards Authority of India **(FSSAI)** is an autonomous body, which was established under the **Ministry of Health and Family Welfare** of the Government of India, under the **Food Safety and Standards Act, 2006.**

- FSSAI is the **regulatory body related to food safety** and **laying down of standards of food in India.**

- FSSAI follow **acts,** like **Fruit Product Order** (FPO), **Meat Food Products Order** (MFPO) and **Prevention of Food Adulteration** (PFA) to assure the quality of produce.
- FSSAI has its **headquarter in New Delhi.** Besides, it has 5 **regional offices** which are located in Delhi, Guwahati, Mumbai, Kolkata and Chennai, 4 referral laboratories and 72 local laboratories located throughout the country.
- The FSSAI is **responsible for protecting and promoting public health** through the **regulation and supervision of food safety.**
- It has been **created for laying down science-based standards** for articles of food and **to regulate their manufacture, storage, distribution, sale and import, to ensure availability of safe** and wholesome **food for human consumption.**

Food Safety and Standards (Licensing and Registration of Food Businesses) Regulation, 2011

According to Food Safety and Standards (Licensing and Registration of Food Businesses) Regulation, 2011, it is **mandatory for all food business operators, manufacturers, importers, distributors, wholesalers, retailers, hotels, restaurants, eateries,** as well as **petty food businesses to have an FSSAI registration/license** so they are in compliance with the FSSAI Act.

- **Food articles imported to India** from foreign countries and distributed in India **also need to conform to the FSSAI regulations** or suffer restrictions on import.
- The FSSAI **also has stringent regulations for packaging and labeling under Food Safety and Standards** (Packaging and Labeling) Regulation, 2011.

Food Safety Issues and Regulations Concerning

- Agriculture and animal husbandry practices
- Food manufacturing practices
- Food additives
- Novel foods
- Genetically modified foods
- Food labels
- Food contamination

FOOD ADDITIVES

Food additives are the **substances which are added to food to preserve its flavor or enhance taste, appearance or other qualities.**

Some of the additives have been used for centuries, such as vinegar and salt for preserving pickles. With the advent of processed foods in recent years, many more additives have been introduced, both, of natural and artificial origin.

GENERAL PRINCIPLES FOR USE OF FOOD ADDITIVES

- Food additives (whether in use or being proposed for use) **should have undergone, or should be subjected to, appropriate toxicological testing and evaluation.** This should take into account (among other things) **any cumulative, synergistic or potentiating effects of its use.**
- Only those food additives should be endorsed for use, which can be judged on the basis of presently available evidence that are known to **cause no health hazards** at the level of proposed use.
- Food additives should be **kept under continuous observation** and should be **re-evaluated,** whenever necessary, **in the light of changing conditions of use and new scientific information.**
- Food additives should, at all times, **conform to approved specifications,** e.g. the specifications of identity and purity **recommended by the Codex Alimentarius Commission.**
- The **use** of food additives **should be justified** and **allowed only to serve one or more of the following four purposes** (which cannot be achieved by other means) that are **economically and technologically**

practicable, and **do not present a hazard to the health of the consumer,** that is:

a. **To preserve the nutritional quality of the food;** an intentional reduction in the nutritional quality of a food would be justified in the circumstances dealt with in sub-paragraph b, and also in other circumstances **where the food does not constitute a significant item in a normal diet;**

b. **To provide necessary ingredients or constituents for foods manufactured for groups of consumers having special dietary needs;**

c. **To enhance the keeping quality or stability of a food or to improve its organoleptic properties,** provided that this does not so change the nature, substance or quality of the food as to deceive the consumer;

d. **To provide aids in the manufacture, processing, preparation, treatment, packing, transport or storage of food,** provided that the additive is not used to disguise the effects of the use of faulty raw materials or of undesirable (including unhygienic) practices or techniques during the course of any of these activities.

- **Approval,** or temporary approval, **for the inclusion** of a food additive **in an advisory list or in a food standard should:**
  - As far as possible be **limited to specific foods for specific purposes and under specific conditions;**
  - Be at the **lowest level of use, necessary to achieve the desired effect;**
  - As far as possible take into account any **"Acceptable Daily Intake"** or equivalent assessment, established for the food additive and the probable daily intake of it from all sources. Where the food additive is to be used in foods eaten by special groups of consumers, account should be taken of the probable daily intake of the food additive by consumers in those groups.

FUNCTIONS OF FOOD ADDITIVES

- **To maintain product consistency:** Additives such as **emulsifiers, stabilizers and thickeners** are used to maintain consistency of food. For example, **emulsifier such as peanut butter** gives a consistent texture to the product and prevents it from separating. **Stabilizers and thickeners** are used **in ice cream to give it a smooth and uniform texture.**
- **To improve or maintain nutritional value:** Such additives are added **to make up for the elements that are likely to be lacking in a diet,** or **replacing those which may be lost during processing.** Such nutrients should be listed in the list of ingredients. For example, thiamine, riboflavin, niacin and iron in flours and cereals; vitamins A and D in milk, vegetable oils and ghee; or iodine in salt, etc.
- **To provide leavening, or control acidity and alkalinity:** Leavening agents release acids, when heated, e.g. **baking soda added to cakes, biscuits** and other baked foods. It is added during baking **to improve the texture.** Some additives also modify acidity or alkalinity of the food.
- **To enhance flavor or impart desired color:** Many **spices and flavoring agents enhance taste of the food.** For example, **color, dye, pigment or any other substance** that imparts color to a food, **enhances appearance of food and make it more appealing.**
- **To maintain palatability and wholesomeness:** Some preservatives **retard spoilage of food,** caused by mold, bacteria, fungi or yeast. Others like **antioxidants are added to prevent fat** (in baked and other foods) **from becoming rancid** and thus, to **develop bad flavor.**

CATEGORIES OF FOOD ADDITIVES

Food additives can be divided into several groups, although, there may be some overlap, because some additives exert more than one effect.

- **Acidity regulators:** Acidity regulators **(pH control agents)** are food additives used for controlling pH (to change or maintain pH, i.e. acidity or alkalinity) of foods for their stability, or to affect activity of enzymes. They can be **organic** or **mineral acids, bases, neutralizing agents,** or **buffering agents.** Typical agents include some of the acids or their sodium salts, e.g. **ascorbic acid, acetic acid, benzoic acid, propionic acid,** etc. Acidity regulators are indicated by their E numbers, such as E260 (acetic acid).
- **Antioxidants:** Antioxidants are **compounds that inhibit oxidation,** a chemical reaction that produces free radicals, which may damage cells of organisms.

  The term antioxidant is used for two groups of substances, i.e.:
  - **Industrial chemicals** that are added to products to prevent oxidation. They have diverse uses, such as **acting as preservatives in food** and cosmetics, or oxidation inhibitors.
  - **Naturally occurring compounds** that are present in foods and tissue such as **glutathione** or **enzymes** (which are produced internally), or **dietary antioxidants** like vitamins C and E.
- **Bulking agents:** Bulking agents such as **starch** are the additives that **increase bulk of the food** without affecting its taste.
- **Food coloring agents:** Food coloring or **color additive** is any **dye, pigment or substance that is added to food to replace the color lost during preparation,** or to **make food look more attractive.** These agents come in many forms such as liquids, powders, gels or pastes. Food coloring agent is used, both, in commercial food production as well as in domestic cooking. Besides, **color retention agents** are used **to preserve the existing color of food.**
- **Fortifying agents:** They are added **to increase nutritional value of food,** e.g. vitamins, minerals, dietary supplements, etc.
- **Emulsifiers:** Emulsifiers, also known as an **emulgents,** are compounds, which typically have a polar, or hydrophilic (i.e. water-soluble) part, and a nonpolar (i.e. hydrophobic or lipophilic) part, e.g. **egg yolk** (which has lecithin as the main emulsifying agent), or **mono- and diglycerides** that are **added in many food products** such as coffee creamers, ice creams, spreads and cakes, etc.
- **Flavoring agents:** Flavor is a quality of food that affects sense of taste. Flavoring agents are added **to give food a particular taste or smell,** and may be derived from natural ingredients or made artificially. For example, **artificially flavored jellies, soft drinks or candies** have various flavors, due to the use of different scents or fragrances.

  Besides, **flavor enhancers,** such as monosodium glutamate (MSG), enhance existing flavor of the food. Some flavor enhancers have their own flavor that is independent of the food.
- **Preservatives:** A preservative is a substance or a chemical that is **added** to products, such as food, beverages, pharmaceutical drugs, biological samples, cosmetics, and many other products, **to prevent decomposition by microbial growth or undesirable chemical changes.** Preservatives include chemicals or physical agents:
  - **Chemical preservation** refers to the addition of certain chemical compounds to the product. They **reduce the risk of food-borne infections, decrease microbial spoilage,** but preserve nutritional quality.
  - **Physical techniques** of food preservation include **dehydration, UV radiation, freeze-drying and refrigeration.**
- **Sweeteners:** Sweeteners **(sugar substitutes)** are food additives that **provide sweet taste** like that of sugar, but **provide**

significantly less calories. Most of them are not produced naturally and are also referred to as **artificial sweeteners,** e.g. **saccharin and aspartame,** etc.

- **Thickeners:** Thickener or **thickening agent** is a substance, which can **increase viscosity of a liquid,** without, substantially, changing its other properties. These are commonly used to thicken **sauces, soups, and puddings,** etc. without altering their taste.
- **Glazing agents:** They **provide a shiny appearance** or protective coating to foods.

NUMBERING OF FOOD ADDITIVES

To regulate the use of food additives, and inform consumers, **each additive is assigned a unique number,** termed as **E number.** This is used in **Europe** for all the approved additives.

This numbering scheme has now been adopted and extended by the ***Codex Alimentarius* Commission, to internationally identify all additives.** For example, **acetic acid** is written as **E260** on products sold **in Europe.** It is simply known as **additive 260** in some other countries.

United States Food and Drug Administration (USFDA) lists these items **generally recognized as safe** (GRAS). These are listed under both, their **Chemical Abstracts Service Number** and **FDA regulation.**

FOOD FORTIFICATION

Food fortification refers to the **addition of a nutrient to the food** so that **its quality is improved,** or maintained, without the quantity being significantly increased.

Food fortification is an important part of nutrition intervention strategy as a means of delivering nutrients to population.

The program of food fortification **was launched in India** to overcome the widespread micronutrients deficiencies in the community, such as those of iodine, vitamin A and iron. For example, **iodination of common salt with potassium iodate** to eliminate iodine deficiency disorders. Similarly, **delivery of iron through common salt** was **launched by National Institute of Nutrition** (NIN) **to mitigate the problem of anemia.**

Vitamins A and D are also commonly used for the fortification of milk and vegetable oils.

DIETARY SUPPLEMENTS

Dietary supplement is the product that is intended to supplement the diet. These are neither drugs nor food or food additives. Their manufacture and sale are also not regulated, differently from foods, food additives and drugs. The word supplement, however, should be clearly stated on the label.

FOOD ADULTERATION

Food adulteration refers to the **addition of some non-food material or the inferior quality product to the food.** In this process, a **spoilt, stale or poor-quality food is made attractive and fresh by adding harmful colors or other chemicals.** Frequently, **adulterated food items include milk and milk products, cereals, pulses and their products, edible oils and spices.**

Types of Food Adulterations

Different classes of food adulterants include:

- Non-permitted colors like metanil yellow,
- Non-edible oils such as castor oil,
- Cheaper agricultural produce like various starches in milk powder,
- Extraneous matter such as husk, sand and sawdust, and
- Metal contaminants like aluminum or iron filings, etc.

Consumption of adulterated foods could lead to disease outbreaks of epidemic proportions.

Buying food from a reliable and reputed source, careful checking of foods before purchase, and **insisting on certified brands** will **minimize the risk of food adulteration.**

PREVENTION OF FOOD ADULTERATION ACT (PFA)

Prevention of Food Adulteration Act (PFA) was enacted by the **Govt. of India,** to ensure protection of health of the consumers. PFA consolidates the laws relating to food being administered by different ministries/departments. Since food is essential for the maintenance of health, the act was enacted with the objective that the food available to the consumers should be nutritious, wholesome and pure.

According to PFA, food is described as any article that is used as food, or drink, for human consumption other than the drugs and water. PFA includes:

- **Any article which ordinarily enters into or is used in the composition or preparation of human food,**
- **Any flavoring matter or condiments,** and
- **Any other article which the Central Government may having regard to its use, nature, substance or quality, declare, by notification in the official gazette as food** for the purpose of the PFA.

Objectives of PFA

Objectives of PFA include:

- To protect the public from poisonous and harmful foods
- To prevent the sale of substandard foods
- To protect the interests of the consumers by eliminating fraudulent practices

Rules and Standards of PFA

Rules and standards framed under PFA are uniformly applicable throughout the country. These include:

- **Enforcement** of the food laws, primarily rests **with the states/UTs.**
- The **implementation** of the Act in most of the states is under the administrative control of the **Directorate of Health Services,** whereas in a few states, the implementation is being combined with Drugs Administration, under the **Joint Food and Drug Administration.**
- The provisions under PFA Rules have been **amended nearly 360 times** and **standards of around 250 articles of food** which are of mass consumption **have been prescribed.**
- By and large, in most of the states, **implementation** in corporation/municipal area **rests with the local bodies,** which employ their own **food inspectors.** Licensing of food industries/establishments is also left to them.
- There are **72 food laboratories** in the country at district/regional or state level, in addition to **four Central Food Laboratories** set-up by the Central Government.
- Almost **every state has got one or more laboratory** depending upon its need.
- About **12 of these laboratories are under the administrative control** of the **local bodies,** whereas the **remaining** ones are **under the administrative control of the State Government.**

SOME IMPORTANT QUESTIONS

1. **What are food additives? Describe various categories of food additives.**
2. **Write notes:**
   i. Food adulteration
   ii. Prevention of food adulteration act (PFA)
   iii. Food fortification
   iv. Food additives
   v. Food standards

CHAPTER

15

Balanced Diet

The food, we all take and enjoy eating, **is essentially required** by all living organisms for the following purposes:

- **For energy:** Food is essentially required and used by the body as a fuel to work our muscles and other body organs.
- **For growth and repair:** Various nutrients and chemicals, present in the food, are used by the body to make new cells, which are required for growth, and to replace old or damaged cells.
- **To stay healthy:** Several chemicals, present in food, are also used in the cellular reactions, in our body to provide energy, to keep us healthy.

In order to maintain healthy body, we, therefore, must eat a healthy and balanced diet, which means variety and moderation in choice of food. It also means matching the amount of energy (calories) intake, via food, with the amount of energy output, in basal conditions, for daily activities and exercise, etc.

A balanced diet may be defined as the one, **which provides, quantitatively as well as qualitatively,** i.e. required amounts and proper proportions, of **all the nutrients** (proximal principles of food), **for maintaining a good health and physiological efficiency.**

The quantities of foods needed to meet the nutrient requirements, however, vary with age, gender, physiological status and physical activity.

ELEMENTS OF BALANCED DIET

As discussed in Chapter 3, a balanced diet should have, both, macro- and micronutrients (chemical constituents), which include:

- Carbohydrates
- Proteins
- Fat
- Vitamins
- Minerals
- Water

A balanced diet comprises the above nutrients, which are essential for daily life. All these nutrients can be obtained from different food groups.

FOOD GROUPS

A food group is a **collection foods** which **share similar nutritional properties** or biological specifications. Foods are grouped together because they provide similar amounts of the key nutrients of that food group. For example, the key nutrients of the milk, yogurt, cheese and alternatives food group include calcium and protein, while the fruit group is a good source of vitamins, especially, vitamin C.

All the required nutrients (as mentioned above), **which form a balanced diet can be obtained from four basic food groups,** which include:

1. Cereals, millets and pulses
2. Vegetables and fruits
3. Milk and milk products, egg, meat and fish, and
4. Oils and fats, and nuts and oilseeds

To meet the requirement of all the nutrients, which are essential for good health, **one need to eat a variety of foods, from each food group,** daily, **in the recommended amounts,** because different foods vary in amounts of the key nutrients that they provide. For example, in the vegetables and legumes food group, orange vegetables (such as carrots and pumpkins) contain significantly more vitamin A than other vegetables (such as white potatoes).

NUTRIENT PROFILE OF FOOD GROUPS

Nutrient profile of some food groups is shown in Table 15.1.

Whole Grain Cereals and Millets

Cereals, such as **rice and wheat,** and **millets,** like jowar, bajra, ragi, etc. are the most widely eaten staple foods in India.

- These are the cheapest **sources of calories** and constitute as much as 70–80% of the calories in the diet of majority of population, in our country.
- Most cereal grains also contain 6–12% **proteins.** In general, cereal proteins are deficient in the essential amino acid lysine. Rice protein, however, is rich in lysine, compared to other cereals.
- Whole grain cereals are also important sources of **B vitamins,** especially, **thiamine** and **nicotinic acid,** which are present in the outer bran layer of the grain. Excessive milling and polishing of rice remove the outer covering and, hence, decreases its thiamine content.
- Cereal grains do not contain vitamin A, except yellow maize, which contains some amount of **β-carotene.**
- Total fat content in cereals varies from 2–5%.
- On an average, 400 g of cereals are consumed per person, per day, in India.
- Commonly used legumes include **grams, peas and beans.**
- Dried **pulses and legumes** are rich in **protein** (about 19–24%). They are good sources of **lysine** and **threonine,** which are deficient in most of the cereals. Pulses are, however, poor source of sulfur-containing amino acids.
- Pulses are also good sources of several B vitamins and minerals, such as **thiamin, riboflavin** and **phosphorus.**

Table 15.1: Nutrient profile of some food groups

Food group	*Nutrient profile*
Cereals and millets	Carbohydrates, proteins, water-soluble vitamins and minerals
Pulses and legumes	Proteins, water soluble vitamins and minerals
Vegetables	Proteins, water soluble vitamins and minerals
Roots and tubers	Carbohydrates, small amount of proteins and vitamin C
Fruits	Carbohydrates and water-soluble vitamins
Fats and oils	Fat and fat-soluble vitamins
Milk and milk products	Proteins, fat, fat-soluble vitamins, water-soluble vitamins and minerals
Meat, fish and eggs	Proteins, fat, fat-soluble vitamins, water-soluble vitamins and minerals

- Legumes, however, contain some **natural toxins** that can be removed by soaking and normal cooking procedures. The cooking procedures, however, result in loss of some B vitamins.
- Legumes are **good for young children** provided these are cooked, finely mashed and mixed with other food items.
- Germination or **sprouting increases vitamin C,** riboflavin and niacin contents of legumes.

Nuts and Oilseeds

Nuts and oilseeds, such as peanut (groundnut), soybean and oilseeds, are rich sources of **protein.** They contain about 18–40% protein. They are also rich sources of **fat,** several **B vitamins and vitamin E.**

- **Groundnut** contains about 20–30% protein and 40–50% oil. Though limiting in lysine, threonine and methionine, groundnut is a good source of **thiamin, niacin, pantothenic acid** and **phosphorus.** When harvested under moist conditions, groundnut gets contaminated with *Aspergillus flavus*, which produces **aflatoxin.** Roasting destroys trypsin inhibitors and improves its nutritive value.
- **Soybeans** contain nearly 35–45% protein and 15–20% fat. Soybean proteins are good sources of all **essential amino acids** except methionine. It is also a good source of **thiamin** and **niacin.** Soybean, however, contains hemagglutinins and trypsin, and certain growth inhibitors, which can be inactivated by pressure-cooking. Soybean is mainly used in soy-flour, milk substitutes and infant foods.

Vegetables

Vegetables are broadly classified into 3 groups, as green leafy vegetables, roots and tubers, and other vegetables.

- **Green leafy vegetables:** Many types of green leaves, such as spinach (palak), amaranth, fenugreek leaves (methi), drumstick leaves, mint, coriander, mustard leaves, colocasia leaves, radish and turnip leaves, and bathua, are rich sources of iron, β-carotene, vitamin C, riboflavin, folic acid and calcium. They also provide dietary fiber and antioxidants, and proteins (about 2–7%). Green leafy vegetables, however, contain oxalic acid, which, in turn, interferes with the absorption of calcium.
- **Roots and tubers:** Roots and tubers, such as potatoes, sweet potatoes, carrots, etc. are good sources of starch. They also contain small amount of protein; some B vitamins and vitamin C. Yellow sweet potatoes and carrots are also rich sources of carotene.
- **Other vegetables:** These include green peas and beans, pumpkin, gourds, okra, brinjal, etc. Green peas and beans are good sources of protein and some B vitamins. They are also fair sources of vitamin C and certain minerals.

Fruits

Fruits are good sources of different carbohydrates, vitamins and minerals.

- Fresh fruits are, generally, good sources of vitamins. **Amla** (gooseberry), is, especially, rich in **vitamin C.**
- **Yellow fruits,** like mango and papaya, contain β-carotene.
- **Dried fruits,** like dates and raisins, are rich sources of **iron.**
- Banana is rich in carbohydrates. Some fruits contain glucose, while others contain fructose or pentose.
- Most of the fruits are also good sources of potassium.
- Fruits also contain pectin, which provide bulk to the diet and helps in bowel movement.
- Drying of fruits results in loss of carotene. Other procedures cause loss of thiamin. Canning of fruit juice results in loss of vitamin C.

Since, fruit and vegetables provide vitamins, minerals and fiber, they should be included in meals and snacks each day. Choose a variety of fruits and vegetables (including different colors, textures and flavors) to provide a wide range of vitamins and minerals.

Milk and Milk Products

Milk is either used as such or in the preparation of several products, such as curd, cheese, ice cream, butter, ghee and a variety of sweets. Milk is an ideal food for infants and children. It is also a good supplementary food for adults. Milk contains good quality proteins (3.2–4.3%). It is also rich in calcium and several other nutrients in proper proportions, and, thus, milk is considered to be a complete food. Milk is, however, deficient in vitamin C and iron. Composition of milk varies widely, from its source. For example, human milk contains more lactose, while buffalo milk contains more fat.

Milk, yoghurt and cheese are the most common dairy foods, and main dietary sources of calcium. Having enough calcium is important for healthy bones and teeth. Full-cream plain milk is recommended for children aged one to two years, while reduced-fat plain milk is suitable for adults.

Pasteurization results in loss of vitamin C, while prolonged boiling results in loss of thiamin, vitamin B_6 and vitamin B_{12}.

Eggs and Poultry

Eggs contain about 13% proteins and 13% fat. Egg proteins are good sources of all essential amino acids and have high nutritive value. Egg is also a rich source of vitamin A and some B vitamins. Egg, however, does not contain vitamin C and is a poor source of calcium. Egg consists of egg white and egg yolk.

- **Egg white** contains about 11% protein, mainly **albumin.** Besides, egg white is also a good source of **riboflavin** but devoid of fat and vitamin A. Raw egg white also contains a heat labile factor, called **avidin,** which binds with biotin and makes it unavailable.
- **Egg yolk** contains about 15% proteins and 30% fat. It is a rich source of riboflavin, vitamin A, iron and phosphorus. Egg yolk is also rich in cholesterol. It is used as a supplement to the diet of infants.
- **Poultry meat** is a good source of proteins, containing all essential amino acids.

Meat and Fish

This group includes red meat (such as beef and lamb), white meat (such as pork and chicken) and fish. They are rich in protein, iron and zinc.

- Protein content of **flesh foods** is around 20%. Meat is also a good source of several B vitamins, particularly, vitamin B_{12}, iron and phosphorus. Flesh foods, generally, are not good sources of vitamin A with the exception of liver, which is very rich in vitamin A.
- **Fish** contains polyunsaturated fatty acids, which protect against cardiovascular diseases. Fish is also rich in protein, but a fair source of B vitamins. Fatty fish also contains vitamins A and D. Small fishes, are good source of calcium, since these are eaten with bones. Large fishes are rich in phosphorus.

Canning of meat and poultry results in loss of various B vitamins, particularly thiamin.

Fat and Oils

Fats and oils are the main sources of energy as well as essential fatty acids and fat-soluble vitamins.

- **Fats of animal origin** contain cholesterol, but poor source of vitamin E and essential fatty acids.
- On the other hand, **fats of vegetable origin,** such as sunflower oil, soybean oil, cottonseed oil, etc. are good sources of essential fatty acids and vitamin E.

- Frying destroys vitamin A, vitamin E and essential fatty acids.
- Rancidity results in the formation of peroxides, which, in turn, affect intestinal flora and have irritating effects on the intestine.

Sugar

Sugar and other carbohydrate-rich foods serve as a source of energy. Honey and jaggery also contain some vitamins and minerals.

Condiments and Spices

Condiments and spices are used as seasoning or flavoring agents in food, to increase its acceptability. Since condiments and spices are used in small quantities, they do not add, substantially, to the nutritive value of the food, but improve taste and flavor of the cooked food. They also act on the mucous membranes of mouth, stomach and intestine, and stimulate secretion of digestive juices.

- Some of the condiments, like chilies and coriander, are good sources of carotene.
- Green chilies supply vitamin C.
- Turmeric and tamarind are fair sources of antioxidants and iron.
- Some of the spices, such as garlic, also have their effect on intestinal flora and prevent flatulence.
- Others, such as chilies and black pepper, etc. are very pungent. Their excessive use can cause irritation of the mucous membrane, resulting in peptic and duodenal ulcers.

Beverages

Various beverages have different effects.

- **Coffee and tea** contain caffeine, which stimulates gastric secretion and may aid in the digestion. Excess of caffeine produces insomnia, causes irritability and rapid heart action, and increases excitability of the nervous system. Tea, however, is also a rich source of oxalic acid. Hence excessive consumption of tea may lead to the development of renal calculi.
- **Fruit juices** contain sugar, vitamin C, small amounts of other vitamins and some of the minerals.
- Beverages, such as **sugarcane juice,** contain nearly 9% sugar, while sweetened carbonated beverages contain about 10–15% sugar.
- **Alcoholic beverages** contain varying amounts of alcohol (from 4 to 40%). Alcohol in moderate doses stimulates gastric secretion and serves as a source of energy. Excessive consumption of alcohol causes severe depression and incoordination of movements, and loss of consciousness, due to its depressant action on the nervous system.

DIETARY GUIDELINES FOR INDIANS

Widespread malnutrition is largely a result of dietary inadequacy and unhealthy lifestyle. Other contributing factors are poor purchasing power, faulty feeding habits, large family size, frequent infections, poor health care, inadequate sanitation and low agricultural production. Population living in the backward and drought-prone rural areas and urban slums, and those belonging to the socially backward groups, like scheduled castes and tribal communities, are highly susceptible to undernutrition. Similarly, landless labourers and destitute are also at a higher risk.

The most rational, sustainable and long-term solution to the problem of malnutrition is ensuring availability, accessibility and consumption of adequate amounts of foods.

Dietary guidelines help to achieve the objective of providing optimal nutrition to the population.

The following 15 **dietary guidelines for Indians** have been suggested by the **National Institute of Nutrition** (and endorsed by the **Ministry of Health, Govt. of India),** for the general public, for different population groups:

1. Eat a variety of foods, to ensure a balanced diet.
2. Ensure provision of extra food and health care to pregnant and lactating women.
3. Promote exclusive breastfeeding for 6 months and encourage breastfeeding until 2 years, or as long as possible.
4. Feed home-based semi-solid foods to the infant after 6 months.
5. Ensure adequate and appropriate diets for children and adolescents, both, in health and sickness.
6. Eat plenty of vegetables and fruits.
7. Ensure moderate use of edible oils and animal foods, and use a minimum of ghee/butter/vanaspati.
8. Avoid overeating to prevent overweight and obesity.
9. Exercise regularly and be physically active to maintain ideal body weight.
10. Restrict salt intake to a minimum.
11. Ensure the use of safe and clean foods.
12. Adopt the right pre-cooking processes and appropriate cooking methods.
13. Drink plenty of water and take beverages in moderation.
14. Minimize the use of processed foods rich in salt, sugar and fats.
15. Include micronutrient-rich foods in the diets of elderly people to enable them to be fit and active.

FOOD PYRAMID

Dietary guidelines suggest that the nutrients must be obtained through a judicious choice and combination of a variety of foodstuffs from different food groups, as per food pyramid (Fig. 15.1).

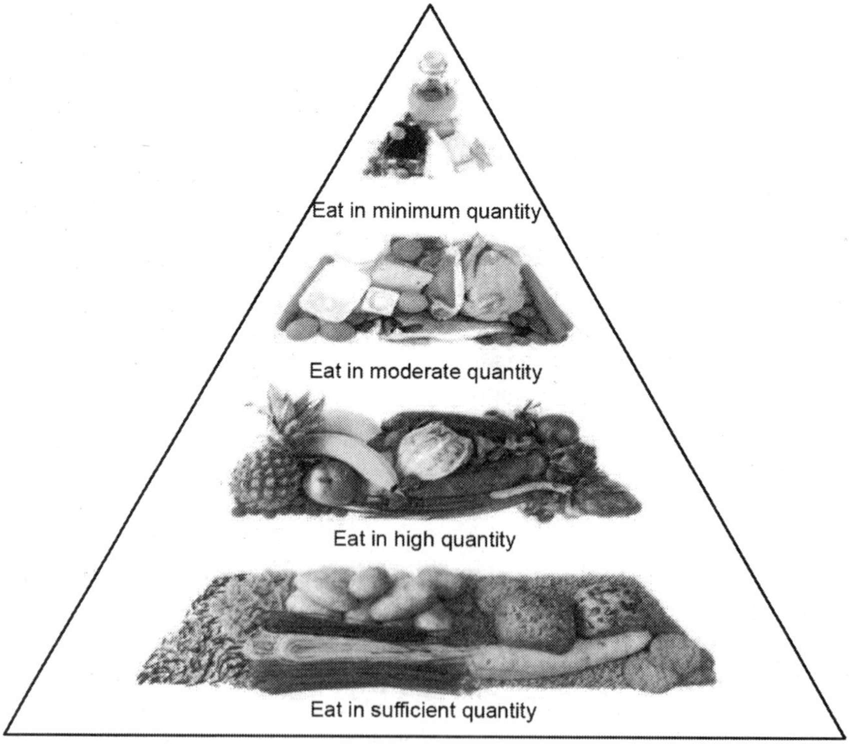

Fig. 15.1: Food pyramid

Food pyramid (Food guide pyramid) is a graphic representation of the number of servings from the four major food groups, needed daily, to form a healthful diet.

The pyramid is divided into four levels of foods, according to recommended consumption, that is:

- **At the base,** the foundation of a healthful diet is the group of **cereals and legumes/ beans,** which should be eaten in sufficient quantity.

  Foods in this group are the **sources of complex carbohydrates** and provide **important vitamins, minerals and fiber.** Dietary fiber delays and retards absorption of carbohydrates and fats, and increases the satiety value. Diets rich in fiber also reduce glucose and lipids in blood, and increase the bulk of the stools. Thus, diets rich in complex carbohydrates are healthier than low-fiber diets based on refined and processed foods.

- **On the second level** (going up the pyramid) are **vegetables and fruits,** which should be eaten liberally.

  Vegetables **provide vitamins** (such as vitamin A, vitamin C and folate) and the **minerals** (like iron and magnesium) and carbohydrates including fiber. Fruits also are good sources of vitamins A and C. Vitamins are essential for numerous body processes and for maintenance of the structure of skin, bone, nerves, eye, brain, blood and mucous membrane. Minerals are required for maintenance and integrity of skin, hair, nails, blood and soft tissues. They also govern nerve cell transmission, acid–base and fluid balance, enzyme and hormone activity as well as the blood-clotting processes.

- Next up, **on the third level,** are dairy foods along with meat and meat alternatives (e.g. nuts, eggs and legumes), i.e. **animal source foods and oils,** which should be eaten moderately.

  Dairy products provide protein, vitamins (especially, riboflavin, vitamin A and vitamin D) and minerals (particularly, calcium and phosphorus). Meat and meat substitutes are good sources of protein, some of the B vitamins, iron and zinc. Animal proteins are of high quality as they provide all the essential amino acids in right proportions, while plant or vegetable proteins are not of the same quality because of their low content of some of the essential amino acids. However, a combination of cereals, millets and pulses provides most of the amino acids, which complement each other to provide better quality proteins.

- **The upper part** of the pyramid (at the apex) contains fat and sweets, i.e. the **highly processed foods,** which should be eaten sparingly.

  Excess of these substances could lead to obesity, diabetes, cardiovascular disease and cancer.

Accompanying the pyramid there is a recommendation to **do regular physical activity,** and **warnings against smoking and drinking alcohol.**

The pyramid, thus, is an easy way to use guideline that helps us to select a variety of foods.

COMPONENTS OF A BALANCED DIET

According to ICMR-NIN (2020), a balanced diet should provide, nearly, 55–60% of the total required calories from **carbohydrates,** preferably from complex carbohydrates, about 10–15% from **proteins** and 20–30% from fat (both visible and invisible fat).

In addition, a balanced diet should also provide other non-nutrients, such as **dietary fiber, antioxidants** and **phytochemicals,** which have positive health benefits.

Dietary fiber includes complex carbohydrates, such as those obtained from whole grains, fruits, vegetables, beans and legumes. Dietary fiber is low or moderate in calories, and devoid of refined grains and sugar. Dietary fiber promotes healthy bowel movement and decreases the risk of chronic diseases, such as coronary heart disease and diabetes.

Antioxidants: Antioxidants are present in green leafy vegetables and plant foods, like papaya, turmeric, palm oil, amla and guava. Dietary antioxidants include nutrients, such as **β-carotene** (provitamin A), **ascorbic acid** (vitamin C), **tocopherols,** tocotrienols, riboflavin, sulfur-containing amino acids (cysteine and methionine) and selenium.

ICMR-NIN (2020) Expert Group has recommended that in addition, to the RDA of various macro- and micronutrients, one should consume at least **500 g of fruits** every day **to meet the daily demand of** antioxidants and certain non-nutrients like **polyphenols and flavonoids** which protect against chronic diseases.

Non-nutrient antioxidants are various carotenoids, flavinoids, anthracyanins and indoles. These agents remove free radicals, such as superoxide (O_2^-), hydrogen peroxide and lipid peroxides. These agents inhibit lipid peroxidation. They also lower cholesterol level and promote HDL levels, prevent cancer, cardiovascular diseases and cataract.

Phytochemicals also help in detoxification, i.e. detoxification of drugs, toxicants, carcinogens and mutagens.

BALANCED DIET FOR INDIANS

Our diet must provide adequate calories, proteins and micronutrients to achieve maximum growth potential. Therefore, it is important to have appropriate diet during different stages of one's life. For example:

- **Breast milk and energy-rich foods:** For growth and appropriate milestones.
- **Energy-rich body building and protective foods:** For growth, development and to fight infections.
- **Body building and protective foods:** For growth spurt, maturation and bone development.
- **Nutritionally adequate diet, with extra food for child bearing and rearing:** For maintaining health, productivity, to prevent diet-related disease, and to support pregnancy and lactation.
- **Nutrient-dense low-fat foods:** For being physically active and healthy.

SOME IMPORTANT QUESTIONS

1. **Define balanced diet. Describe various components of a balanced diet.**
2. **Write notes on:**
   i. Balanced diet
   ii. Food groups for a balanced diet
   iii. Nutrient group for a balanced diet
   iv. Food pyramid
   v. Balanced diet for Indians
   vi. Dietary guidelines for Indians

CHAPTER

16

Recommended Daily Allowances

A proper diet is essential from the very early stages of life, for proper growth, development and to remain active. **Dietary standards** define healthful diets in terms of specific amounts of the nutrients. These standards are the **sets of recommended intake values** for nutrients or the way to tell that how much of each nutrient we should have in our diet. These dietary standards help set nutrition policy as well as guide in the planning and evaluation of diets for groups as well as individuals, practically all healthy people.

Recommended Dietary Allowance **(RDA) refers to the daily dietary nutrient intake level** that is sufficient **to meet the nutrients requirement of nearly all (97–98%) the healthy individuals, in a particular life stage and gender group.** RDA is derived from the EAR, as the mean plus 2 SD of the distribution of requirements.

RDA is the safe and adequate level, which incorporates margin of safety, intended to be sufficiently generous to encompass the presumed variability in requirements among individuals and meet the needs of almost all the healthy people in a given population.

Most of the countries are using a set of recommended daily intake values, called the **Recommended Dietary Allowances** or **RDA** (sometimes, also referred to as **Recommended Daily Allowances**).

- RDAs (RDA) are the estimates of nutrients, to be consumed daily, to ensure the requirements of all individuals in a given population.
- The recommended level depends upon the bioavailability of nutrients (the proportion what is absorbed and utilized by the body) from a given diet.
- In addition, RDA includes a margin of safety, to cover variation between individuals, dietary traditions and practices.
- They are nutrient-centred and technical in nature.
- The RDAs are suggested for physiological groups, such as infants, pre-schoolers, children, adolescents, pregnant women, lactating mothers, and adult men and women, taking into account their physical activity.

SIGNIFICANCE OF RDA

RDA represents level of the nutrient, to be consumed daily, to meet all the requirements of most of the individuals in a given population. RDA is important:

- **In modifying nutrient requirements in clinical management** of diseases.
- **To help public health nutritionists to compose diets** for schools, hospitals, prisons, etc.

- **For health care policymakers and public health nutritionists** to design and develop nutrition intervention programs and policies.
- **For planning and procuring food supplies** for population groups.
- **For evaluating adequacy of food supplies** in meeting national nutritional needs.
- **For interpreting food consumption records** of individuals and population.
- **For establishing standards for the national feeding programs** implemented by the Government for its vulnerable population.
- **For designing nutrition education programs** for the masses.
- **For developing new food products and dietary supplements** by the industry.
- **For establishing guidelines for the National labelling of the packaged foods** by the Food Standards Safety Authority of India (FSSAI).

The **Food and Nutrition Board** of the **National Academy of Sciences, National Research Council, USA,** is the recognized authority for setting standards of nutrition in the United States. The Board had set up a table of recommended daily dietary allowances for Canada and US, which became the first RDA values. The recommendations were listed for infants, preschool and schoolchildren, older boys and girls, men and women of varying ages, and for pregnancy and lactation. The table is a guide for the entire healthy population. For each age category, specific allowances are listed for protein, vitamins and minerals. The table is revised, periodically, to include new research, as and when becomes available. Recent recommendations have been given for 2020–2025.

DIETARY GUIDELINES (2020–2025) FOR AMERICANS

1. **Follow a healthy dietary pattern at every life stage:** Every life stage means **infancy, toddlerhood, childhood, adolescence, adulthood, pregnancy, lactation and older adulthood.** It is suggested that it is never too early or too late to eat healthfully.
   - **For about the first 6 months of life exclusively feed the infants with human milk. Continue to feed** infants human milk through **at least the first year of life,** and longer if desired. Feed infants **iron-fortified infant formula during the first year** of life when human milk is unavailable. Provide infants with **supplemental vitamin D beginning soon after birth.**
   - **At about 6 months introduce** infants to **nutrient-dense complementary foods.** Introduce infants to potentially allergenic foods along with other complementary foods. **Encourage infants and toddlers to consume** a variety of **foods from all food groups.** Include foods **rich in iron and zinc,** particularly for infants fed human milk.
   - **From 12 months through older adulthood** follow a **healthy dietary pattern** across the lifespan to meet nutrient needs, **help achieve a healthy body weight,** and **reduce the risk of chronic disease.**
2. **Customize and enjoy food and beverage choices to reflect personal preferences, cultural traditions, and budgetary considerations:** A healthy dietary pattern can benefit all individuals **regardless of age, race, or ethnicity, or current health status.** The dietary guidelines provides a framework intended to be customized to individual needs and preferences, as well as the foodways of the diverse cultures in the United States.
3. **Focus on meeting food group needs with nutrient-dense foods and beverages, and stay within calorie limits:** An underlying premise of the

dietary guidelines is that **nutritional needs should be met primarily from** foods and beverages, specifically, **nutrient-dense foods and beverages.** Nutrient-dense foods **provide vitamins, minerals, and other health-promoting components** and have **no or little added sugars, saturated fat, and sodium.** A healthy dietary pattern consists of nutrient-dense forms of foods and beverages **across all food groups, in recommended amounts, and within calorie limits.**

The core elements that make up a healthy dietary pattern include:

- **Vegetables of all types,** i.e. dark green; red and orange; beans, peas and lentils; starchy and other vegetables.
- **Fruits,** especially whole fruit.
- **Grains,** at least half of which are whole grain.
- **Dairy,** including fat-free or low-fat milk, yogurt and cheese, and/or lactose-free versions and fortified soy beverages and yogurt as alternatives.
- **Protein foods,** including lean meats, poultry, and eggs; seafood; beans, peas and lentils; and nuts, seeds and soy products.
- **Oils,** including vegetable oils and oils in food such as seafood and nuts.

4. **Limit foods and beverages higher in added sugars, saturated fat, and sodium, and limit alcoholic beverages: At every life stage,** meeting food group recommendations, even **with nutrient dense choices,** requires most of a person's **daily calorie needs and sodium limits.** A healthy dietary pattern does **not have much room for extra added sugars, saturated fat or sodium, or for alcoholic beverages.** A small amount of the added sugars, saturated fat, or sodium can be added to nutrient-dense foods and beverages to help meet food group recommendations, but foods and beverages high in these components should be limited to:
   - **Added sugars: Less than 10 percent of calories per day starting at age 2.** Avoid foods and beverages with added sugars for those younger than age 2.
   - **Saturated fat: Less than 10 percent of calories per day** starting at age 2.
   - **Sodium: Less than 2,300 milligrams per day** and even less for children younger than age 14.
   - **Alcoholic beverages:** Adults of legal drinking age can **choose not to drink or to drink in moderation** by limiting intake to 2 drinks or less in a day for men and 1 drink or less in a day for women, when alcohol is consumed. Drinking less is better for health than drinking more. There are some **adults who should not drink alcohol such as women who are pregnant.**

DIETARY RECOMMENDATIONS FOR VARIOUS NUTRIENTS FOR AMERICANS

Based on the 2020–2025 guidelines, **dietary recommendations for various nutrients for Americans** are as follows:

- **Calories:** It is recommended that daily calories intake for moderately active children should be **1000 kcal at 2 years** of age, for **both the sexes.**
  - Thereafter, it is recommended that the moderately active **females should take 1400 kcal/d during 3–5 years of age, 1600 kcal/d during 6–8 years, 1800 kcal/d during 9–11 years and 2800 kcal/d during 16–25 years. Thereafter, it should be reduced to 2400 kcal/d after 46 years of age.**
  - Accordingly, moderately active **males should take 1400 kcal/d during 3–5 years of age, 1800 kcal/d during 9–13 years, 2200 kcal/d during 14–18 years** and **2400 kcal/d during 19–30 years.** Thereafter, calories intake should be reduced to **2200/d kcal**

during 31–50 years and to **2000 kcal/d after 51 years.**

- **Carbohydrates:** Carbohydrates should provide **45–65% of the total calories** for the age 2 years and above.
  - Accordingly, **carbohydrate intake** should be **95 g for the age group of 6–11 months/d** and **130 g/d for 1 year and above.**
  - **Dietary fiber:** Total dietary fiber intake should be **14 g/1000 kcal/d.**
  - **Added sugars should not be** included in the diet of **infants and children below 2 years of age.** For the **other age groups,** the **added sugars** should be **below 10% of the total calorie intake.**
- **Fat:** Fat should provide **30–40% of the total calories up to 2 years of age.** Thereafter, fat intake should be **reduced to provide 25–35% of the calories between 14–18 years** and **20–35% to 19 years and elder** of both the sexes.
  - **Saturated fatty acids should provide below 10% of the total calorie intake.**
  - **Omega-6 fatty acid (18:2 linoleic acid)** intake **should be 4.6 g/d between 6–11 months of age and 7.0 g/d between 1–3 years. For adults, 51 years and above,** its intake has been suggested to be **11 g/d for females and 14 g/d for males.**
  - **Omega-3 fatty acid (18:3 linolenic acid)** intake should be **0.5 g/d between 6–11 months of age and 0.7 g/d between 1–3 years. For adults, 51 years and above,** its intake has been suggested as 1.1 g/d for females and 1.6 g/d for males.
- **Protein:** Protein should provide **10–30% calories for the age group of 4 to 18 years of age** and **10 to 35% for the older groups.**
  - Accordingly, **protein intake should be 11 g/d for the age group of 6–11 months and 13 g/d for age group between 12–23 months.**
  - **Total protein intake should be 46 g/d for the females** and **56 g/d for males of 14 years and above.**
- **Minerals**
  - **Calcium:** Calcium intake should be **1300 mg/d from 9 years and above.**
  - **Phosphorus**—Phosphorus intake should be **275 mg/d between 7–11 months of age.**
  - **Iron:** Iron intake should be **8 mg/d between 9–13 years** and **15 mg/d between 14–18 years.** For **adults above 51 years** iron intake should be **8 mg/d for both females** and **males.**
  - **Magnesium:** Magnesium intake should be **75 mg/d between 7–11 months of age and 80 mg/d between 1–3 years.**
  - **Zinc:** Zinc intake should be **3 mg/d between 7 months and 3 years of age.**
  - **Sodium:** Sodium intake should be **370 mg/d between 7–11 months of age.** For **adults above 51 years** sodium intake should be **2300 mg/d for both females** and **males.**
  - **Potassium:** Potassium intake should be **860 mg/d between 7–11 months of age.** During lactation, potassium intake should be **2800 mg/d.**
- **Vitamins**
  - **Vitamin A:** Vitamin A intake should be **500 µg/d** (retinol activity equivalents, **RAE**) **between 7–11 months** and **300 µg/d between 1–2 years of age.** During lactation vitamin A intake should be **1300 µg/d.**
  - **Vitamin D:** Vitamin D intake should be **400 mg/d (between 7–11 months of age** and **600/d IU** for **adults above 51 years,** for both **females** and **males).**
  - **Vitamin E:** Vitamin E intake should be **5 mg/d (α-tocopherol) between 7–11 months of age.** During pregnancy its intake should be 15 mg/d.
  - **Vitamin K:** Vitamin K intake should be **25 µg/d between 7–11 months of age and 30 µg/d between 1–3 years.** Its intake should be **75 µg/d** during 14–18 years.
  - **Thiamine:** Thiamine intake should be **0.3 mg/d between 7–11 months of age** and **0.5 mg/d between 1–3 years.**

Table 16.1: Dietary nutrition goals for Americans per day*

Population/ group (age)	*Calories (kcal)*	*Carbo-hydrates (g)*	*Dieraty fiber (g)*	*Fat (g)*	*Protein (g)*	*Thiamine (mg)*	*Riboflavin (mg)*	*Niacin (mg)*	*Vitamin B_6 (mg)*	*Choline (mg)*	*Folate DFE (μg)*	*Vitamin B_{12} (μg)*	*Vitamin C (mg)*	*Vitamin A RAE (μg)*	*Vitamin K (μg)*	*Calcium (mg)*	*Mag-nesium (mg)*	*Sodium (mg)*	*Iron (mg)*
6–11 months	800	95				0.3			0.3	150	80	0.5	50	500	25		75	370	
12–23 months	1000	130		30–40	13	0.5	0.5		0.5		150		15	300	30		80		
2–3 years	1000	130		30–40	13						150				30				
Females																			
4–8 years	1400	130		25–35				8		250					55				
9–13 years		130		25–35	34					375		1.8				1300			8
14–18 years		130	25	25–35											75	1300			15
19–30 years		130	28	20–35					1.3	425	300								18
51+	2400	130		20–35	46				1.5	425									8
Pregnant (19–30 years)		175	36					18		450			85				350	2300	
Lactating (19– 30 years)			34		45-65					550	500	2.8		1300			310	2300	8
Males																			8
4–8 years		130		25–35				8		250					55				
9–13 years		130	25	25–35	34					375	300	1.8				1300			8
14–18 years		130	31	25–35	52		1.3		1.3	550					75	1300			8
19–30 years		130	34	20–35	56		1.3		1.3	550									
51+		130	28	20–35	56					550									

*Dietary Guidelines for Americans (2020–2025)

- **Riboflavin:** Riboflavin intake should be **0.5 mg/d between 7–11 months of age.** Between **14–30 years** of age, its intake has been suggested as **1.3 mg/d.**
- **Niacin:** Niacin intake should be **8 mg/d between 4–8 years of age.** During pregnancy, its intake should be **18 mg/d.**
- **Vitamin B_6:** Vitamin B_6 intake should be **0.3 mg/d between 7–11 months of age.** During **14–18 years** of age its intake has been suggested as **1.3 mg/d** and **1.5 mg/d for** age **above 19 years.**
- **Choline:** Choline intake should be **150 mg/d between 7–11 months of age** and **200 mg/d between 1–3 years.** For **adults above 51 years** its intake should be **425 mg/d for females** and **550 mg/d for males.**
- **Folate:** Folate intake should be **80 µg/d (dietary folate equivalent) between 7–11 months of age and 150 µg/d between 1–3 years.** During pregnancy its intake should be 300 µg/d.
- **Vitamin B_{12}:** Vitamin B_{12} intake should be 0.5 µg/d between 7–11 months of age and 1.8 µg/d between 9–13 years. During pregnancy its intake should be 2.8 µg/d.

As per Dietary Guidelines (2020–2025), dietary nutrition goals set for Americans are shown in Table 16.1

RECOMMENDED DIETARY ALLOWANCES FOR INDIANS

In India, first attempt to define nutrient requirements and desirable dietary intakes of nutrients for Indians to maintain good health **was made by** the Nutrition Advisory Committee of the Indian Research Fund Association, now **Indian Council of Medical Research** (ICMR) **in 1944.**

- Thereafter, **in the wake of reports by** the Food and Agriculture Organization **(FAO) on energy and protein, requirements for these were revised** by the Committee **in 1958.**
- Subsequently, the Committee **revised requirements for all the nutrients except energy in 1968 and 1978.**
- Further, based on the international data provided by FAO/WHO/UNU 2004 expert committee, the ICMR **Committee further revised and upgraded** the Required Dietary Allowances **(RDA)** recommendations for Indians **in 2010.**

At this stage, the Committee, however, derived only the RDA and not the Estimated Average Requirement (EAR).

- **Recently,** the Indian Council of Medical Research—National Institute of Nutrition (ICMR-NIN) Expert Group has further **revised and defined nutrient distribution and requirements** for normal individuals of all age and physiological groups along with the different physical activity groups of Indian population **in 2020.**

The Group has given recommendations for all the nutrients including **energy, carbohydrates, dietary fiber, fats and oils, proteins, fat-soluble vitamins** (vitamins A, D, E and K), **water-soluble vitamins** (vitamin B complex, i.e. thiamine, riboflavin, niacin, pantothenic acid, pyridoxine, biotin, folate and cyanocobalamin, and vitamin C), **minerals** (calcium and phosphorus, iron, magnesium, sodium and potassium, zinc, copper, chromium, manganese, selenium and iodine), **water and antioxidants.**

GENERAL CONSIDERATIONS TO ESTIMATE NUTRIENT REQUIREMENTS FOR INDIANS

ICMR-NIN (2020) Expert Group considered following points for giving its recommendations for various nutrients for Indians:

- **Recent data on energy expenditure and protein metabolism**
- **Available data on minerals and vitamins losses, and absorption.**

- In order to derive a single value for the requirement of various nutrients, the Group **used two features of the distribution of requirements,** i.e. either the median of the distribution of requirements (referred to as **Estimated Average Requirement,** EAR) or the 97.5th percentile of the distribution (called **Recommended Daily Allowance,** RDA).
- **Requirements** of various nutrients **have been suggested for different age** and **physiological categories, based on sex, body weight** and **physical activity level.**
- Taking several factors into consideration, **energy requirements** have been **calculated with respect to the BMR values for normal healthy individuals** and have been **expressed in terms of kcal** (kilocalories) per day.
- **Carbohydrates intake** has been suggested **based on the minimum level of glucose required for utilization by the brain** and have been expressed **in grams per day.**
- For the first time, the Group has recommended the **requirement of dietary fiber. Based on energy intake,** the **safe intake of dietary fiber** has been suggested **in grams per day**.
- We know that **fat provides essential fatty acids** and **is necessary for** the **absorption of fat-soluble vitamins.**

The Group has suggested the **upper limit for visible fat intake in grams per day.** Further, it is also recommended that **a minimum of 20% of the dietary energy should be derived from fat,** out of which 10% of the dietary energy should be **from visible fat.** The Group further suggested that as a source of visible fat, a **correct combination of oils should be used.**

- The Group has calculated the **protein requirement** according to the value of net-protein utilization (NPU) of dietary proteins **by taking the NPU values of the mixed vegetable proteins** contained in Indian diets and the safe intake has been expressed in grams per day. This is due to the reason that although, both, animal foods (milk, meat, fish and eggs) and plant foods (pulses and legumes) are rich sources of proteins, but the **animal proteins are of high quality** (as they provide all the essential amino acids and in right proportions) **compared to the proteins from the plant** or **vegetable sources** (which are not of the same quality because of low contents of some of the essential amino acids). But **a combination of proteins from cereals, millets and pulses provides all the essential amino acids,** i.e. they **complement each other so as to provide better quality protein.**

So, **to define protein requirement the Group has introduced** a newer protein quality index referred to as **Digestible Indispensable Amino Acid Score** (DIAAS).

Further, RDA for protein has been suggested based on body weight and varies for different age categories.

- **RDA for vitamins B_1, B_2, niacin, pantothenic acid, vitamin B_6 and vitamin C** have been **expressed in mg** (milligrams) per day; for **biotin, folate, vitamin B_{12} and vitamin A in µg** (microgram) per day; while for vitamin D in IU (international units) per day.

Further, **RDA for niacin has been calculated in terms of niacin equivalent (NE)** by taking into account the **contribution of tryptophan** and assuming that 60 mg of tryptophan forms 1 mg of niacin in the body.

RDA **for folate** has been given **in terms** of the **dietary folate equivalent** (DFE).

The Group has also suggested that **vitamin B_{12} is derived, entirely, from the foods of the animal origin.**

The requirement for **vitamin A has been expressed in terms of retinol equivalents (RE),** considering a **conversion factor of 12:1 for α-carotene and 6:1 for β-carotene.**

Based on the consumption of extra calories, additional requirements for vitamins B_1, B_2 and B_6 have been suggested during pregnancy and lactation.

- **RDA for calcium, phosphorus, magnesium, sodium, potassium, iron, zinc, copper** and **manganese** are expressed **in mg/day** while for **chromium, selenium and iodine in µg** (micrograms) per day.

  Due to the increasing incidence of hypertension, intake of sodium has been recommended as safe intake.

  RDA for iron has been suggested **based on the consideration that nearly 8% of iron is absorbed from food** in healthy adults, and **menstrual losses in women** during the reproductive age.
- **RDA during pregnancy and lactation has been suggested as additional intakes.** This requirement is **over and above** the **normal requirement of the non-pregnant adult women.**
- **For infants and children,** RDA values for energy, protein, iron, thiamine, riboflavin and niacin have been **expressed in terms of per kg body weight per day.**
- **Total water requirement** has been suggested **based on energy requirement** (estimated average ratio, 2020) **and the WHO guidelines of 1.5 ml per kcal ingested.**

ICMR–NIN 2020 DIETARY RECOMMENDATIONS

As per recommendations of the ICMR-NIN (2020), RDA for Indians for various nutrients, for different age and sex groups are shown in Tables 16.2 to 16.4.

Table 16.2: RDA of macronutrients for Indians (ICMR-NIN, 2020)

Population/ group	*Category of worker/ period*	*Carbohydrates (g)*	*Dietary fiber* (g)*	*Visible fat (g)*	*Protein (g)*
Adult men (19+)	Sedentary	100	30	25	
	Moderate	100	40	30	54
	Heavy	100	50	40	
Adult women (19+)	Sedentary	100	25	20	
	Moderate	100	30	25	46
	Heavy	100	40	30	
Pregnant women	2nd trimester	135		30	(+) 9.5
	3rd trimester	135		30	(+) 22
Lactating women	0–6 months	155		30	(+) 16.9
	7–12 months	155		30	(+) 13.2
Infants	0–6 months**	55*		25	8
	7–12 months	95*			10.5
Children	1–3 years	100	15	25	12.5
	4–6 years	100	20	25	16
	7–9 years	100	26	30	23
Adolescents	Boys 10–12 years	100	33	35	32
	Boys 13–15 years	100	43	45	45
	Boys 16–18 years	100	50	50	55
	Girls 10–12 years	100	30	35	33
	Girls 13–15 years	100	36	40	43
	Girls 16–18 years	100	38	35	46

* EAR (estimated average requirement)
** AI (adequate intake)

Table 16.3: RDA of vitamins for Indians (ICMR-NIN, 2020)

Population/ group	*Category of worker/period*	*Thiamine (mg)*	*Riboflavin (mg)*	*Niacin (mg)*	*Pantothenic acid* (mg)*	*Pyridoxine (mg)*	*Biotin* (μg)*	*Folate* (μg)*	B_{12} *(μg)*	*Vitamin C (mg)*	*Vitamin A (μg)*	*Vitamin D (IU)*
Adult men (18+)	Sedentary	1.4	2	14	5	1.9	25	300	2.2	80	1000	600
	Moderate	1.8	2.5	18	5	2.4	25	300	2.2	80	1000	600
	Heavy	2.3	3.2	23	5	3.1	25	300	2.2	80	1000	600
Adult women (18+)	Sedentary	1.4	1.9	11	5	1.9	25	220	2.2	65	840	600
	Moderate	1.7	2.4	14	5	1.9	25	220	2.2	65	840	600
	Heavy	2.2	3.1	18	5	2.4	25	220	2.2	65	840	600
Pregnant women	2nd trimester	2	2.7	(+) 2	5	2.3	25	570	(+) 0.25	(+)15	900	600
	3rd trimester	2	2.7	(+) 2	5	2.3	25	570	(+) 0.25	(+) 15	900	600
Lactating women	0–6 months	2.1	3	(+) 5	(+) 2	(+) 0.26	(+) 5	330	(+) 1	(+) 50	950	600
	7–12 months	2.1	2.9	(+) 5	(+) 2	(+) 0.17	(+) 5	330	(+) 1	(+) 50	950	600
Infants	0–6 months*	0.2*	0.4*	2*	2	0.1*	4	25*	1.2	20*	350*	400*
	7–12 months	0.4*	0.6*	5*	2	0.6*	5	85	1.2	30*	350	400*
Children	1–3 years	0.7	1.1	7	2	0.9	7	120	1.2	30	390	600
	4–6 years	0.9	1.3	9	3	1.2	9	135	2.2	35	510	600
	7–9 years	1.1	1.6	11	4	1.5	12	170	2.2	45	630	600
Adolescents	Boys 10–12 years	1.5	2.1	15	5	2	15	220	2.2	55	770	600
	Girls 10–12 years	1.4	1.9	14	5	1.9	16	225	2.2	50	790	600
	Boys 13–15 years	1.9	2.7	19	5	2.6	20	285	2.2	70	930	600
	Girls 13–15 years	1.6	2.2	16	5	2.2	20	245	2.2	65	890	600
	Boys 16–18 years	2.2	3.1	22	5	3	25	340	2.2	85	1000	600
	Girls 16–18 years	1.7	2.3	17	5	2.3	25	270	2.2	70	860	600

*Adequate intake

Table 16.4: RDA of minerals for Indians (ICMR-NIN, 2020)

Population/ group	*Category of worker/period*	*Calcium (mg)*	*Phosphorus (mg)*	*Magnesium (mg)*	*Sodium* (mg)*	*Potassium* (mg)*	*Iron (mg)*	*Zinc (mg)*	*Copper (mg)*	*Chromium (µg)*	*Manganese (mg)*	*Selenium (µg)*	*Iodine (µg)*
Adult men (18+)	Sedentary	1000	1000	440	2000	3500	19	17	1.7	50	4	40	140
	Moderate	1000	1000	440	2000	3500	19	17	1.7	50	4	40	140
	Heavy	1000	1000	440	2000	3500	19	17	1.7	50	4	40	140
Addult women (18+)	Sedentary	1000	1000	370	2000	3500	29	13	1.5	50	4	40	140
	Moderate	1000	1000	370	2000	3500	29	13	1.5	50	4	40	140
	Heavy	1000	1000	370	2000	3500	29	13	1.5	50	4	40	140
Pregnant women	2nd trimester	1000	1000	440	2000	3500	27	14.5					220
	3rd trimester	1000	1000	440	2000	3500	27	14.5					
Lactating women	0–6 months	1200	1200	400	2000	3500	23	14.1					280
	7–12 months	1200	1200	400	2000	3500	23	14.1					
Infants	0–6 months	300**	450**	30**	500	900							100**
	7–12 months	300**	450**	75**	650	1100	3	2.5					130**
Children	1–3 years	500	500	90	1000	1750	8	3.3	0.6	22	1.8	16–18	90
	4–6 years	550	550	125	1300	2250	11	4.5	0.9	28	2.9	29–32	90
	7–9 years	650	650	175	1600	2825	15	5.9	1	31	3.6	36–42	90
Adolescents	Boys 10–12 years	850	850	240	2000	3500	16	8.5	1.28	36	4.7	51	100
	Girls 10–12 years	850	850	250	2000	3500	28	8.5	1.15	34	4.1	45	100
	Boys 13–15 years	1000	1000	345	2000	3500	22	14.3	1.43	41	5.1	58	140
	Girls 13–15 years	1000	1000	340	2000	3500	30	12.8	1.3	37	4.6	52	140
	Boys 16–18 years	1050	1050	440	2000	3500	26	17.6	1.8	44	6.1	71	140
	Girls 16–18 years	1050	1050	380	2000	3500	32	14.2	1.54	38	4.7	55	140

*Safe intake
**Adequate intake

RDA FOR NORMAL HEALTHY ADULT MODERATE WORKERS

Based on the recommendations of the ICMR-NIN (2020), RDA for various nutrients, for adult moderate workers are described below:

- **Energy: RDA for calories for adult moderate workers** has been suggested as **2710 kcal/day for males and 2130 kcal/d for females.**

  It is further suggested that since 70–80% of the total dietary calories in India are derived from carbohydrates that are present in plant foods such as cereals, millets and pulses, the recommendation for **cereals and millets is 400 g** and for **pulses 80 g/day.**
- **Carbohydrates:** It is recommended that a **minimum of 100–130 g of carbohydrates should be consumed per day.**
- **Dietary fiber: Safe intake of dietary fiber** has been suggested as **15 g per 1000 kcal/d.**
- **Fats:** The **upper limit for visible fat intake for healthy adult moderate workers has been suggested as 30 g for males** and **25 g/d for females.**
- **Protein: Safe intake of protein** has been suggested as **0.83 g/kg/d.**
- **Vitamins:**
  - **Thiamin: RDA for thiamine for** adult moderate workers has been suggested as **1.8 mg/d for males and 1.7 mg/d for females.**
  - **Riboflavin: RDA for riboflavin** for adult moderate workers has been suggested as **2.5 mg/d for males and 2.4 mg/d for females.**
  - **Niacin: RDA for niacin (NE)** for adult moderate workers has been suggested as **18 mg/d for males and 14 mg/d for females.**
  - **Pyridoxine: RDA for pyridoxine** for adult moderate workers has been suggested as **2.5 mg/d for males** and **1.9 mg/d for females.**
  - **Folate: RDA for folate** for adult moderate worker has been suggested as **300 µg/d for males** and **220 µg/d for females.**
  - **Vitamin B_{12}:** RDA for vitamin B_{12} for adult moderate male and female workers has been suggested as **2.2 µg/d.**
  - **Vitamin C: RDA for vitamin C** for adult moderate workers has been suggested as **80 mg/d for males and 65 mg/d for females.**
  - **Vitamin A: RDA for vitamin A** (RE) for adult moderate workers has been suggested as **1000 µg/d for males and 840 µg/d for females.**
- **Minerals:**
  - **Calcium and phosphorus:** RDA for calcium for adult moderate workers has been suggested as **1000 mg/day** for males and females.

    Additional 200 mg per day has been suggested **for women during post-menopause.**

    Similar values have been recommended for phosphorus.
  - **Magnesium: Estimated average requirement** for magnesium for adult moderate workers has been recommended as **440 mg/d for males and 370 mg/d for females.**
  - **Sodium and potassium: Safe intake of sodium** has been suggested as **2000 mg/day.** Accordingly, the **salt intake** has been recommended as **5 g/day.**

    Potassium intake has been suggested as **3500 mg/day.**
  - **Iron: RDA for iron** for adult moderate workers has been suggested as **19 mg/d for males and 29 mg/d for females.**
- **Water: Total water requirement** for adult moderate workers has been suggested as **4050 ml/d for males** and **3200 ml/d for females.**

RDA FOR PREGNANT AND LACTATING WOMEN

Pregnancy is the time of **tremendous physiological changes** that **demands healthful dietary** and **lifestyle choices.** This is also a **process of growth and development that affects both, the mother as well as the fetus.**

Guided by the changing levels of hormones, **body of the mother undergoes various changes** during pregnancy. Various maternal tissues, including the **breast, uterus and adipose stores increase in size,** and **blood volume is expanded.** At the same time, **gastrointestinal motility is slow,** as a result of which food moves more slowly through the intestinal tract. Further, **due to vomiting and loss of appetite during the early months of pregnancy, food intake is** also, generally, **reduced.**

Thus, **additional food is required for gestational weight gain of** nearly 10–14 kg **and** the **full-term birth weight** of the **fetus of about 3.3 kg.** Besides some micronutrients **(vitamins and minerals) are also required in extra amounts** during these physiological stages.

Accordingly, the **daily diet of a pregnant woman should contain additional amounts of:**

- **Energy:** Due to change in body weight during pregnancy, the Group has suggested a proportionate increase in energy requirement.

  In case of lactation, an increase in energy requirement has been suggested because of utilization of energy in milk production. Accordingly:
  - **Additional 350 kcal/d** have been suggested **during pregnancy**.
  - **Additional** energy requirement of a women who exclusively breast feed, has been recommended as **600 kcal/d during the first 6 months of lactation** and **520 kcal/d during 7–12 months of lactation.**
- **Carbohydrates:** Carbohydrate intake has been suggested as **135 g/d during pregnancy** and **155 g/d during lactation**.
- **Fat: Total visible fat intake** has been suggested as **30 g/d during pregnancy** as well as **lactation.**
- **Protein: Additional requirement** of protein has been recommended as **9.5 g/d during the second trimester** and **22 g/d during the third trimester of pregnancy.**

  Additional protein requirement for lactating women has been recommended as 16.9 g/d during the first 6 months and 13.2 g/d during 7–12 months of lactation.
- **Vitamins:**
  - **Thiamine:** RDA for thiamine has been suggested as **2.0 mg/d during pregnancy, and 2.1 mg/d during lactation.**
  - **Riboflavin:** RDA for riboflavin has been suggested as **2.7 mg/d during pregnancy.**

    RDA during lactation has been suggested as 3.0 mg/d during the first 6 months and **2.9 mg/d during 7–12 months.**
  - **Niacin: Additional 2 mg/d** of niacin has been suggested **during pregnancy.**

    Additional 5 mg/d of niacin has been suggested during lactation.
  - **Pantothenic acid:** RDA for pantothenic acid is suggested as **5.0 mg/d during pregnancy.**

    Additional 2.0 mg/d has been recommended **during lactation.**
  - **Vitamin B_6:** RDA for vitamin B_6 has been suggested as **2.3 mg/d during pregnancy.**

    Additional recommendations of **0.26 mg/d during 0–6 months of lactation** and **0.17 mg/d during 7–12 months of lactation** have been made.
  - **Biotin: RDA** for biotin has been suggested as **25 μg/d during pregnancy.**

    Additional 5.0 μg/d has been suggested **during lactation.**
  - **Folate: Additional** intake of dietary folate has been suggested as **270 μg/d during pregnancy.** Further, it is recommended that to reduce the risk of congenital malformations and increase in birth weight of the fetus,

folate should be taken throughout the pregnancy.

Additional intake of dietary folate has been suggested as **110 μg/d during lactation.**

- **Vitamin B_{12}: Additional** intake of vitamin B_{12} has been suggested **0.25 μg/d during pregnancy** and **1.0 μg/d during lactation.**
- **Vitamin C: Additional** intake of vitamin C has been suggested as **15 mg/d during pregnancy** and **50 mg during lactation.**
- **Vitamin A: RDA** of vitamin A has been suggested as **900 μg/d during pregnancy** and **950 μg/d during lactation.**

  It is further suggested that during pregnancy and lactation a **minimum 50% of the vitamin A** (retinol equivalent, RE) requirement should be met from animal sources.
- **Vitamin D: RDA** of vitamin D has been suggested as **600 IU/d during pregnancy and lactation.**

• **Minerals:**

- **Calcium:** It is well known that calcium is essential, both during pregnancy as well as lactation for proper formation of bones and teeth of the offspring, besides its secretion in breast milk as well as to prevent osteoporosis in mothers.

  RDA for calcium has been suggested as **1000 mg/d during pregnancy.**

  An **additional 200 mg/d** has been suggested **during lactation.**
- **Phosphorus:** Recommendations for phosphorus is **similar to that for calcium.**
- **Magnesium: RDA for magnesium has been suggested as 440 mg/d during pregnancy and 400 mg/d during lactation.**
- **Iron:** Extra iron is required by the mother as well as the growing fetus to meet the increased demand for erythropoiesis (formation of RBC).

  Accordingly, RDA for iron has been suggested as **27 mg/d during pregnancy** and **23 mg/d during lactation.**
- **Zinc: RDA** for zinc has been suggested as **14–15 mg/d during pregnancy as well as lactation.**
- **Iodine: RDA** for iodine has been suggested as **220 μg/d during pregnancy** and **280 μg/d during lactation.**
- **Water:** Total water requirement has been suggested as 3700 ml/d during pregnancy and 4100 ml/d during lactation.

The Group has further suggested that, **to meet the above requirements, pregnant and lactating women should eat a wide variety of foods** to make sure that her own nutritional needs as well as those of the growing fetus are met. Though, there is no particular need to modify the usual dietary pattern, the quantity and frequency of usage of different foods should be increased. Furthermore, it is suggested that:

- Maximum amount of **energy can be derived from rice, wheat and millets.**
- A **proper combination of cereals, pulses and nuts can be used to provide adequate protein.**
- **Mineral and vitamin requirements can be met by consuming** a variety of seasonal vegetables, particularly, **green leafy vegetables, milk and fresh fruits.**
- In addition, they are also advised to take daily **supplement of iron, folic acid, vitamin B and calcium.**
- These women should also choose **foods rich in dietary fiber,** like whole grain cereals, pulses and vegetables, to avoid constipation.
- Besides, they should take **plenty of fluids,** including 8–12 glasses of water per day.
- **Salt intake should also be restricted** to prevent pregnancy-induced hypertension and pre-eclampsia.

RDA FOR INFANTS

RDA for 0–6 months of age:

- **Energy:** For infants with the average body weight of 5.8 kg, **adequate intake** of energy has been suggested as **530 kcal/d.**
- **Fat:** Minimum level of total fat has been suggested as **40–60% of the total energy intake.**
- **Protein: RDA** for protein has been suggested as **8.0 g/d.**
- **Vitamins:**
  - **Thiamine:** RDA for thiamine has been suggested as **0.2 mg/d.**
  - **Riboflavin: RDA** for riboflavin has been suggested as **0.4 mg/d.**
  - **Niacin: RDA** for niacin has been suggested as **2.0 mg/d.**
  - **Vitamin B_6:** RDA for vitamin B_6 has been suggested as **0.1 mg/d.**
  - **Folate: RDA** for folate has been suggested as **25 µg/d.**
  - **Vitamin B_{12}:** RDA for vitamin B_{12} has been suggested as **1.2 µg/d.**
  - **Vitamin C: RDA** for vitamin C has been suggested as **20 mg/d.**
  - **Vitamin A: RDA** for vitamin A has been suggested as **350 µg/d.**
  - **Vitamin D:** RDA for vitamin D has been suggested as **400 IU/d.**
- **Minerals:**
  - **Calcium: RDA** for calcium has been suggested as **300 mg/d.**
  - **Magnesium: RDA** for magnesium has been suggested as **30 mg/d.**
  - **Iodine: RDA** for iodine has been suggested as **100 µg/d.**
- **Water:** Total water requirement has been suggested as 600 ml/d, which is available from breast milk.

  Further, it has also been suggested that, since **breast milk contains all these nutrients** which are essentially required for infants, and that the **requirements of these nutrients, for infants between 0–6 months of age, can be met from breast milk,** thus, breast-feeding should, essentially, be promoted at least for six months.
  - Breast milk also **provides several special components** such as **growth factors, enzymes, hormones** and **anti-infective factors.**
  - It also has a **high content of DHA** (docosahexaenoic acid) which plays an important role in brain development.
  - Breast milk also provides **IgA** (immunoglobulin A), **lactoferrin, lacto-peroxidase and complements** which provide immunity and protects the infant from several types of infections.
  - Besides breast milk, **colostrum** (the milk secreted during the first 3–4 days after child birth) **is also rich in proteins, minerals, vitamins** (especially vitamin A) and **antibodies.**

RDA for 6–12 Months of Age

- **Energy:** For infants above 6 months of age, with the average body weight of 8.5 kg, **adequate intake** of energy has been suggested as **680 kcal/d.**
- **Fat:** Minimum level of total fat has been suggested as **35% of energy.**

  It is further suggested that **visible fat intake should be 25 g/d.**
- **Protein: RDA** for protein has been suggested as **10.5 g/d.**
- **Vitamins:**
  - **Thiamine: RDA** for thiamine has been suggested as **0.4 mg/d.**
  - **Riboflavin: RDA** for riboflavin has been suggested as **0.6 mg/d.**
  - **Niacin: RDA** for niacin has been suggested as **5.0 mg/d.**
  - **Vitamin B_6: RDA** for vitamin B_6 has been suggested as **0.6 mg/d.**
  - **Folate: RDA** for folate has been suggested as **85 µg/d.**
  - **Vitamin B_{12}: RDA** for vitamin B_{12} has been suggested as **1.2 µg/d.**
  - **Vitamin C: RDA** for vitamin C has been suggested as **30 mg/d.**

- **Vitamin A: RDA** for vitamin A has been suggested as **350 μg/d.**
- **Vitamin D: RDA** for vitamin D has been suggested as **400 IU/d.**

- **Minerals:**
  - **Calcium: RDA** for calcium has been suggested as **300 mg/d.**
  - **Magnesium: RDA** for magnesium has been suggested as **75 mg/d.**
  - **Iron: RDA** for iron has been suggested as **3 mg/d.**
  - **Zinc: RDA** for magnesium has been suggested as **2.5 mg/d.**
  - **Iodine: RDA** for iodine has been suggested as **130 μg/d.**
- **Water:** Total water requirement has been suggested as 1000 ml/d. It can be met from breast milk, water and other fluids.

Further it has been suggested that these requirements should, partially, be met from breast milk. Accordingly, along with the breast milk, these infants, after six months of age, should be given home-based semi-solid foods. For this purpose:

- In addition to breast milk, **they should be provided the supplementary or complementary foods such as** liquids (like **milk**), semisolids (like **khichdi and kheer**) and solid preparations like rice, etc.
- **These can be low-cost food supplements which can be prepared, at home, from commonly used ingredients,** such as cereals (wheat, rice, ragi. jowar, bajra, etc.), pulses (grams and dals), nuts and oilseeds (groundnut, sesame, etc.), vegetable oils (groundnut oil, sesame oil, etc.), and sugar and jaggery. These foods, in turn, will provide **good quality protein, adequate calories and several protective nutrients.**
- In addition, these infants should also be **given fruits and green leafy vegetables** which are rich sources of vitamins and minerals. However, these should be well-cleaned before cooking.

RDA FOR CHILDREN AND ADOLESCENTS

Childhood and adolescence are the **periods of continuous growth and development.**

- **During the second-year,** a **child increases in height by 7–8 cm** and **gains body weight,** approximately, **to 4 times of its birth weight.**
- **During the pre-adolescent period,** a **child grows, on an average. by 6–7 cm in height** and **1.5–3.0 kg in body weight, every year** and simultaneously, development and maturation of the various tissues and organs takes place.
- **Adolescent period** (teenage) **is spread almost over a decade** and is **characterized by rapid increase in height** and weight along with the hormonal changes, sexual maturation and wide swing in emotions.
  - Adolescent **growth spurt starts at about 10–12 years in girls** and **two years later in boys.**
  - **Annual peak rates for increase in height and weight are 9–10 cm and 8–10 kg,** respectively.
  - During this period, development of the critical bone mass is essential as this forms the ground for maintaining mineral integrity of bone in later life.
  - Pattern and proportion of various body components, like body water, muscle mass, bone and fat, increase during the entire childhood and adolescence to reach adult values by about 18 years.
  - **Adolescent girls** are at greater physiological stress than boys because of menstruation. Their **nutritional needs are of particular importance** as they have to prepare for motherhood. All these rapid anabolic changes require more nutrients per unit body weight.

Accordingly, it is advised that:

- **Growing children and adolescents require more calcium.** It is recommended that they **should consume calcium rich foods** like **milk and milk products, ragi** (fox tail millet) and **til** (sesame seed), etc.

- **Young children,** below 5 years of age, **should be given** less bulky **foods** but are **rich in energy and protein,** such as **legumes, pulses, nuts, edible oil/ghee, sugar, milk and eggs.**
- **Vegetables,** including **green leafy vegetables, and** locally available **seasonal fruits** should be a part of their daily menu.
- Older children and adolescents **should also consume plenty of milk** to fulfil high calcium requirements.
- They should consume, nearly, **25–50 g of cooking oils/ghee.**
- **Excessive salt intake should be avoided,** particularly, by children having a family history of hypertension.

RDA FOR ELDERLY PERSONS

As one grows old, his/her **body composition changes.** In general:

- Elderly person **loses lean body mass** and **gains fat mass.**
- **Loss of lean tissue compromises strength, reduces resting energy expenditure** and increases the **risk of osteoporosis.**
- **Perception of taste** also **declines with age,** which also contributes to **loss of appetite** and **poor food intake.**
- **Reduction in acid and enzymes secretions** further affect nutrient absorption.
- **Immune functions also decline** with age.
- **Absorption, transport, storage and metabolism of fat-soluble vitamins are also affected** by aging.

Thus, aging causes **multiple physiological changes,** which, accordingly, **affect our nutrients need as well as nutritional status.**

Accordingly, **ICMR-NIN (2020)** has recommended that, **to maintain regular physical activity, elders should consume nutrient-dense foods,** such as **nuts, oilseeds, fruits, vegetables, legumes and flesh-foods,** to meet their daily requirements of vitamins and minerals.

Recommendations of the Group for various nutrients for the elderly persons (more than 60 years of age) are shown in Table 16.5.

Table 16.5: RDA of macro and micronutrients for the elderly

Dietary nutrient	*Male (60+)*	*Female (60+)*
Energy (kcal)	1700	1500
Dietary fiber (g)	32	25
Proteins (g)	54	46
Thiamine (mg)	1.4	1.4
Riboflavin (mg)	2	1.9
Niacin (mg)	12	9
Vitamin B_6 (mg)	1.9	1.9
Folate (µg)	300	200
Vitamin B_{12} (µg)	2.2	2.2
Vitamin C (mg)	80	65
Vitamin A (µg)	1000	840
Vitamin D (IU)*	800	800
Calcium (mg)	1200	1200
Magnesium (mg)	440	370
Iron (mg)	19	19
Zinc (mg)	17	13
Iodine (µg)	150	150

* Adequate intake

- **Energy:** Due to a reduction in BMR and the sedentary lifestyle, the Group has **suggested** RDA for energy in terms of **estimated average requirement** (EAR).

  EAR for energy has been suggested as **1700 kcal/day for elderly males** (with average body weight of 65 kg) and **1500 kcal for elderly females** (with average body weight of 55 kg).
- **Dietary fiber:** RDA for dietary fiber has been suggested as **30 g/d for elderly males** and **25 g/d for elderly females.**
- **Protein:** RDA for protein has been suggested as **54 g/d for elderly males** and **46 g/d for elderly females.**

- **Vitamins:**
  - **Thiamine:** RDA for thiamine has been suggested as **1.4 mg/d for elderly males as well as females.**
  - **Riboflavin:** RDA for riboflavin has been suggested as **2.0 mg/d for elderly males** and **1.9 mg/d for elderly females.**
  - **Niacin:** RDA for niacin (NE) has been suggested as **14 mg/d for** elderly **males** and **11 mg/d for elderly females.**
  - **Vitamin B_6:** RDA for vitamin B_6 has been suggested as **1.9 mg/d for elderly males as well as females.**
  - **Folate:** RDA for dietary folate has been suggested as **300 µg/d for elderly males** and **200 µg/d for elderly females.**
  - **Vitamin B_{12}:** RDA for vitamin B_{12} has been suggested as **2.2 µg/day for elderly males as well as females.**
  - **Vitamin C:** RDA for vitamin C has been suggested as **80 mg/d for elderly males** and **65 mg/d for elderly females.**
  - **Vitamin A:** RDA for vitamin A (RE) has been suggested as **1000 µg/d for elderly males** and **840 µg/d for elderly females.**
  - **Vitamin D:** RDA for vitamin D has been suggested as **800 IU/d for** elderly **males as well as females.**
- **Minerals:**
  - **Calcium:** RDA for calcium has been suggested as **1200 mg/d for elderly males as well as females.**
  - **Magnesium:** RDA for magnesium has been suggested as **440 mg/d for elderly males** and **370 mg/d for elderly females.**
  - **Iron:** RDA for iron has been suggested as **19 µg/d for elderly males as well as females.**
  - **Zinc:** RDA for zinc has been suggested as **17 mg/d for elderly males** and **13 mg/d for elderly females.**
  - **Iodine:** RDA for iodine has been suggested as **140 µg/d for elderly males as well as females.**
- **Water:** Water is essential for various body functions. In elderly persons, decreased thirst response and reduced concentrating capacity of the kidney may lead to dehydration. Moreover, use of diuretics, alcohol and caffeine increase fluid excretion and further contribute to dehydration. With the increasing dietary fiber intake, it is also essential to consume adequate fluid, ideally water, to avoid dehydration and constipation.

  Accordingly, total water requirement has been suggested as 2800 ml/d for elderly males and 2550 ml/d for elderly females.

DIETARY REQUIREMENTS DURING EXERCISE

A proper well-balanced diet is an essential component of any fitness or sports program. As the performance of a racing car depends upon a high-performance engine and the energy dense fuel it uses. Accordingly, the physical activity and sports performance of an individual depends upon energy production in the body.

The food we consume is processed as fuel by our muscles in the form of chemical energy, to produce power for physical performance. Thus, requirement depends upon the duration, intensity and type of exercise. Optimal nutrition for most includes a variety of nutrient dense food. Food should be high in carbohydrate (providing about 60–70% of calories), low in fat (providing about 20–30% of calories) and moderate in protein (providing about 10–15% of calories). General recommendations include:

1. Consumption of adequate energy and nutrients to support health and performance, and
2. Maintenance of hydration status with normal fluid intake.

- **Energy:** Adequate energy intake is critical for athletic performance and to maintain lean body mass. Though all proteins, fat and carbohydrates can be used as the possible sources of fuel for muscle contraction, the requirement however, varies with weight, height, age, sex and intensity and duration of the exercise.

- **Carbohydrate:** Carbohydrate-rich diet helps maximize muscle and liver glycogen stores before exercise and promotes faster recovery after exercise. It is suggested that minimum of 60–70% of total calories should come from carbohydrates. The type of exercise, level of intensity and time of the day, however, influence choice.

  Pre-exercise meal keeps the athlete away from feeling hungry before and during the exercise, and maintains optimal levels of blood glucose for the exercising muscle. A pre-exercise meal, thus, can improve performance compared with exercising in a fasted state. Accordingly, 1–4 hours prior to intense exercise one should consume 1.0 to 4.5 g of carbohydrate per kg body weight.

  Since it takes 24 to 48 hours, after an event, to replenish glycogen stores, timing and type of carbohydrates are also important in the refueling process, during recovery after exercise. The best way to replenish glycogen stores after intense exercise is to consume 1.0 to 1.5 g of carbohydrate per kg body weight, within 30 minutes after a workout, followed by additional 1.0 to 1.5 g per kg body weight after every two hours.

  Carbohydrate loading is recommended for athletes who compete in events that last for 90 minutes or longer, e.g. marathon, long-distance swimming, etc.

- **Fat:** Fat is a most concentrated source of food energy and supplies more than twice the calories as compared to each gram of the protein or carbohydrate. Fat also provides essential fatty acids that are necessary for cell membrane, synthesis of some hormones as well as for fat-soluble vitamins. For a general population, dietary recommendations promote a diet with less than 30% of calories from fat. Although fat is an important fuel for exercise, a high fat diet is not necessary. It is generally advised that athletes should consume 15–25% of calories as dietary fat. Any extra fat calories may come from monounsaturated and polyunsaturated fatty acids.

  Endurance training increases body's capacity to use fat as a fuel. In trained athletes, relative contribution of fatty acids as a fuel declines as the intensity of exercise increases. A low fat diet is also important for health reasons because high fat diet is associated with cardiovascular disease, obesity, diabetes and some types of cancer.

- **Protein:** Besides a source of energy, dietary protein also serves as a source of essential amino acids for the synthesis of body proteins. RDA for protein, for adults, is 0.8 g/kg body weight per day. People who are regularly engaged in low-intensity exercise do not need additional protein but athletes who are engaged in vigorous activities have slightly higher protein needs.

  The need for protein in exercise depends upon energy intake since calories play an important role in sparing protein. Protein is also used as an energy source if calories are insufficient. Consuming more protein, than the body can use, is not necessary and should be avoided. High-protein intake can result in diuresis and potential dehydration.

  Endurance athletes, involved in heavy training, require 1.2 to 1.4 g of protein/kg body weight/day. Amino acids contribute 3 to 6% of the fuel for energy metabolism during exercise. Branched chain amino acids are preferred for oxidative metabolism in skeletal muscle and are used for energy production as muscle glycogen stores decline during prolonged exercise.

Athletes need to be in positive nitrogen balance in order to gain muscle mass and strength. The best way to obtain protein is from high quality protein foods. Along with carbohydrates, protein is also important for post-exercise recovery. Low fat dairy products, egg white, chicken, fish and legumes are good sources of protein.

- **Vitamins and minerals:** Vitamins and minerals are important components of an athlete's diet. The B vitamins are essential for energy metabolism. The athletes are at risk for B vitamin deficiencies. If they consume adequate calories and plenty of complex carbohydrates from fruits and vegetables in the diet, they need high levels of B vitamins.

Other micronutrients of concern in athletes are calcium and zinc. Iron and vitamin B_{12} may also be a problem for athletes who follow a veggan diet.

Calcium is essential for normal muscle function and strong bones. As inadequate calcium may increase risk of stress fractures in athletes, hence adequate calcium intake coupled with regular exercise is necessary. This in turn also delays the onset of osteoporosis, which is a major health problem, especially in women. Teen athletes should take about 1300 mg of calcium/day. Low-fat dairy products, calcium fortified fruit juice and other fortified foods are good sources of calcium.

Iron is vital to oxygen delivery and energy production. It is also a key component of several enzymes vital to the production of ATP by the oxygen energy system. Female athletes are at higher risk of iron deficiency as a result of menstrual loss. Heavy training also causes a transient decrease in serum ferritin and hemoglobin. These are a result of an increase in plasma volume, which causes hemodilution. This may also be referred to as **sports anemia.** It, however, has no effect on performance. All athletes, especially females, long-distance runners and vegetarians, should be screened periodically to assess their iron status. If iron depletion is present, iron supplementation along with vitamin C to enhance its absorption, is essential.

Strenuous exercise also taxes the body's reserves of **copper** (essential for red blood cell synthesis) and **zinc** (vital for proper functioning of many enzymes, particularly related to energy production). Exercise also increases oxidative processes in the muscle leading to increased generation of lipid peroxides and free radicals.

The **antioxidant nutrients,** such as vitamins A, E and C, β-carotene and selenium, play an important role in protecting the cell membrane from oxidative damage. Supplementation of antioxidant nutrients also has a role in enhancing recovery from exercise and maintaining immune response.

- **Fluid:** Exercise generates heat. Heat production can increase by 15 to 20 folds during heavy exercise. Most body heat is lost through evaporation of fluid from the skin, as sweat. Sweating rate of elite athletes can range from 1 to 2 L/hr. Sweat rate is affected by environmental temperature, humidity, type of clothing, fitness level and initial fluid balance. During exercise, adequate fluid consumption helps offset fluid loss, minimize cardiovascular changes, reduce perception of effort and maintain a supply of fuel to working muscles. Active people must consume adequate amount of fluid before, during and after exercise.

ICMR-NIN (2020) suggested that adequate amounts of fluids, carbohydrates and electrolytes should be consumed before, during and after exercise.

SOME IMPORTANT QUESTIONS

1. **Define recommended daily allowances (RDA). What is the significance of RDA?**
2. **Describe dietary requirements for Indians.**
3. **Briefly describe:**
   i. RDA for pregnant and lactating women
   ii. RDA for infants
   iii. RDA for children and adolescents
   iv. Dietary recommendations for Indians
   v. Dietary requirements for the elderly persons

CHAPTER

17

Nutritive Value of Foods

Nutritive values are the average of many samples of foods, analyzed in laboratories. Several factors determine the nutritive value of foods, which include:

- Conditions of growing the crop,
- Handling of the produce from farm to market to consumer,
- Care given to food in home, and
- Manner in which the food is cooked.

AVERAGE NUTRITIVE VALUE OF DIFFERENT TYPES OF FOODS

Average nutritive value of different types of foods is given in Table 17.1.

CALCULATION OF THE NUTRITIVE VALUE OF FOOD

Nutritive value of food can be calculated by making the list of the kind and amount of every foodstuff, including sugar, butter, coffee, etc., as well as the foods that are eaten in between the meals. The value can be calculated for all of its nutrients from Table 17.1.

Nutritive values of some of the common foods are shown in Table 17.2.

NUTRITIVE VALUE OF AN AVERAGE INDIAN DIET

An average Indian diet is highly cereal-based, particularly, of the weaker economic sections, where cereals form bulk of the diet and provide 80% of the calories. They are, however, deficient in pulses, green leafy vegetables, oils and fats, and fruits. Most staple foods used are rice in Southern parts and wheat in North India. The trend of mixed cereals consumption is, however, emerging.

- These predominant cereal diets have little or no visible fats. They, however, consist of significant quantity of invisible fat, which contributes to nearly 6% energy, in an adult diet with 2400 kcal.
- These diets can be improved by eating mixed cereals or by adding coarse cereals (millets), locally grown leafy vegetables, butter milk and increased use of pulses and local fruits.
- Another improvement which can be affected, is improvement of cooking practices, e.g. not to discard cooking water. It is advisable to use minimum of water or to utilize cooking liquid in either soups or gravies.
- It is not advisable to peel and cut the vegetables long before they are ready for boiling.
- Excessive washing of rice should be avoided to save vitamin B1 (thiamin). The rice kanjee, which is strained away during cooking, also carries with it, thiamin and nicotinic acid.
- Tamarind can be added to cooking water to preserve vitamins.

Table 17.1: Average nutritive values of some of foods (per 100 g)*

Foodstuffs	*Protein (g)*	*Fat (g)*	*Carbohydrates (g)*	*Calories (kcal)*
Cereals	9.9	2.3	71.0	344
Bread	7.8	0.7	51.9	245
Salt biscuits	6.6	32.4	54.6	534
Sweet biscuits	6.4	15.2	71.9	450
Pulses	22.6	2.0	58.4	342
Green leafy vegetables	3.8	0.6	6.0	45
Roots and tubers	1.2	0.2	16.0	70
Other vegetables	2.2	0.3	6.3	36
Nuts and oilseeds	15.2	46.6	20.4	578
Condiments and spices	9.8	6.6	40.6	261
Fruits	1.1	0.4	7.6	79
Meat	21.0	4.9	0.8	131
Eggs	13.3	13.3	0.0	173
Milk	3.6	5.8	4.7	85
Curd	3.1	4.0	3.0	60
Butter	0.0	81.0	0.0	29
Ghee	0.0	100.0	0.0	900
Oil	0.0	100.0	0.0	900
Sugar	0.1	0.0	99.4	398
Honey	0.3	0.0	79.5	319
Jagery	0.4	0.1	95.0	383
Sago	0.2	0.2	87.1	351

* NIN-ICMR (1998)

SOME IMPORTANT QUESTIONS

1. **Describe nutritive value of foods.**
2. **Describe the procedure for the calculation of the nutritive value of foods**

Table 17.2: Nutritive values of some of the common foods

Nutrients	*Food groups*	*Foodstuffs*	*Nutrient content* (per 100 g of the edible portion)*
Energy (kcal)	Cereals and tubers	Rice, wheat and tapioca	340
	Nuts and oilseeds	Almonds, cashew nuts, coconut (dry) and groundnut	600
	Oil and ghee	Vegetable oil, ghee and vanaspati	900
Protein (g)	Pulses and legumes	Bengal gram, black gram, green gram, lentil and red gram	22
	Nuts and oilseeds	Groundnuts, cashew nuts and almonds	23
	Fish		20
	Meat and poultry	Meat	22
		Egg white	11
	Milk products	Cheese, khoa, skimmed milk powder and whole milk powder	30
Vitamin A (µg)	Fasts and edible oils	Butter, ghee and hydrogenated oil (fortified)	700
β-Carotene (mg)	Leafy vegetables	Coriander leaves, spinach, mint and radish leaves	2–6
		Other leafy vegetables such as amaranth, curry leaves and fenugreek leaves	7–15
	Other vegetables	Pumpkin and green chilies	1.0
		Carrots	6.5
	Fruits	Ripe mango	2.0
		Papaya	0.9
Vitamin C (mg)	Green leafy vegetables	Cabbage, coriander leaves, drumstick leaves and knol-khol (green)	112–220
	Other vegetables	Giant chilies (capsicum)	137
		Green chilies	117
		Amla	600
	Fruits	Guava	212
Riboflavin (mg)	Cereal grains and grain products	Bajra, barley, ragi wheat-germ and wheat bread (brown)	0.2
	Pulses and legumes	Bengal gram, black gram, green gram, lentil, red gram and soybean	0.2
	Leafy vegetables	Amaranthus, carrot leaves, colocasia leaves, curry leaves, fenugreek leaves, mint, radish leaves and spinach	0.25
	Nuts and oilseeds	Mustard seeds, sunflower seeds, almonds and walnuts	0.3
		Chillies (dry), chillies green, coriander and cumin seeds	0.35
	Condiments and spices	Apricot dried and papaya	0.23
	Fruits	Sheep liver	1.7
	Meat and poultry	Egg	0.26
	Milk and milk products	Skimmed milk power and whole milk powder	1.5

Contd.

Table 17.2: Nutritive values of some of the common foods (*Contd.*)

Folic acid	Green leafy vegetables	Amaranth, mint and spinach	120 (μg)
	Pulses	Bengal gram, black gram, green gram and red gram	130
	Oilseeds	Soybean	180
Iron (mg)	Green leafy vegetables	Amaranth, Bengal gram leaves, cauliflower (green) and radish leaves	18–40
Calcium (mg)	Cereals and legumes	Ragi, Bengal gram (whole), horse gram (whole), rajmah and soybean	200–340
	Green leafy vegetables	Amaranth, cauliflower (green), curry leaves and knol-khol leaves	500–800
		Colocasia leaves	1540
	Nuts and oilseeds	Coconut (dry), almonds, mustard seeds and sunflower seed	130–490
		Cumin seed	1080
	Fish	Bacha, katla, mrigal, pran and rohu	320–650
	Milk and milk products	Buffalo milk, cow milk, goat milk and curd	120–210
		Cheese, khoa, skimmed milk powder and whole milk powder	790–1370

CHAPTER

18

Planning Menu and Budgeting of Food

A **menu** is a list of specific foods offered for a specific period. It includes a list of dishes to be served in a given meal.

Menu planning refers to the practice of deciding what one would like to eat for each meal, including main dishes, side dishes, and desserts. It is the process of listing down the foods which can be served for breakfast, lunch, dinner or snacks. Menu plans may be for a day, week or month. It is also a way to make sure that one is eating a balanced diet, meeting ones nutritional needs.

SIGNIFICANCE OF PLANNING MENU

Planning the menu is important due to the following reasons:

- It enables the planner to think ahead and assures what to prepare in advance.
- It maximizes the use of available resources, like food supplies, fuels, tools, equipment and food in season.
- It enables one to predict the expected cost/budget for food.

PRINCIPLES OF PLANNING MENU

- **It should meet nutritional requirements:** A good menu should include recommended amounts of food from each major food groups. The complete menu should supply not only adequate calories, fat and protein but also minerals, vitamins, water and roughage, essential for the physical well being of each member of a family. Loss of nutrients during processing and cooking can be minimized, e.g. sprouted grains and fermented foods enhance the nutritive value. Pressure cooker can be used to conserve the nutrients.
- **It should fulfil needs of all family members:** As requirements of several nutrients vary with age, occupation and lifestyle of the family members. A family meal should cater to the needs of all the family members, such as for infants and children of various ages, the pregnant and lactating women, the elderly, and for the specific health needs. For example, enough fat and flexibility in caloric density is essential to meet the energy needs of children. A young child requires soft and bland diet, whereas adolescents need rich food to satisfy appetite. Pregnant women require more greens in the diet. A heavy worker requires more calories and B vitamins. It should also provide suitable nutrients for different situations, like during sickness, deficiencies or diabetes, etc.
- **Considerate food habits and variety:** During menu planning one must also consider psychological and cultural habits of the family members. Also, within each food group, one must select

as wide a variety of food as possible, with respect to the:

- **Color:** Use food that complement each other in color, and avoid all meals of one color.
- **Texture:** Combine soft food with crisp and chewy food.
- **Flavor:** Combine bland and highly flavored food. Herbs and spices may be used with a light touch.
- **Preparation methods:** Different methods of food preparation, such as boiling, steaming, baking, broiling, roasting and frying, must be incorporated.
- **Season:** The food may be planned according to the season, yet retaining same nutritive value, particularly, with respect to fruits and vegetables.
- **Number and sequence of course:** Menu should cover appetizer, main dish, dessert, etc.
- **Occasions:** Menu planning should also include special occasions, such as festivities, etc.
- **Environmental conditions:** Specific dishes offered, should consider the environmental temperatures, e.g. special hot foods can be offered on cold rainy days and vice versa.

- **It should save time and energy:** Planning of meals should be done in such a way that the recipes should be simple and nutritious. Labor and time saving devices can be used. Proper storage of food is also essential.
- **Economic considerations:** Meals that are not within budget should not be put into practice. The cost of meals can be reduced by bulk purchasing and using seasonal fruits and vegetables.

BUDGETING OF FOOD

A **budget** is the sum of money allocated for a particular purpose and the summary of intended expenditures along with proposals for how to meet them. A family budget is a predetermined amount of money set aside and spent for certain categories of living expenses.

Determine the amount of money you have in your household **budget** to spend on **food.** Knowing how much money is available to spend on food is important for menu planning.

According to US Department of Agriculture, 10 percent represents the typical amount consumer's budget for food.

As per recent report, richer countries spend a smaller fraction of their income on food, e.g. the average American spends just 6.5 percent of his/her household budget on food consumption. On the other hand, poorer countries spend a much larger share of their budget on food.

The average Indian family spends between 30–40 percent of the household budget on food.

FACTORS INFLUENCING FOOD BUDGETING

Several factors influence amount of money that needs to be allocated for food expenditure. Some of these relate to the individual and family, while others relate to food availability and cost. These include:

1. Income of the family
2. Size of the family
3. Food prices
4. Production and processing of foods
5. Relative interest of family members in food compared to other commodities.

SUGGESTIONS TO REDUCE FOOD BUDGET

- **Plan a menu:** Decide which recipes you will make for lunch and dinner. Take a look at these ideas from your family and friends for some time (sample menu plan), and then make your own menu. Plan menu in advance and prepare a market order. Modify according to market cost and availability of the food.
- **Purchase foods when they are on sale:** Take advantage of special advertisements to know which foods are plentiful and

lower in cost. For this purpose, check store flyers, newspaper inserts and coupon sites online. Just be sure to buy and plan for foods that you will actually use, so that they do not go to waste. Also, look for the expiry dates of the foods and ingredients. Also, look for recipes in the menu that use those foods and ingredients.

- **Look for cheaper substitutes:** Avoid buying food on impulse. Although the meat group is a good source of protein, iron and other minerals, and some B vitamins, substitution of pulses and legumes are not only good sources of protein at a low cost but also reduces fat and cholesterol intake. Grains, such as rice, pasta, barley, etc. are less expensive and can be used in many recipes.
- **Avoid recipes that need special ingredients:** Avoid recipes that need a special ingredient that you may not have. Look for it to know that how much does that ingredient cost? Does it come in a small or big package? Can you use it in any other recipes before it goes bad? It may not be worth the money to buy an ingredient, if you are only going to use it once. Leave the ingredient out or try the recipe with an ingredient that you already have at home.
- **Look for seasonal recipes:** Fresh fruits and vegetables, especially, those locally grown, are often less expensive in season. Thus, buy seasonal fresh foods, since out of season foods are, usually, more expensive.
- **Know your family's likes:** Encourage your family to share their favorites and help with menu planning. That way you can look for favorite ingredients and foods when they are on sale.
- Consider the nutritive value of the food and compare its cost with the home prepared food, e.g. yogurt, cream, cheese and ice cream, etc.
- Purchase only the quantities that are likely to be used by the family, and store food properly.
- Think about how you can use leftovers. Do not let a big bunch of foods, such as carrots or celery, to go waste. Use it all up by making an extra dish.

SOME IMPORTANT QUESTIONS

1. **What is menu planning? What is the importance of menu planning? Describe principles of menu planning.**
2. **What do you mean by budgeting of food? Describe various factors influencing of budgeting of food.**
3. **Describe various ways to reduce food budget.**
4. **Write notes on:**
   i. Planning menu
   ii. Planning budgeting of food

CHAPTER

19

Introduction to Therapeutic Diets

In nutrition, **diet** is the sum of food consumed by a person, or other organism. The word diet often implies the use of specific intake of nutrition for health or weight management reasons.

A **therapeutic diet** is a meal plan that controls the intake of certain foods or nutrients. It is part of the treatment of a medical condition and are, normally, prescribed by a physician, and planned by a dietician. Therapeutic diet can be defined as the modification of normal meal to treat the indiscriminate health state of an individual.

TYPES OF THERAPEUTIC DIETS

As mentioned above, a therapeutic diet is, usually, a modification of the regular diet. It is modified or tailored to fit nutrition needs of a particular person. Therapeutic diets are modified for nutrients or texture.

Nutrients Modifications

- Decreased calories intake for weight reduction, or provide extra calories for weight gain
- Balance the amounts of carbohydrates, fat and protein
- High fiber diet
- Low fat and/or low cholesterol diet
- Decreased amount of a nutrient, such as low sodium diet
- To exclude a particular food, due to allergy or intolerance

Texture Modifications

- Mechanical soft diet
- Liquid diet
- Semi-solid diet

COMMON THERAPEUTIC DIETS

- **High fiber diet:** It is prescribed in the prevention or treatment of a number of gastrointestinal, cardiovascular and metabolic diseases. Increased fiber should come from a variety of sources, including fruits, legumes, vegetables, whole breads and cereals.
- **Low fat/low cholesterol diet:** It is low in total fat (limits to 50 g) and saturated fats, and contains approximately 250–300 mg cholesterol. It is used to reduce fat levels and/or treat medical conditions that interfere with the use of body fat, such as diseases of the liver, gallbladder or pancreas.
- **Low sodium diet:** It has 2 g sodium, e.g. sausage, cured meats, canned soups, salty seasonings, pickled foods, salted crackers, etc. It is used for people who have oedema (may be holding water), or those who have high blood pressure, heart disease, liver disease or first stage of kidney disease.

- **Food allergy modifications:** Food allergies are due to an abnormal immune response to an otherwise harmless food. The most common food allergens are milk, egg, soy, wheat, peanuts, tree nuts, fish and shellfish. Foods implicated with allergies are strictly eliminated from the diet and appropriate substitutions are made to ensure that the meal is adequate in nutrients. For example, a gluten-free diet would include the elimination of wheat, rye and barley, or corn and rice products with potato, etc.
- **Food intolerance modifications:** The most common food intolerance is intolerance to lactose, called lactose intolerance due to milk sugar (lactose) because of a decreased amount of the enzyme lactase, in the body. Other common types of food intolerance include adverse reactions to certain products added to food, may be to enhance taste, color or protection against bacterial growth. Common symptoms involving food intolerances are vomiting, diarrhea, abdominal pain and headaches.
- **Mechanically altered diet:** Mechanically altered diet, or soft diet, is used when there are problems with chewing and swallowing. It includes chopped or ground meats and chopped or ground raw fruits and vegetables. It is for people with poor dental conditions, missing teeth, no teeth or a condition known as dysphasia.
- **Liquid diet:** It has minimum residue fluids that can be seen through, e.g. juices without pulp. It is often used as the first step to the restarting of oral feeding after surgery or an abdominal procedure. It can also be used for fluid and electrolyte replacement in people with severe diarrhea. As it does not provide enough calories and nutrients, such a diet should not be used for an extended period.
- **Semi-solid diet:** It includes diets that are not clear in nature, e.g. ice cream, pudding (kheer), thinned hot cereal (khichri), custard, strained cream soups and juices with pulp. It is used as the second step to restart oral feeding, once clear liquids are tolerated. It should not be used for extended periods.
- **Tube feeding:** Tube feedings (nutrition support) are used for people, who cannot take adequate food or fluids by mouth.

DIETARY MODIFICATIONS FOR SOME COMMON AILMENTS

FOR DIABETICS

Diabetes mellitus is a group of diseases characterized by high blood glucose concentration, resulting from defects in insulin secretion and/or its action.

Therefore, the ideal diet for diabetic patients depends on the presence or absence of obesity, the response to a weight-reduction diet and the stage of progression of β-cell dysfunction. Dietary modifications include:

- **Calories:** To lose weight, one need to eat fewer calories and replace less healthy foods, with foods lower in calories, fat and sugar.
- **Carbohydrate:** Carbohydrates have a big impact on blood sugar levels, so one need to be smart about what types of carbohydrate to eat. One should limit refined carbohydrates, like white bread, pasta, and rice, as well as soda, candy, packaged meals and snack foods. One should also focus on high-fiber complex carbohydrates. They are digested more slowly; thus, prevent the body from producing too much insulin.
- **Proteins:** Persons with diabetes and normal renal function can have usual protein intake of 10% to 20% of energy. The proteins consumed should primarily come from plant sources.
- **Fats:** Intake of fried foods, and other foods high in saturated and trans fat should be limited.
- **Vitamins and minerals:** Whole grains, and fruits and vegetables, consumed by the diabetics can meet the required amounts of vitamins and minerals.

- **Dietary patterns and food selection:** The goal of nutrition therapy for diabetes also emphasizes the role of lifestyle in improving glucose control, lipid and lipoprotein profiles, and blood pressure.

FOR HYPERTENSION

Diet for a person with hypertension, also referred to as the Dietary Approaches to Stop Hypertension (DASH diet), is a diet that should be followed by a person with high blood pressure. For such individuals, dietary modifications include:

- **Fat:** One should limit the consumption of foods with saturated fat from animals (such as fatty meats, whole milk, butter, cream, and other dairy foods made with whole milk), palm, palm kernel, or coconut oil (tropical oils) and all foods made with hydrogenated oil (trans fat). Unsaturated fat from soybean, canola, olive or sunflower oil, and omeg-3 fatty acids fatty from coldwater fish (such as salmon and tuna), flaxseed and flaxseed oil should be consumed more.
- **Minerals:** One should eat foods that contain high amounts of potassium, magnesium and calcium to help lower blood pressure. It is also recommended that one should limit the intake of sodium between 1500–2400 mg per day.
- **Dietary patterns and food selection:** The diet should include high amounts of fruits, vegetables and whole grains, along with lean sources of protein, low-fat dairy foods, nuts, seeds and legumes. Several lifestyle changes, such as weight control and physical activity help in lowering blood pressure.

FOR A PERSON WITH FEVER

Fever is due to elevation of body temperature above normal. Dietary modifications include:

- **Energy:** Calories and energy requirement is increased by 4–7% for every degree rise in temperature.
- **Proteins:** Easily digestible protein foods, like dal, soup or soft-cooked dal, are required, which help in the repair of worn out tissues.
- **Fat:** Requirement of fat increases, due to increased need of fat-soluble vitamins by the body.
- **Vitamins:** Requirement of B vitamins increases in relation to increased energy needs. Increased intake of vitamins A and C helps in preventing infections.
- **Minerals:** Extra quantity of electrolytes, like sodium and potassium, are needed in high fever, diarrhoea and vomiting. Zinc is beneficial for immunity and iron is required in case of any blood loss.
- **Dietary patterns and food selections:** Small frequent meals with easily digestible bland foods and judicious use of sugar, fat, cream and milk powder to help increased protein content.

FOR A PERSON HAVING DIARRHOEA

Diarrhoea can be defined as the frequent passage of stools. Dietary modifications include:

- **Energy:** The requirement of energy is increased to replace losses and can be met from foods like fruit juices, suji kheer, etc.
- **Protein:** For proteins, foods that are easy to digest can be given to the patients, e.g. washed moong dal, paneer, etc.
- **Fats:** Fats rich foods are restricted, because the intestine is incapable of absorbing them. Butter and light fats like cream, can be given after the improvement in the condition.
- **Vitamins:** Deficiency of water-soluble vitamins (B and C) is caused by the loss of water in diarrhea, hence, juices must be added in the diet.
- **Minerals:** Loss of sodium and potassium leads to their deficiency, like loss of appetite, restlessness and loss of flexibility in muscles. Their deficiency can be made by giving up fruit juices, after adding salt.

- **Water:** As lot of water is excreted, hence, water (fluid) should be given in the form of juices, lemon water, barley water, mineral water, etc.
- **Dietary patterns and food selection:** Small frequent meals should be given. Since milk is poorly tolerated, curd may be the better option. Strongly flavored foods, fried and fatty foods, and nuts and rich desserts should be avoided. Fiber intake should be restricted. Instead, low fiber cereals and de-husked pulses should be included.

FOR A PERSON HAVING CONSTIPATION

Constipation is a state when one finds difficult to pass the stools. Dietary modifications include:

- **Carbohydrates:** Carbohydrates should be given in the form of fibres, e.g. fibrous fruits, vegetables, flour with bran, whole cereals, guava, apples, grapes, vegetables salad, etc.
- **Proteins:** Protein foods, like soyabeans and legumes, provide good dietary proteins.
- **Fats:** Fats should be given in reasonable amount, to stimulate the flow of bile needed for digestion and keep the tract well lubricated. Spicy, fried foods irritate the tract.
- **Vitamins:** It is necessary to give B-complex vitamins, as it enhances the muscular movement of intestine.
- **Water:** Water is required for flushing out the body waters. Person must consume 8–10 glasses of water.
- **Dietary patterns and food selection:** One should have regular meal timings. Vegetables should be given in the form of salad, fruits with skin and seeds, besides, whole pulses and sprouts. In addition, bulking agents, such as psyllium husk (isabgol) and other natural laxative agents, must be used.

FOR A PERSON WITH JAUNDICE

Jaundice is a very common liver disorder occurring specially in summers. Dietary modifications include:

- **Carbohydrates:** Calorie requirement can be gradually regulated depending on the health of the individual. Fruit juices with sugar, glucose, honey, sugarcane juice and jam, etc. can be given in the diet, to provide energy.
- **Protein:** Diet high in complete proteins should be given, to speed up the regeneration of liver cells.
- **Fats:** All kinds of fats must be avoided for at least two weeks.
- **Vitamins:** Vitamins B and C, in the form of fresh juices and fruits, stimulate the regeneration of liver cells.
- **Minerals:** Sodium and potassium loss take place due to vomiting. Adding salt to the juices and soup should be practiced.
- **Water and roughage:** Plenty of water and less of fiber is desirable. Grapes, apples, sugarcane, barley water, coconut water, fresh fruit juices, spinach, fenugreek, carrot and radish with leaves are useful. Saturated fats (like ghee and butter), eggs, whole pulses, fiber-rich cereals, papad, chutney, pickles and ice-cream should be avoided.

LIFESTYLE CHANGES

Lifestyle change is a type of therapy advised to help an individual to decrease blood cholesterol levels and reduce the risk of a heart disease. According to the American Heart Association, it is also used to treat coronary artery disease and diabetes. It was designed by experts of the National Heart, Lung and Blood Association's National Cholesterol Education Program. The diet requires one to limit saturated fat intake to less than 7 percent of total daily calories and to limit cholesterol intake to less than 200 mg a day. It also encourages one to consume 10 to 25 g of soluble fiber, and

2 g of plant sterols and stanols a day, to help lower blood cholesterol levels. Calories on such diets are also controlled to help weight management.

NATUROPATHY

Naturopathy is a system of alternative medicine based on the theory that diseases can be successfully treated or prevented without the use of drugs, by techniques such as control of diet, exercise and massage.

In **naturopathy,** a **diet** works to prevent illness, increase energy and improve overall health. It relies on food as close to its natural state as possible. This means eating foods that do not contain artificial ingredients and are free of chemical preservatives and additives. Foods typical of a naturopathic diet include raw vegetables that are organic and seasonal, and meat from animals that are pesticide, hormone and antibiotic-free.

Guiding Principles of Naturopathy

In naturopathy, diet follows six guiding principles, i.e.:

- Trust that the body can heal itself,
- Identify and treat the cause,
- Treat the person as an integrative whole,
- Use non-harming and non-invasive techniques,
- Focus on overall health, wellness and disease prevention, and
- Use education to allow people to take responsibility for their health.

According to the principle of naturopathy, the food must be taken in natural form. Fresh seasonal fruits, fresh green leafy vegetables and sprouts are excellent.

These diets are broadly classified into three types, which are as follows:

- **Eliminative diet:** Liquids such as lemon, citric juices, tender coconut water, vegetable soups, butter milk, wheat grass juices, etc.
- **Soothing diet:** Fruits, salads, boiled/ steamed vegetables, sprouts, vegetable chutney, etc.
- **Constructive diet:** Wholesome flour, unpolished rice, little pulses, sprouts, curd, etc.

Being alkaline, these diets help in improving health, purifying the body and rendering it immune to disease. To this end, a proper combination of food is necessary. Our diet should consist of 20% acidic and 80% alkaline food for maintaining health. A balanced food is a must for any individual seeking good health.

Food is regarded as a medicine in naturopathy. With this in mind, a typical naturopathic meal includes a combination of, approximately, 50% organic vegetables, 25% whole grains and 25% protein made up of organic dairy products or free-range meats.

Conditions that are treated and eliminated with a naturopathic diet include digestive issues, food sensitivities and allergies, immune disorders, reproductive imbalances, high cholesterol, insomnia, stress and anxiety.

SOME IMPORTANT QUESTIONS

1. Define a therapeutic diet. Describe various types of therapeutic diets.

2. Describe therapeutic diet for:

i. Diabetes
ii. Fever
iii. Constipation
iv. Jaundice
v. Diarrhoea
vi. Hypertension

3. Write notes on:

i. Therapeutic diet
ii. Therapeutic lifestyle changes
iii. Naturopathy

CHAPTER

20

National Programs Related to Nutrition

National programs related to nutrition have been categorized into two categories which included **direct programs** and **indirect programs.**

DIRECT PROGRAMS

Through National Nutritional Programs in late1960s and early 70s, with the inception of 5-year plans, a number of short-term measures were suggested to combat problems of malnutrition. Direct programs included:

1. Integrated child development services (ICDS) scheme,
2. Nutrition programs for the adolescent girls,
3. Nutrition advocacy and awareness general programs for food and nutrition board, and
4. Follow-up action for national nutrition policy:

- By the Ministry of Health and Family Welfare, which included:
  - Iron and folic acid supplementation to pregnant women,
  - Vitamin A supplementation to children of 9–36 months age group, and
  - National iodine deficiency disorder control program.
- By the Department of elementary school and literacy, which included:
  - Mid-day meal for primary school children.

INDIRECT PROGRAMS

Indirect programs were started by various departments, viz.:

- Department of Agriculture and Cooperation, which included:
  - Increased food production, and
  - Horticulture interventions.
- By food and public distribution, which included:
  - Targeted public distribution system,
  - Antodaya anna yojana, and
  - Annapurna scheme
- By the Rural and Urban Development, which included:
  - Food for work program,
  - Safe drinking water and alleviation program, and
  - National rural employment guarantee scheme.
- By the Ministry of Health, which included:
  - National rural health mission, and
  - Poverty alleviation program
- By the Department of Women and Child Development, which included:
  - Various women's welfare and support programs
- By the Department of Education and Literacy, which included:
  - Sarva siksha abhiyan, and
  - Adult literacy program

NUTRITION INTERVENTION PROGRAMS

Direct nutrition intervention programs which are operative in the country to improve nutritional status of the vulnerable groups are as under and broadly divided into two categories, viz.:

- **Food supply and supplementary nutrition programs**
- **Specific nutrient supplementation programs**

SUPPLEMENTARY NUTRITION PROGRAMS

Supplementary nutrition programs include Balwadi Nutrition Program, National Mid-day Meal Program (NMMP), Applied Nutrition Program (ANP) and Integrated Child Development Services (ICDS).

BALWADI NUTRITION PROGRAM

Balwadi nutrition program (BNP) was **launched by the Ministry of Social Welfare in 1970,** with the **focus on pre-school children** (2–5 years of age), and **pregnant and lactating women.** For this purpose, Balwadis were set-up in rural areas and the program is implemented by the Department of Social Welfare, in collaboration with CARE (Cooperative of American Relief Everywhere).

Aim of the Program

Food supply and supplementary nutrition, with the focus on pre-school children (2–5 years of age), in rural areas.

Beneficiary

Pre-school children 2–5 years of age.

Services

- Diet supplementation–300 kcal and 10 g protein per day par child, for 270 days a year, and
- Pre-school education

NATIONAL MID-DAY MEAL PROGRAM

National Mid-day Meal Program (NMMP), also known as **school lunch program,** is in operation **since 1961** with the objective **to attract more children for admission to schools.**

The program was **initiated by the Government of India in 1962–63,** as a follow-up measure of the school health committee report (1961–62). The supplies for this were donated by the Cooperative of American Relief Everywhere (CARE).

Aim of the Program

To provide food supplement to **school going children** (age 6–11 years) **to meet** at least **one-third of calories** and **half of the protein** requirements for the day.

Beneficiary

School going children, age 6–11 years (classes 1–8th).

Services

Supplement to home diet—at least 1/3 of the energy and 1/2 of the protein requirements for the day (cereals 75 g, pulses 30 g, oils and fats 8 g, leafy vegetables 30 g and non-leafy vegetables 30 g/day/child).

APPLIED NUTRITION PROGRAM

Applied nutrition program (ANP) was one of the earliest nutrition programs maintained by **the Ministry of Rural Development,** with the help of UNICEF, FAO and WHO.

Applied nutrition program was **introduced as a pilot scheme in Orissa in 1963** and was later extended to Tamil Nadu and UP. It was, thereafter, **extended to the entire country in 1973.**

Aim of the Program

- To raise the level of nutrition and standard of living of the vulnerable population, i.e. the **pre-school children,** and **pregnant and lactating mothers** through education in nutrition, and

- To **increase production and consumption of protective foods** by the above-mentioned vulnerable groups.

Beneficiary

- Children between 2–6 years, and
- Pregnant and lactating mothers.

Services

- **Nutrition education,** to teach rural communities through demonstration, about how to produce food for their consumption through their own efforts.
- **Focus on local production of protective foods** through poultries, fisheries, community and school-kitchen gardens, and community dairies, etc. and
- **To ensure their consumption by pregnant and nursing mothers,** and **children.**

SPECIAL NUTRITION PROGRAM

Special Nutrition Program (SNP) was **launched in** the country in **1970** by the **Ministry of Social Welfare,** in urban slums, tribal areas and backward rural areas, **under Minimum Needs Program** (MNP), with the aim **to improve nutritional status of the targeted group.**

Aim of the Program

To provide supplementary feeding to preschool children, and **expectant and nursing mothers, in urban slums, tribal areas and backward rural areas** to improve nutritional status of the targeted group.

Beneficiary Group

- Children below 6 years
- Pregnant and lactating women

Services

To provide supplementary feeding for a total of **300 days in a year to:**

- Preschool children—300 kcal and 10 g protein, and
- Pregnant and lactating mothers—500 kcal and 25 g protein,

INTEGRATED CHILD DEVELOPMENT SERVICES

Integrated child development service (ICDS) scheme was **launched on 2nd October, 1975** (under 5th Five-year Plan), under **Ministry of social welfare,** in pursuance of the National policy for children in 33 experimental blocks. Success of the scheme led to its expansion to 2996 projects by the end of March 1994 and, subsequently, with the goal of universalization, throughout the country.

Administration of the scheme at the central level is under the Department of Women and Child Development, Ministry of Human Resource Development; at the state level under the Department of Social Welfare; and at the district level under CDPO, Medical Officer, Mukhya Sevika, Multipurpose Worker and Anganwadi Workers.

Aim of the Program

- **Improve the nutrition and health status of children,** in the age group of **0–6 years,**
- Lay the foundation for proper **psychological, physical and social development of the child,**
- Effective coordination and implementation of policy among the various departments, and
- **Enhance the capability of the mother** to look after the normal health and nutrition needs through proper nutrition and health education.

Beneficiaries

- Children below 6 years,
- Pregnant and lactating women,
- Women in the reproductive age group (15–44 years), and
- Adolescent girls (in selected blocks).

Services

- Supplementary nutrition, vitamin A, iron and folic acid,

- Immunization,
- Health check-ups,
- Referral services,
- Treatment of minor illnesses,
- Nutrition and health education to women,
- Pre-school education of children in the age group of 3–6 years, and
- Convergence of other supportive services, like water supply, sanitation, etc.

SPECIFIC NUTRIENT SUPPLEMENTATION PROGRAMS

Specific nutrient supplementation programs are the programs related to the prevention of specific deficiency states. These include National Program for Control of Blindness (NPCB), National Nutritional Anemia Prophylaxis Program (NNAPP), National Iodine Deficiency Disorders Control Program (NIDDCP) and National program for prevention and control of fluorosis (NPPCF).

NATIONAL PROGRAM FOR CONTROL OF BLINDNESS

National Program for Control of Blindness (NPCB) or **vitamin A prophylaxis for prevention of nutritional blindness** was started with the aim to prevent **vitamin A deficiency** (VAD).

As discussed in Chapter 9, vitamin A is essential for normal vision. It also helps to maintain integrity of the epithelial cells and is important for many metabolic functions.

Vitamin A deficiency (VAD) delays dark adaptation and lowers resistance to infections. Prolonged deficiency of the vitamin may produce blindness, a permanent disability.

In India, VAD is most common, particularly, in under-privileged population. Young children, below the age of 3 years, and pregnant and lactating women are most vulnerable to VAD. VAD was recognized as a major public health problem in 1970, when it was estimated that nearly 30,000–40,000 children could lose their eyesight, due to VAD. Prevalence of VAD is more pronounced in several states like Rajasthan, Bihar, Madhya Pradesh, Orissa, UP, Tamil Nadu, Karnataka and Andhra Pradesh.

To overcome the problem of VAD, Ministry of Health and Family Welfare launched Vitamin A Prophylaxis for Prevention of Nutritional Blindness or Vitamin A Deficiency Program in 1970, as a component of **National Program for Control of Blindness** (NPCB).

Aim of the Program

To prevent nutritional blindness due to VAD, leading to keratomalacia in children under 5 years of age.

The program has two strategies:

- **Short-term strategy** includes the administration of vitamin A (vitamin A supplementation) to young children (below 5 years of age), and
- **Long-term strategy** as ultimate solution for the prevention of vitamin A deficiency by the regular consumption of vitamin A-rich foods, which are cheap and locally available **(food-based approach)**.

Beneficiaries

All children in 6 months to 5 years age

Services

- **Administration of supplemental dose of vitamin A:**
  - At 6–11months, a single dose of 1 lac IU of vitamin A, and
  - During 1–5 years, 2 lac IU, biannually.
- **Long-term strategy:**
  - Promotion of regular intake of vitamin A-rich foods,
  - Particularly feeding locally available foods, and
  - Kitchen gardening of vitamin A-rich foods

- **Treatment of vitamin A deficiency:**
  - Immediately after diagnosis to administer 2 lac IU, followed by another dose of 2 lac IU after 1–4 weeks.

NATIONAL NUTRITIONAL ANEMIA PROPHYLAXIS PROGRAM

National Nutritional Anemia Prophylaxis Program (NNAPP) is a program with the aim to control **nutritional anemia,** which is a disease syndrome caused by the malnutrition in its widest sense.

Nutritional anemia is defined by WHO as a condition in which **hemoglobin content of the blood is lower than normal,** as a result of the deficiency of one or more essential nutrients. By far the most frequent cause of nutritional anemia is iron deficiency and less frequently the deficiency of folate or vitamin B_{12}.

Iron deficiency anemia is the most common form of nutritional anemia, commonly, observed in pregnant and lactating mothers, infants, preschool children and adolescent girls. It **may be caused,** when **iron intake is inadequate, insufficient iron is absorbed, bioavailability of dietary iron is reduced, need of iron is increased,** or there is **chronic blood loss.** Besides iron deficiency, **malaria, hookworm infestation and other infections** play important role in tropical climates (Chapter 10).

National nutritional anemia prophylaxis program was launched in 1970, by the Ministry of Health and Family Welfare, as a part of **National Family Planning Program for the prevention of nutritional anemia in mothers and children.**

The target **beneficiaries included expectant and nursing mothers,** acceptors of family planning methods (like IUCD users and tubectomised women) and **preschool children.**

The program was renamed in 1991, as National nutritional anemia control program and the beneficiaries were redefined, as the program was extended to both anemic and non-anemic lactating, and expecting mothers and 1–5 years children.

The **dosage** of iron given vary from **60 to 100 mg of elemental iron daily.** Since 2005, it is integrated with **National Rural Health Mission (NRHM).**

Aim of the Program

To significantly **decrease the prevalence and incidence of anemia in women in reproductive age group,** especially, pregnant and lactating women, and **preschool children.**

Beneficiaries

- Children 1–5 years of age
- Expecting and lactating mothers
- Family planning (IUD) acceptors

Services

- **Distribution of iron and folic acid:**
  - **Expecting and lactating mothers as well as IUD acceptors:** Sixty mg of elemental iron plus 0.5 mg of folate, everyday, for 100 days.
  - **Children (1–5 years):** Twenty mg of elemental iron plus 0.1 mg of folate, everyday, for 100 days.
- Commercial production of **iron-fortified common salt.**

NATIONAL IODINE DEFICIENCY DISORDER CONTROL PROGRAM

Iodine is an essential micronutrient necessary for the synthesis of thyroid hormones which regulate vital physiological processes, such as early growth and development of the brain and the body, in man (Chapter 10).

Iodine deficiency has serious consequences for human beings.

In children, it results in **impaired mental functions, poor intellectual performance, lowered IQ, muscular disorders, and impaired coordination** and **sluggishness.**

In pregnancy, iodine deficiency causes **spontaneous abortions, stillbirth and**

infant deaths. Deficiency of iodine in pregnant women also **interferes with brain development of the fetus and** results in **cretinism** (birth of iodine deficient babies, those characterized by mental deficiency, hearing defects, squint and stunted growth).

Iodine deficiency disorders (IDD) are prevalent worldwide. In India, IDD was earlier thought to be a problem in the sub-Himalayan region, however, surveys, carried out subsequently, showed that no state in the country is completely free from IDD. In 1994, it was estimated that around 1500 million people were at risk of IDD and that 225 million had goiter, 0.6 million were cretins and 20 million had mild neurological disorders. Realizing the magnitude of the problem, **Government of India** launched **National goiter control program (NGCP) in 1962,** and a policy decision of **universal iodization of edible salt** was taken **in 1984.**

NGCP was **renamed National iodine deficiency disorders control program** in August 1992, taking into consideration the control of wide-spectrum of IDD, like mental and physical retardation, deaf mutism, cretinism, stillbirth, abortion, etc.

Aim of the Program

- **Surveys to assess the magnitude** of the IDD,
- **Universal iodization of salt** and supply of iodized salt all over the country,
- Resurvey after every 5 years to assess the extent of IDD and impact of iodized salt
- Laboratory monitoring of iodized salt and urinary iodine excretion, and
- **Health education and publicity.**

Services

- Replacement of common salt with **iodized salt,**
- Use of **iodized tablets to schoolchildren,**
- Use of **iodized oil** (1 ml injection of iodized oil to those suffering from IDD) for oral administration, as prophylaxis in IDD severe areas, and
- **Mass communication for public awareness** through mass media and public health programs.

NATIONAL PROGRAM FOR PREVENTION AND CONTROL OF FLUOROSIS

Excess intake of fluoride in drinking water leads to a condition referred to as **endemic fluorosis.** Fluoride, once impregnated in tooth and bone, stays there for lifetime.

This, in turn, affects all parts of the body, predominantly, skeletal system **(skeletal fluorosis)** and teeth **(dental fluorosis).** These are irreversible conditions and cannot be cured by any drug or medicine. Further, fluorosis produces crippling effects, permanent disability, discoloration and loss of teeth. Children under 10 years of age are most vulnerable (Chapter 10).

Endemic fluorosis has been reported to be an important health problem in certain parts of the country, where drinking water contains excessive amount of fluoride. It is endemic in 19 states of India. Over 70–100% of the districts are affected in the state of Rajasthan, Gujarat and Andhra Pradesh, where the problem is very severe.

Realizing that there is no cure of skeletal and dental fluorosis, and that prevention is the only means to tackle the problem, Government of India initiated **National program for prevention and control of fluorosis (NPPCF),** as a preventive measure against fluorosis, as a part of safe water supply. WHO has set the standard of fluoride in drinking water at 1.5 mg/L. These guidelines further state that climatic conditions, volume of water consumed and intake of fluoride from other sources are to be considered while setting national standards.

Aim of the Program

Preventive measure against fluorosis, as a part of safe water supply.

Services

Safe water supply.

SOME IMPORTANT QUESTIONS

1. Describe various nutrition intervention programs which are operative in the country.

2. Describe:

i. Supplementary nutrition programs
ii. Specific nutrient supplementation programs

3. Write notes on:

i. National nutrition programs
ii. Balwadi nutrition program
iii. National mid-day meal program
iv. Applied nutrition program
v. Integrated Child Development Services (ICDS)
vi. National program for control of blindness
vii. National iodine deficiency disorders control program
viii. National nutritional anemia prophylaxis program
ix. National program for prevention and control of fluorosis

CHAPTER 21

International and National Agencies Working Towards Food/Nutrition

Several international and national agencies are working in the field of food and nutrition with the aim to improve nutritional status of the population by providing better food technology, high yielding varieties, food supplementations and better health care.

INTERNATIONAL AGENCIES

FOOD AND AGRICULTURE ORGANIZATION

The **Food and Agriculture Organization (FAO) of the United Nations** is a **specialized agency** of the United Nations that leads international efforts **to defeat hunger and improve nutrition and food security.**

FAO was **founded in 1945** with its first conference in Quebec City, Canada. It has its **head office in Rome** (Italy). FAO **has 195 members** (194 countries and the European Union) and works in over 130 countries, **including India.**

Priorities outlined by FAO

Some of the priorities outlined by FAO in its fight against hunger include:

- Help eliminate hunger, food insecurity and malnutrition
- Make agriculture, forestry and fisheries more productive
- Enable inclusive and efficient agricultural and food systems

INTERNATIONAL FUND FOR AGRICULTURAL DEVELOPMENT

The International Fund for Agricultural Development **(IFAD)** is an **international financial institution.**

It is **a specialized agency of the United Nations** which was **formed in 1974** as an **outcome of the World Food Conference.**

Aims

- IAFD is dedicated for the eradication of poverty and hunger in rural areas of the developing countries.
- It supports the innovative projects that target extremely poor and food-insecure population in the rural areas, inclusive of youth and women.

UNITED NATIONS INTERNATIONAL CHILDREN'S EMERGENCY FUND

United Nations International Children's Emergency Fund **(UNICEF)**, now called as **United Nations Children's Fund,** is a specialised agency of the United Nations. It was **established in 1946** with the aim **to rehabilitate children in war ravaged countries.** UNICEF has its **headquarter in New York.**

- UNICEF **works in 190 countries** and territories **to save children's lives, to defend their rights and to help them fulfil**

their potential, from early childhood through adolescence.

- UNICEF works in collaboration with FAO, UNDP, WHO and UNESCO, and provides assistance in varied fields of MCH, environment and sanitation. Its funding is derived voluntarily, from Governmental and non-Governmental organisations.
- UNICEF staffers fight for the rights of every child seeking safe shelter, nutrition, protection from disaster and conflicts, and equality.

Services Provided by UNICEF

Some of the services provided by UNICEF include:

- Provides vaccines
- Child health and nutrition,
- Safe water and sanitation
- Quality education and skill building
- HIV prevention and treatment for mothers and babies
- Protection of children and adolescents from violence and exploitation

WORLD FOOD PROGRAM

The World Food Program **(WFP)** was **established in 1961.** It is the biggest humanitarian agency for saving lives during emergencies. It has its **presence in 120 countries.**

The WFP provides food assistance to build a pathway to peace, stability and prosperity to the people those who are recovering from conflicts, disasters and the impact of climate change.

WFP was Awarded the Noble Peace Prize in 2020

Areas of Work

- WFP work to **enhance nutrition in women and children**
- **Support smallholder farmers** in **improving productivity** and reducing losses,
- Help **countries and communities prepare for and cope with climate-related shocks**
- **Boost human capital** through school feeding programs
- In conflict situations, WFP also **bring relief to exhausted populations** and **use food assistance** to build pathways to peace and stability

WORLD HEALTH ORGANISATION

World Health Organization (WHO) is a specialized agency of the United Nations. It was founded in 1948 and is responsible for international public health. It has 6 regional offices and 152 field offices in countries with the aim to connect nations, partners and people to promote health, and keep the world safe and attain the highest level of health.

Aims

- WHO leads global efforts to expand universal health coverage.
- To direct and coordinate the world's response to health emergencies.
- To promote healthier lives, from pregnancy care through old age.

UN-NUTRITION

UN-Nutrition is a **United Nations inter-agency coordination mechanism for nutrition.** It was **founded in 2020 by its above five constituent members,** i.e.:

- The Food and Agriculture Organization of the United Nations (FAO);
- The International Fund for Agricultural Development (IFAD)
- The United Nations Children's Fund (UNICEF)
- The World Food Program (WFP)
- The World Health Organization (WHO).

Vision of UN-Nutrition is—"A World without malnutrition"

Mission: Mission of the UN-Nutrition is **"to coordinate and leverage the response of the United Nations agencies to address**

malnutrition in all its forms along with its root causes".

Presently, the joint efforts are focused on the following priorities:

- Facilitate UN agencies' coordination in countries
- Healthy diets from sustainable food systems
- Private sector engagement
- Nutrition in fragile contexts
- Accelerate coordinated work on internationally-agreed nutrition targets

Besides, UN-Nutrition also promote its members for the follow-up to major Nutrition Conferences such as United Nations Food Systems Summit, International Conference on Nutrition, etc.

COOPERATIVE FOR ASSISTANCE AND RELIEF EVERYWHERE (CARE)

Cooperative for Assistance and Relief Everywhere **(CARE)** was **established** in the wake of the Second World War, **in 1945, in New York,** as the **Cooperative for American Remittances to Europe.**

CARE is one of the World's largest independent, non-profit, non-sectarian international relief and development organization. It provides emergency aid and long-term development assistance.

In India its operation started in 1950.

By 1953, E **(Europe)** in CARE **became Everywhere,** thus, **naming it as Cooperative for American Remittances to Everywhere.**

In 1992, CARE moved its **headquarter** from New York to **Atlanta** and **changed its name** to **Cooperative for Assistance and Relief Everywhere.**

Presently, CARE and its partners work **in 109 countries,** reaching 167 million people **through more than 1600 projects.**

Program Areas where CARE Works

Some of the program areas where CARE works include:

- Food and water
- Health
- Education and work
- Climate

INTERNATIONAL UNION OF NUTRITIONAL SCIENCES

The International Union of Nutritional Sciences **(IUNS)** represents the global family of nutritional scientists. It was started in 1946, in London, where a meeting was convened by the British Nutrition Society, with the principal objects of:

- Exchange of information,
- Organization of International Congresses, and
- Publication of the results of scientific investigation.

Commissions and Committees were established to accomplish more extensive international cooperation among Scientists, in nutrition-related research and education. IUNS is best known for the periodic **International Congress of Nutrition (ICN)** that brings together professionals in nutrition, to exchange the latest findings from, both, basic research and applications for the betterment of human livelihood.

The mission and objectives of IUNS include:

- To promote advancement in nutrition science, research and development through international cooperation at the global level.
- To encourage communication and collaboration among nutrition scientists as well as to disseminate information in nutritional sciences through modern communication technology.

UNITED NATIONS FOOD SYSTEMS SUMMIT

The first ever, UN Food Systems Summit was held in New York in 2021 for transforming global food systems to achieve the Sustainable Development Goals by 2030. With the participation of, nearly, 300 Indigenous Peoples Organizations, 148 commitments have been registered to action for Nourish all people.

Action Areas

- Food is Never Waste Initiative
- Healthy Diets Initiative
- Agroecology Initiative
- Decent Work and Living Wage Initiative
- Local Food Supply Alliance

INTERNATIONAL NUTRITION FOUNDATION

International Nutrition Foundation **(INF)** was founded in 1982, to mobilize support for training, research, communication and policy related to food and nutrition in developing countries. INF's collaboration has steadily expanded to other agencies, such as IUNS, several UN and bilateral agencies, and non-Government organizations. In honor of Dr. Nevin Scrimshaw and his tireless contributions to international nutrition research, programming and capacity building, the INF was renamed in 2009 as, the **Nevin Scrimshaw International Nutrition Foundation.**

The mission of the INF is to raise the priority and profile of nutrition, within developmental goals of low-income populations, by identifying critical issues, shaping debate, educating future leadership and, therefore, promoting dissemination of critical knowledge.

Vision of the INF

INF's vision is to contribute to the realization of a world, which every person has the right:

- To good nutrition,
- To support infant, and childhood growth and development,
- Educational performance,
- Economic productivity and
- Health.

NATIONAL AGENCIES

NATIONAL COUNCIL OF INDIA'S NUTRITION CHALLENGES

National Council of India's Nutrition Challenges (NCINC-NITI Aayog) is the apex body formed by the Ministry of Women and Child Development. It is chaired by the Vice Chairperson of the NITI Aayog.

- NCINC formulates overall policies and guidelines
- Monitors all nutrition-based schemes, highlighting a life-cycle approach.
- Coordinates and reviews convergence among Ministries for providing policy directions to address India's nutritional challenges.

NATIONAL INSTITUTE OF PUBLIC COOPERATION AND CHILD DEVELOPMENT

National Institute of Public Cooperation and Child Development (NIPCCD) was established in 1966, under the Ministry of Women and Child Development. In order to cater the region-specific requirements of the country, NIPCCD, over a period of time, has established four regional centres at Guwahati (1978), Bangalore (1980), Lucknow (1982) and Indore (2001).

NIPCCD functions as an apex institution for the training of the functionaries of the Integrated Child Protection Scheme (ICDS) program. As a nodal resource agency, it has also been entrusted with the responsibility of training and capacity-building of functionaries at the national and regional levels, under the ICDS. It has also been designated by the Ministry of Women and Child Development as a nodal institution for imparting training on issues of Child Rights and Prevention of trafficking of women and children for SAARC countries.

NIPCCD is devoted to the promotion of voluntary action, research, training and documentation in the overall domain of women and child development.

FOOD AND NUTRITION BOARD

Food and Nutrition Board (Ministry of Women and Child Development, Govt. of India) was set up in 1964. It is an attached office of the Ministry of Women and Child

Development, and has a countrywide set up. Originally with Ministry of Food, the FNB was shifted to Ministry of Women and Child Development (then Department of WCD) in 1993. Nutrition is the focal point of health and well-being. Nutrition is directly linked to human resource development, productivity and ultimately to the national growth.

Food and Nutrition Board comprises a technical wing at the Centre, 4 Regional Offices and Quality Control Laboratories at Delhi, Mumbai, Kolkata and Chennai and 43 Community Food and Nutrition Extension Units (CFNEUs) located in 29 States/UTs. However, there is no CFNEU in the States Uttarakhand, Tripura, Nagaland, Trivandrum and UTs of Lakshadweep and Daman and Diu.

Activities of Food and Nutrition Board

Activities of Food and Nutrition Board include:

- Nutrition Education and Training, both for the masses and for ICDS functionaries,
- Mass Nutrition Awareness Campaigns,
- Development, production and distribution of nutrition education and training material,
- Training in Home Scale Preservation of Fruits and Vegetables, and Nutrition,
- Development and Promotion of locally available Nutritious Foods,
- Food Analysis and Standardization,
- Follow-up action on National Nutrition Policy.

NATIONAL INSTITUTE OF NUTRITION

The National Institute of Nutrition **(NIN)** is an Indian Public Health, Nutrition and Translational Research Center, located in Hyderabad, India. The institute is one of the oldest research centers in India, and the largest center, under the **Indian Council of Medical Research.**

- The Institute was founded in 1918, for the study of Beriberi, and was called the **Beriberi enquiry unit.**
- The scope of the laboratory was expanded to include all deficiency diseases, and in 1928-29, it became the **Nutrition Research Laboratories** (NRL).
- The facility moved to Hyderabad in 1958, and in 1969 it was renamed the **National Institute of Nutrition.**
- The institute carries out research and patent development in various fields, including clinical nutrition.
- WHO and FAO have recognized NIN as a **Centre for excellence** in food quality, safety and nutrition research.
- NIN also offers **advanced education courses** and PhD program(s) for nutrition, biochemistry, dietetics and laboratory animal sciences, and is recognized by various Universities for pursuing higher education in various streams of Life Sciences, especially, Nutrition and Biochemistry.

Some of the Achievements of NIN Include

- **Assessed dietary intake** of individuals, households and nutritional profiles of different communities, **through periodic surveys** of NNMB in various states.
- **Commercially delivered** double fortified Salt, Tata Salt Plus, is an **iodine plus iron fortified salt,** developed by double fortification technology.
- **Exploded the protein myth** and **highlighted calorie gap,** as the major bottleneck **for healthy growth of children.**
- **Developed** simple and **sensitive biochemical indicators,** for assessment of vitamin nutritive and pathogenic mechanisms, **of various nutritional deficiency syndromes.**
- **Emphasized the importance of growth monitoring,** for early diagnosis and appropriate management of protein energy malnutrition.

- **Generated database on nutritive values of** over 650 **Indian foods,** which is used by various national organizations, planners and academic research institutions.
- **Formulated** Recommended Dietary Allowances **(RDA) for Indians.**
- **Developed** food based **Dietary Guidelines for Indians.**
- **Developed National Nutrition Surveillance system** (NSS - Triple A cycle of Assessment, Analysis and Action), to serve as an early warning system about nutrition problems.

NATIONAL NUTRITION MONITORING BUREAU

The National Nutrition Monitoring Bureau **(NNMB)** was established under the aegis of Indian Council of Medical Research in the year 1972, with the Central Reference Laboratory at the National Institute of Nutrition (NIN), Hyderabad. The Bureau is currently in operation in the States of Andhra Pradesh, Gujarat, Karnataka, Kerala, Madhya Pradesh, Maharashtra, Orissa, Tamil Nadu, Uttar Pradesh and West Bengal.

The Bureau **carries out surveys** under the guidance of a Steering Committee and has been **generating dynamic database on diet and nutritional status** of the communities, regularly, since 1975.

Objectives of the NNMB

- **To collect,** on a continuous basis, on representative segments of population in each of the states, **data on dietary pattern and nutritional status,** adopting standardized and uniform procedures and techniques, and
- **To periodically evaluate the ongoing National Nutrition Programmes,** to identify their strengths and weaknesses, and to recommend appropriate corrective measures.

CENTRAL FOOD TECHNOLOGICAL RESEARCH INSTITUTE

Central Food Technological Research Institute (CFTRI) is one of the constituent laboratories under the aegis of the **Council of Scientific and Industrial Research (CSIR),** established in 1950, in Mysore, Karnataka. There are sixteen research and development departments, including laboratories focusing on food engineering, food biotechnology, grain sciences, Biochemistry, Molecular Nutrition and food safety.

- CFTRI is one of the prime leaders to **generate and apply knowledge of food science and technology** for optimal conservation and utilization of nation's food resources.
- The institute is engaged in **research in the production and handling of grains, pulses, oilseeds, spices, fruits, vegetables, meat, fish and poultry.**
- The institute **develops technologies to increase efficiency and reduce post-harvest losses,** add convenience, increase export, find new sources of food products, integrate human resources in food industries, reduce costs, and modernize.
- CFTRI has **developed over 300 products,** processes including equipment designs, and most of these technologies have been released to over 4000 licensees for commercial exploitation.
- The institute has played an **important role in areas of human resource development** and R&D partnerships, by having international linkages with institutions, such as the Institute of Food Technologists (USA), UN University (Tokyo), European Economic Commission (Belgium) and National Science Foundation (USA).
- The institute offers **Master of Science (Food Technology) course.**

SOME IMPORTANT QUESTIONS

1. **Describe various International and National agencies working for food and nutrition in India.**
2. **Describe:**
   i. International agencies working for food and nutrition in India.
   ii. National agencies working for food and nutrition in India.
3. **Describe the role of the following agencies towards food and nutrition in India:**
   i. Food and Agriculture Organization (FAO)
   ii. United Nations Children's Fund (UNICEF)
   iii. UN-Nutrition
   iv. Co-operative for assistance and relief everywhere (CARE)
   v. International Union of Nutritional Sciences (IUNS)
   vi. International nutrition foundation (INF)
   vii. Food and Nutrition Board
   viii. National Institute of Nutrition
   ix. National Nutrition Monitoring Bureau (NNMB)
   x. Central Food Technological Research Institute (CFTRI)

CHAPTER

22

Assessment of Nutritional Status

The **nutritional status** of an individual is usually a result of multiple factors that interact with each other at different levels. These include:

- The consumption of adequate amount of food, both, in terms of quantity and quality is one of the key determinants, which has a significant impact on the nutritional status.
- Furthermore, the eating pattern of an individual is a crucial factor that dictates the occurrence of a disease, especially, some chronic conditions, such as coronary heart disease, hypertension, stroke, diabetes mellitus and cancer.
- In addition, adverse outcomes, such as low birth weight, malnutrition, disability, poor quality of life and mortality, are also related to poor eating pattern, in both developed and developing countries.

Recognizing the role of diet at onset of many diseases and assessing nutritional status of an individual, family and community are important for public health.

Assessment of nutritional status involves measurement of nutritional health of the body. It is a routine part of nutritional care of the individual, since both, undernutrition and overnutrition may affect health. It is done to obtain information about the prevalence and geographic distribution of nutritional disorders within a community or a specified population group. Nutrition assessment can also be used to identify high-risk groups and to assess the role of different epidemiological factors in nutritional deficiencies.

Significance of Assessment of Nutrition Status

Assessment of nutritional status serves a variety of purposes:

1. Nutrition assessment helps **to evaluate nutrition-related risks** that may affect current, or future, health of an individual
2. It is a routine part of **nutrition care of the hospitalized patients,** including effectiveness of treatment.
3. Nutrition assessment helps **identify people in need of nutrition-related interventions** and to monitor effectiveness of such programs.
4. It also determines **nutritional health of population,** to identify common health risks in a population group.

METHODS OF ASSESSMENT OF NUTRITIONAL STATUS

Nutritional assessment can be done using the **ABCD** methods. These refer to the following, i.e.:

- A (Anthropometry)
- B (Biochemical methods)

- C (Clinical methods)
- D (Dietary methods)

ANTHROPOMETRIC MEASUREMENTS FOR ASSESSMENT OF NUTRITIONAL STATUS

The word **anthropometry** comes from two words, i.e. *Anthropo* means **human** and *metry* means **measurement**. Thus, anthropometry allows for assessment of different component parts of the human body, i.e. the anatomical makeup of the body in terms of bone, muscle, water and fat. Since a single measure will not provide a comprehensive overview of an individual's condition, so a number of measurements are done to make a reasonable assessment.

Anthropometric measurements include measurement of physical characteristics of the body, such as weight, length/height, mid upper arm circumference and skin fold thickness. In young children, head and chest circumference are also measured, to assess patterns of growth and development.

Weight

A weighing sling (spring balance), also called the **Salter scale,** is used for measuring the weight of children under two years old, to the nearest 0.1 kg. In adults and children over two years a beam balance is used and the measurement is to the nearest 0.1 kg. Weight is a measure to assess child's growth, predict energy expenditure and protein needs and determine body composition. Sudden change in weight, in growing children, reflects a disease and monitors progress in fat loss, e.g. in cancer or thyroid disorders.

Height

This is measured with the child, or adult, in a standing position (usually children who are two years old or more; for infants and young children, it is the measurement of recumbent length). The head should be in a position where the line passing from the external ear hole to the lower eye lid is parallel to the floor (referred to as the **Frankfurt position**) during measurement, and the shoulders, buttocks and the heels should touch the vertical stand. Either a stadiometer or a portable anthropometer can be used for measuring the height and measurements are recorded to the nearest millimetre. Comparison with the standard growth charts shows how growth of the child is comparable to that of others of the same age and sex.

Upper Mid-Arm Circumference

Upper mid-arm circumference is an accurate way to measure fat-free mass (muscle mass). It is the circumference of the upper arm at the midway between the shoulder tip and the elbow tip on the left arm. The mid-arm point is determined by measuring the distance from the shoulder tip to the elbow and dividing it by two. A low reading indicates a loss of muscle mass. A special tape is used for measuring the mid-upper arm circumference of a child. The tape has three colours, with the red indicating severe acute malnutrition, the yellow indicating moderate acute malnutrition and the green indicating normal nutritional status.

Skin-fold Thickness

Measurement of skin-fold thickness is a method to estimate thickness of a fold of skin and subcutaneous fat with a caliper. It provides an indication of fatness of the body, since a significant amount of body's fat store lies just beneath the skin.

Head Circumference

The head circumference is the measurement of the head along the forehead **(supra-orbital ridge),** anteriorly, and the prominent area on the back part of the head **(occipital prominence),** posteriorly. It is measured to the nearest millimetre using flexible, non-stretchable measuring tape, around 0.6 cm wide. Head circumference is useful in assessing chronic nutritional problems in children under two years old, as the brain grows faster during the first two years of life.

Body Mass Index

Body mass index (BMI) is the weight of a person in kg divided by their height in metres squared, i.e.

$$BMI = Weight (kg)/(Height in metres)^2$$

An adult is considered to have a normal BMI, when it falls between 18.5 and 25 kg/m^2 (Table 22.1).

Table 22.1: Nutritional status based on BMI

BMI (kg/m^2)	*Nutritional status*
<16.0	Severe chronic energy deficiency
16.0–18.49	Chronic energy deficiency
18.5–24.9	**Normal**
25–29.9	Overweight
30.0–40.0	Obese
>40.0	Very obese

If an adult person has a BMI of less than 16 kg/m^2, they will have very poor energy stores. If BMI increases to over 25 kg/m^2, the person is overweight.

BIOCHEMICAL METHODS FOR ASSESSMENT OF NUTRITIONAL STATUS

Assessment of nutritional status by biochemical methods refers to laboratory estimations that measure the quantity of a particular nutrient, or its metabolite, in one or more body fluids, such as blood, urine or feces, e.g. estimation of serum albumin concentration, as an indicator of protein status of the body. Biochemical measurements of the metabolites, storage or transported compounds, or enzymes are better indicators of nutritional status, than directly measuring the blood level of a particular nutrient, such as vitamin A or calcium.

Biochemical investigations are extremely helpful in detecting early changes in body metabolism and nutritional status, before the appearance of overt clinical signs. In addition, the biochemical test results are precise, accurate and reproducible. Common laboratory investigations, include:

- Routine examination of stool, urine and blood, and X-ray.
- Estimation of haemoglobin (Hb), serum proteins and enzymes
- Blood level of nutrients, such as vitamins, iron, amino acids, etc.

CLINICAL METHODS FOR ASSESSMENT OF NUTRITIONAL STATUS

Clinical observations mean assessment by evaluating characteristics of well being that can be seen in a physical examination. Some nonspecific clinical signs provide clue to nutrient deficiency, or excess, that can be confirmed, or ruled out, by further biochemical tests, e.g. wasting of muscle or obesity.

Clinical methods of assessing nutritional status are essential feature of all nutritional surveys, as their primary goal is to assess the health status of individuals, or groups, within a population, in accordance with the type of food consumed. Presence of two or more clinical signs, of a specific nutritional deficiency, increases the diagnostic significance. However, its limitation is that it cannot quantify the exact level of nutrient deficiency, because most of the clinical signs, for nutrient deficiency, are nonspecific and require biochemical analysis to know the nutritional status of the particular nutrient.

Clinical methods of assessing nutritional status involve checking signs and symptoms of deficiency, at specific places on the body, or asking the patient whether they have any symptoms, that might suggest nutrient deficiency. Clinical observations assess changes in skin color and health, hair texture, finger nail shape, eyes, lips, mouth, bones, muscles and joints. There may be some specific clinical findings depicting the deficiency of a particular nutrient, e.g. hemorrhages on the skin (indicative of vitamin C deficiency), cracking at corners of mouth (suggestive of riboflavin, B6 and niacin deficiency), etc. Clinical signs of nutrient deficiency include pallor (on the palm of the hand or the conjunctiva of the eye), pitting oedema, severe visible wasting, Bitot's spots on the eyes or swelling on the neck, etc. (Table 22.2).

Table 22.2: Clinical signs and symptoms of some common nutritional problems

Nutritional deficiency disease	*Signs/symptoms*
Anaemia, may be due to the deficiency of iron, folic acid, vitamin B_{12}, copper, protein of vitamin B_6	Pale palms, conjunctiva and tongue, gets tired easily, loss of appetite and shortness of breath
Vitamin A deficiency	Bitot's spots (whitish patchy triangular lesions on the side of the eye)
Iodine deficiency disorder	Goiter (swelling on the front of the neck)

Bitot's spots: These are the sign of vitamin A deficiency. These spots are a creamy color and appear on the white portion of the eye (Fig. 9.3).

Goitre: Goitre is a swelling on the neck and is the only visible sign of iodine deficiency (Fig. 10.4).

Clinical examination also includes **assessment of associated problems,** like tuberculosis, malabsorption syndrome, any infection or infestation, etc.

DIETARY METHODS FOR ASSESSMENT OF NUTRITIONAL STATUS

Dietary methods of nutritional assessment include asking for information about past or current intake of nutrients from food by individuals, or a group. An estimation of the total daily calorie intake as well as overall quality of diet, thus, can be assessed. For this purpose, information from patients (or their family, if the patient is unable to explain) about their daily dietary intake helps understand patterns of eating, portion sizes, cooking methods, and types of food and drink is collected. The collected information, thereafter, is evaluated for a lack, or excess, of some dietary component, a nutrient or total food intake. It is a record of food intake and eating behavior that includes recent and long-term habits of food consumption. It is done to evaluate a diet for nutrients (e.g. fat, calcium or protein) or consumption of a particular type of food (e.g. number of fruits and vegetables). Dietary intake data may be collected from diet history and/or food records.

- **Diet history:** Dietary history, done by a skilled interviewer, is a most comprehensive form of dietary intake's data collection.
- **Food records:** It provides detailed information about day-to-day eating habits, which, typically, include all foods and beverages consumed during a defined period, usually, for a few consecutive days.

Such data are compared to the established standards, to diagnose nutritional deficiencies, identify dietary inadequacies or evaluate progress as a result of dietary changes. One can seek the information about what the family, or the mother and the child, have consumed over the past 24 hours and, thereafter, use the data to calculate dietary diversity score.

Assessment of dietary intake includes:

- Detailed history of dietary pattern
- Specific food consumed and its amount
- Quality and adequacy of food, in relation of nutrient value

Dietary survey is a scientific assessment of eating pattern that could detect nutrient deficiency. There are many methods to do dietary surveys:

- The **food balance sheet** could aid the program managers to decide the dietary needs of a region or a state or a country. It is obtained by subtracting the amount of food provided for a specified group of population on a specific date and the amount remaining after a previously set time limit, to finally establish the consumption/requirement of food commodities for the earmarked population in that specified arbitrary period.

- The **inventory method** is based on a similar rationale as food balanced sheet except the study population is usually a group of a homogenous population, such as hostel.
- The **weighed food records method** is employed at household level to estimate the food requirement, by weighing either raw food or cooked food for 7–10 days, for a particular family, in a specified period.
- The **24 h recall method** is employed at household level to assess the type of food and the quantities consumed in the last 24 h.
- The **food frequency questionnaire method** helps in assessing meal patterns and dietary habits of people by identifying number of times a specific food item is consumed in a defined time span.

Food balance sheet method and inventory method are similar and the only difference is the settings, e.g. food balance sheet at the state/national level, whereas inventory method at the institutional level, are, generally, considered applicable. However, the other three methods are used at household level, to assess the amount of food consumed/dietary patterns of members of a family in a specified period.

SOME IMPORTANT QUESTIONS

1. Define nutrition status. Describe various methods of the assessment of nutritional status.

2. Write notes on:

i. Nutritional status
ii. Assessment of nutritional status
iii. Anthropometric methods of assessment of nutritional status
iv. Biochemical methods of assessment of nutritional status
v. Clinical methods of assessment of nutritional status
vi. Dietary methods of assessment of nutritional status
vii. Body mass index

CHAPTER

23

Nutrition Education and Role of a Nurse

People in the community show their lack of knowledge about nutrition, when they make poor food choices. Besides, a large proportion of the patients, in the community, suffer from malnutrition. Malnutrition occurs when an individual's nutrients intake falls short of metabolic requirements. This, in turn, can cause weight loss, heart dysfunction, a weak immune system or decreased wound healing. Thus, everyone should be encouraged to eat nutritionally balanced meals, throughout the day.

Nutrition education is essential for everyone. It is a key issue for healthcare professionals in every setting, may be in a hospital, nursing home or community, since the nutritional state of the patient can affect his/her outcome from illness and during recovery. Thus, it should be viewed as an integral and central component of patient's care, irrespective of the patient's physical diagnosis, condition, age or psychological status. To effectively manage and prevent malnutrition, it is important to recognize the barriers to nutritional care for patients, since inadequate nutrition can lead to an increase in hospitalization and mortality.

ROLE OF A NURSE IN NUTRITION EDUCATION

Role of a nurse in nutritional care of patients is extremely diverse.

- The nurse, as a nutrition educator, has a vital role in the overall healthcare system.
- Nurses working in all branches, encounter people requiring nutritional screening, assessment, planning and implementation. For example, a number of people with learning disabilities require eternal feeding, via a gastric tube. Similarly, obesity management is a significant part of the learning disability of a nurse.
- In the mental health setting, poor appetite and dietary intakes are associated with many mental health problems.
- The nurse's role in nutrition is also to educate patient about good nutrition to promote health. A failure to address the issue of nutrition is failure of duty of the nurse to protect health of the patient.
- Pre-hospital nursing has the opportunity to provide nutrition education and can help to preserve health of all populations, particularly, older adults.
- In hospital environment, nurses are also obliged to make observations about physical status, food intake, weight change and response to therapy.

SOME IMPORTANT QUESTION

1. Describe the role of a nurse in nutrition education.

Definitions

Absorption: Movement of substances into or across the tissues, in particular the passage of nutrients and other substances into the walls of the GIT and from there into the bloodstream.

Acceptable Macronutrient Distribution Ranges: AMDR refers to a range of macronutrient intake that is associated with the reduced risk of chronic diseases but provides adequate intakes of essential nutrients. It is usually expressed as a percentage of energy.

Active Transport: Movement of substances into, or out of cell, against a concentration gradient. It requires energy in the form of ATP and a carrier (transport) protein that is present in the cell membrane.

Adequate Intake (AI) or Safe Intake (SI) refers to the recommended average daily intake level based on observed or experimentally determined approximations or estimates of nutrient intake by a group of apparently healthy people that are assumed to be adequate.

Aflatoxins: Toxic and may be carcinogenic factors that are produced by molds that may be present in food.

Alpha-linolenic acid (α-linolenic acid): An 18-carbon fatty acid with three double bonds. Since the first double bond is present on the third carbon atom from the methyl-end (ω-carbon), therefore, α-linolenic acid is called as ω-3 (n-3) fatty acid.

Amino acids: Fundamental building block of proteins.

Anabolism: The process by which complex materials in tissues and organs are built up from simple substances.

Anemia: A clinical condition with abnormally low concentration of hemoglobin in blood stream. It may be a result of impaired synthesis of red blood cells, their increased destruction or significant loss of blood from the body.

Anorexia nervosa: An eating disorder marked by prolonged decrease of appetite and refusal to eat, leading to self-starvation. It results, in part, from a distorted body image and intense fear of becoming fat, often linked to social pressure.

Anorexia of aging: Loss of appetite and muscle wasting associated with old age.

Anthropometric measurements: Physical characteristics of the body such as height, weight, head circumference, girth and skin-fold thickness. These parameters are, particularly, useful in evaluating growth of infants, children and adolescents, and in determining their body composition.

Antioxidants: A group of substances that prevent the damage caused by the oxidation of fatty acids and proteins by oxygen free radicals.

Anti-rachitic factor: An agent, which is used to treat rickets, i.e. vitamin D.

Appetite: A psychological desire to eat. It is related to pleasant sensations often associated with food.

Artificial sweeteners: Substances which impart sweetness to food but supplies a little or no energy to the body, e.g. aspartame, saccharin, sucralose, etc.

Atherosclerosis: Gradual deposition of fatty material and fibrous tissues in the inner lining of arteries with eventual obstruction of blood flow.

Atrophic gastritis: An age-related condition in which stomach loses its ability to secrete acid. In severe cases, its ability to make intrinsic factor is also impaired.

Avidin: A protein found in raw egg-white that binds biotin, thereby preventing the absorption of biotin. Avidin can be destroyed by heat.

Balanced diet: A diet containing all the essential (macro and micro) nutrients in optimum quantities and appropriate proportions that meets the requirement.

Basal metabolic rate (BMR): A clinical measure of resting energy expenditure that is performed upon awakening, usually, after 10 to 12 hours of eating and 12 to 18 hours after significant physical activity. It is often used interchangeably with resting metabolic rate (RMR).

Beriberi: Thiamin deficiency disease with symptoms of muscle weakness, loss of appetite, nerve degeneration and edema in some cases.

Beta-carotene (β-carotene): A yellow-orange plant pigment which yields vitamin A after its oxidation in the body.

Beta-oxidation (β-oxidation): The process of breakdown of fatty acids into two-carbon compound called acetyl coenzyme A (acetyl-CoA).

Bifidus factor: A substance present in human milk which stimulates growth of a micro-organism (*Lactobacillus bifidus*) in infants' intestine.

Bile: An alkaline yellow-green fluid produced in the liver and stored in the gall bladder. Primary constituents of bile include bile acids, phospholipids, cholesterol and bicarbonate. It emulsifies dietary lipids and helps in digestion and absorption of fat.

Biological value of protein: It refers to the extent to which dietary protein can be incorporated into body proteins. Biological value is expressed as percentage of the absorbed dietary nitrogen to that retained in the body.

Body mass index (BMI): Body weight in relation to height, i.e. the body weight in kilograms divided by the square of height in meters. Its value is expressed as kg/m^2.

Bolus: Chewed-moistened lump of food that is ready to be swallowed.

Bomb calorimeter: An instrument which is used to measure energy content of food.

Calorie: A unit which is used to indicate energy value of food. Quantitative requirement of energy is expressed in terms of calories (kilocalories or kcals). Newer unit for energy is kilojoules (kJ).

Calorimeter: A device used to measure quantity of heat generated by the various processes.

Calorimetry: Measurement of the amount of heat given off by an organism. It is used to determine total energy expenditure.

Carotenoids: A group of yellow, orange and red pigments found in plant foods. Many of these compounds are precursors of vitamin A.

Catabolism: The process of the breakdown of complex organic constituents in smaller fragments in the body.

Cataract: Opacity of the lens of the eye, resulting in impaired vision.

Celiac disease: A disease that involves inability to digest gluten (a protein found in wheat, rye, oat and barley). If untreated, it causes flattening of the villi in the intestine leading to severe malabsorption of nutrients. Its symptoms include diarrhea, fatty stool, swollen belly and extreme fatigue.

Cellulose: A straight-chain polysaccharide composed of large number of glucose units which are linked together by β-glycosidic bonds. It is indigestible by human and is a component of insoluble dietary fiber.

Cheilosis: Refers to cracking of skin at the corners of the mouth and inflammation of the lips.

Cholesterol: A lipid constituent of blood and tissues that may be obtained from diet as well as is synthesized in the body.

Cirrhosis: Inflammation and scarring of liver tissues resulting in impaired liver function.

Collagen: A most abundant fibrous protein present in the body and is a major constituent of the connective tissue. It forms foundation for the bone and teeth, and helps in maintaining structures of the blood vessels and other tissues.

Colostrum: Milk produced by mammals during the first few days after delivery.

Complementary proteins: Two or more incomplete food proteins whose assortment of amino acids makeup for, or complement each other, lack of specific essential amino acids in the way that the combination provides sufficient amounts of all the essential amino acids to the body.

Complete protein: A protein that supplies all the essential amino acids to the body.

Coronary heart disease: A disease of the heart due to inadequate blood supply as a result of narrowing/obstruction of the coronary arteries which nourish heart muscle.

Congenital anomalies: Deformities existing at birth or even before.

Cretinism: A congenital condition often caused by the severe deficiency of iodine during gestation. It is characterized by retarded physical and mental development.

Cystic fibrosis: An inherited disorder that causes widespread dysfunction of the exocrine glands, resulting in a chronic lung disease, with abnormally high levels of electrolytes (Na^+, K^+ and Cl^-) in sweat, and the deficiency of pancreatic enzymes needed for digestion.

Dental caries: Destruction of the enamel surface of teeth caused by acids, resulting from bacterial breakdown of sugar in the mouth.

Diabetes mellitus: A clinical condition in which blood glucose concentration is increased and the body tissues cannot utilise glucose properly.

Dietary fiber: Dietary fiber refers to indigestible carbohydrates, such as cellulose and hemicellulose, pectin, lignin, etc. which cannot be digested by human beings due to absence of the required digestive enzymes. Dietary fiber promote healthy bowel movement and decreases risk of several chronic diseases such as coronary heart disease and diabetes.

Dietary supplement: A product taken orally that contains a dietary ingredient which may include vitamins, minerals, herbs or amino acids as well as other substances such as enzymes, organ tissues, metabolites, extracts or concentrates.

Digestion: The process of transforming the food we eat into smaller units for absorption.

Digestive secretions: Substances released in different parts in the GIT to speed up breakdown of ingested carbohydrates, fats and proteins, into smaller components which can be easily absorbed by the body.

Direct calorimetry: Estimation of energy consumption by the body, by measuring the quantity of heat released from an organism enclosed in an insulated chamber that is surrounded by water. In this technique rise in the temperature of water is directly proportional to the quantity of energy consumed by that organism.

Diverticular disease: Presence of several pouches or sac-like protrusions on the wall lining the intestine.

Eating disorder: A spectrum of abnormal eating pattern that eventually may endanger a person's health, or increase the risk of some other disease.

Edema: Swelling caused by the build-up of fluid between the cells.

Empty calories: Foods which provide only energy without any other nutrient, e.g. white sugar and alcohol.

Energy: It is the capacity to do work. Energy in food is the chemical energy which our body converts into mechanical, electrical or heat energy.

Energy balance: The balance in the body between the amount of the energy consumed to that what is expended.

Energy intake: Caloric or energy content of the food provided by all the dietary sources of energy, i.e. carbohydrates (4 kcal/g), proteins (4 kcal/g) and lipids (9 kcal/g).

Energy output: Use of calories or energy by the body for basic body functions, physical activities and processing of the food consumed.

Enzymes: Biological catalysts which enhance rate of the chemical reactions in the body.

Essential fatty acids (EFA): Polyunsaturated fatty acids (PUFA), i.e. linoleic acid and alpha linolenic acid, which are not synthesized by the human body. These have to be supplied through the diet.

Estimated Average Requirement: Estimated Average Requirement **(EAR)**, also called Average Nutrient Requirement (ANR) **refers to the average daily nutrient intake level** estimated **to meet the requirements of half of the healthy individuals in a particular life stage and gender group.** It is the nutrient requirement used in public health nutrition to evaluate the nutrients intakes of a population or group. EAR has been recommended, in alignment with global recommendations, **for population requirement/adequacy estimations and menu or diet planning for individuals.**

Fasting hypoglycemia: A type of hypoglycemia that occurs because the body produces too much of insulin even when no food is eaten. Pancreatic tumor can cause fasting hypoglycemia.

Fat substitutes: These are the compounds that imitate functional and sensory properties of fat but contain less available energy than fat.

Fatty acids: Fundamental constituents of many lipids such as triacylglycerols (triglycerides), phospholipids, etc.

Fatty liver: A clinical condition due to the accumulation of fat (triacylglycerols) in the liver due to the increased synthesis of triacylglycerols.

Ferritin: A complex of iron and apoferritin. It is a major storage form of iron.

Flavonoids: Pigments widely distributed in nature in flowers, fruits and vegetables.

Fluorosis: Mottled discoloration and pitting of tooth enamel caused by prolonged ingestion of excessive fluoride.

Food: Food supply all the essential nutrients and provides a host of other components (non-nutrient phytochemicals) which have a positive impact on health.

Food additives: Substances which are added to the food to perform various functions, such as the addition of some preservative, color, flavor, sugar or fat to improve shelf-life, texture or nutritional value of the food.

Food exchange: Food is classified into different groups which can be exchanged depending upon the availability and needs. Each exchange list includes a number of measured foods of similar nutritive value that can be substituted interchangeably in a meal plan.

Food guide pyramid: A graphic representation of the number of servings from the five major food groups which should be consumed daily, to form a healthy diet. However, the group consisting of fat and oils, and desserts should be consumed sparingly.

Free radicals: Highly reactive oxygen species that are formed in the body during normal metabolic processes. These have the capacity to damage cellular macromolecules by oxidation.

Galactosemia: An inherited disorder of galactose metabolism marked by high level of galactose in blood.

Gestational diabetes: A clinical condition that results in high blood glucose concentration during pregnancy.

Glossitis: Glossitis refers to the inflammation of the tongue, primarily, a symptom of riboflavin deficiency.

Glycemic index: Glycemic index of a food refers the blood glucose response after consuming a carbohydrate consuming food relative to the consumption of the carbohydrate containing reference food, usually 50 g of available carbohydrate from glucose or white bread.

Glycemic load: Glycemic load refers to the glycemic index in relation to total amount of the available carbohydrate present in the food which is to be consumed.

Goiter: A chronic enlargement of the thyroid gland which is visible as a swelling at the front of the neck, primarily, associated with iodine deficiency.

Goitrogen: A compound that produces goiter by blocking synthesis of the thyroid hormones or increasing excretion of iodide.

Haemorrhoids: Commonly known as piles.

Head circumference: Measurement of the largest part of the infant's head (just above the eyebrow and ears). It is used to determine brain growth.

Hemicellulose: A group of large polysaccharides in dietary fiber that are fermented more easily than cellulose.

Hemochromatosis: A hereditary metabolic disorder where excessive absorption of iron results in its abnormal deposition in the liver and other tissue.

Hemosiderin: An insoluble form of storage of iron.

High-density lipoprotein (HDL): These transport cholesterol from extra-hepatic tissues to the liver. HDL is anti-atherogenic.

Hyperlipidemia: Increased concentration of blood lipids (triglycerides and cholesterol).

Hormones: Substances produced by a gland (endocrine) which are secreted directly into the blood stream, to produce specific effect on another organ.

Hunger: Internal physiological drive to find and consume food, i.e. the urge to eat. Unlike appetite, hunger is often experienced as a negative sensation generally manifesting as an uneasy or painful sensation.

Hypercalcemia: Increased level of blood calcium that causes deposition of calcium in soft tissues and affects the nervous system. It is caused by various conditions including excess vitamin D intakes.

Hypoglycemia: Abnormally low concentration of blood glucose, generally below 40 to 50 mg/dl.

Incomplete protein: Protein that lacks one or more essential amino acids. It is found in cereal grains and is also called a poor-quality protein.

Indirect calorimetry: Estimation of energy consumption by the body, without directly measuring the production of heat. Various methods used for include gas exchange, the measurement of oxygen uptake and/or carbon dioxide output, and the doubly-labeled water method.

Infancy: Infancy refers to the period from birth to 12 month of age.

Insensible water loss: It refers to the continual loss of body water by evaporation from the respiratory tract and diffusion through the skin.

Insoluble fiber: These are dietary fiber components that do not dissolve in water, including cellulose, lignin and some hemicelluloses.

Intermediate density lipoprotein (IDL): The lipoprotein formed when lipoprotein lipase strips some of the triglycerides from VLDL. It contains about 40% triglycerides. This is denser than VLDL but less dense than LDL. It is also called VLDL remnants.

Interstitial fluid: Interstitial fluid refers to the fluid between cells in tissues.

Intracellular fluid: Intracellular fluid refers to the fluid in the body's cells. It is usually high in potassium and phosphate but low in sodium and chloride. It constitutes about two-thirds of total body water.

Intravascular fluid: The fluid portion of the blood (plasma) contained in arteries, veins and capillaries. It accounts for about 15% of the extracellular fluid.

Intrinsic factor: A glycoprotein released from parietal cells in the stomach wall that binds to and aids in the absorption of vitamin B_{12}.

Invisible fats: Fat present as an integral component of plant and animal foods such as in cereals, legumes and spices.

Iodine deficiency disorders (IDD): These include a wide range of disorders that affect growth and development due to iodine deficiency.

Iodospin: Color-sensitive pigmented molecules in cone cells that consist of opsin like proteins combined with retinal.

Ischaemia: Lack of blood supply to an organ or tissue resulting in reduced oxygen supply, caused either by constriction or obstruction of the blood vessel.

Kilocalorie: Kilocalorie is a unit of energy. Food energy is measured in kilocalories (1 kilocalorie = 1000 calories).

Kwashiorkor: This is a type of malnutrition that occurs primarily in young children who have an infectious disease and whose diets supply very little protein. Common symptoms include poor growth, edema, apathy, weakness and susceptibility to infections.

Lactoferrin: Minor protein of milk containing iron.

Lactose intolerance: Disorder resulting from improper digestion of milk sugar called lactose, due to lack of an enzyme, lactase, in the intestinal mucosa.

Laxative: Laxative is a substance that promotes evacuation of the bowel by increasing the bulk of the feces, lubricating the intestinal wall and softening the stool.

Lean body mass: This is the portion of the body, exclusive of stored fat, including muscle, bone, connective tissue, organs and water.

Leptin: A hormone produced by adipose cells that signals the amount of body fat content and influences food intake.

Limiting amino acid: A limiting amino acid is an amino acid that is in shortest supply during protein synthesis. It is the amino acid in the lowest quantity when evaluating protein quality.

Linoleic acid: Fatty acid containing 18 carbon atoms and two double bonds. The first double bond is on the sixth carbon atom from the methyl end. Therefore, it is called n-6 fatty acid and is abbreviated as 18:2 n-6.

Lipids: A technical term for fats. They are important dietary constituents. The group includes triglycerides, steroids, cholesterol and other complex lipids.

Lipoproteins: Lipids are not soluble in blood; they are therefore transported as lipid and protein complexes.

Low birth weight infant: Low birth weight infant is a newborn who weighs less than 2500 g, as a result of either premature birth or inadequate growth *in utero*.

Low density lipoprotein (LDL): These transport cholesterol from the liver to tissues. High blood levels indicate that more cholesterol is being transported to tissues.

Lower reference nutrient intake (LRNI) or lower threshold intake (LTI) refers to a value derived from ANR/EAR and is calculated as the ANR/EAR minus 2SD of the distribution of requirements. This value is sufficient to meet the need of the bottom 2% of the individuals.

Macrocytic anemia: Anemia characterized by red blood cells which are larger than normal.

Macronutrients: Nutrients like carbohydrates, proteins and fats which are required in large quantities.

Malnutrition: Malnutrition means failure to achieve nutrient requirements, which can impair physical and/or mental health. It may result from consuming too little food or a shortage or imbalance of key nutrients.

Marasmus: Marasmus is a type of malnutrition resulting from chronic protein energy undernutrition. It is characterized by wasting of muscle and other body tissues.

Megaloblastic anemia: Excess amounts of megaloblasts in the blood caused by deficiency of folate or vitamin B_{12}.

Menke's syndrome: Menke's syndrome is a genetic disorder that results in copper deficiency.

Metabolism: Includes catabolism and anabolism.

Microcytic anemia: Anemia characterized by red blood cells which are smaller than normal.

Micronutrients: Nutrients which are required in small quantities, such as vitamins and trace elements.

Monounsaturated fatty acids: Unsaturated fatty acids with one double bond.

Negative energy balance: Periods of time in which energy intake is lower than energy expenditure, resulting in depletion of the body's energy stores.

Negative nitrogen balance: Nitrogen intake is less than the sum of all routes of nitrogen excretion.

Net protein utilization (NPU): It refers to the percentage of ingested protein nitrogen retained by the body. It measures the amount of dietary protein, the body uses.

Niacin equivalent (NE): A measure that includes preformed dietary niacin as well as niacin derived from tryptophan. Sixty mg of tryptophan yields 1 mg of niacin.

Night blindness: This is the inability of the eyes to adjust to dim light or to regain vision quickly after exposure to a flash of bright light.

Nitrogen balance: Nitrogen balance means nitrogen intake minus the sum of nitrogen excretion.

Nonheme iron: The iron in plants and animal foods that is not part of hemoglobin or myoglobin

Nutrients: Nutrients are the chemical substances in food that are needed by the body. They are divided into six classes, namely carbohydrates, fats, proteins, vitamins, minerals and water. Body can use them to obtain energy, synthesize tissues or regulate functions.

Nutrition: Nutrition refers to the processes in the body for making use of food. It includes eating the correct kind and amounts of food for the needs of the body, digestion of foods, so that the body can use the nutrients, their absorption into the bloodstream, their use by the cells in the body for the production of energy, maintenance and growth of cells, tissues and organs and elimination of waste.

Nutritional care: Nutritional care is the application of the art and science of nutrition to the feeding of people. It deals with the assessment of nutritional status, the planning of meals according to needs and its implementation, etc.

Nutrition assessment: Nutrition assessment is a measurement of nutritional health of the body. It can be determined by anthropometric measurements, biochemical tests, clinical observations and dietary intake as well as medical histories and socioeconomic factors.

Nutritional status: It is the condition of health and is related to the use of food by the body. Measures of nutritional status include changes in body weight, physical examination and biochemical tests.

Obesity: Obesity means excessive accumulation of body fat leading to a body weight in relation to height that is substantially greater than some accepted standards. Obesity that is characterized by body weight exceeding 100% of normal is referred to as morbid obesity. It is so severe a condition that it often requires surgery. Obesity due to an above average number of fat cells is called hypercellular obesity. Obesity due to an increase in the size of fat cells is known as hypertrophic obesity.

Omega-3 fatty acids: Polyunsaturated fatty acid in which the first double bond, starting from the methyl (CH_3^-) end of the molecule, lies between the third and fourth carbon atom, e.g. alpha-linolenic acid and its longer-chain polyunsaturated fatty acids. They are also referred to as n-3 PUFA.

Omega-6 fatty acids: Polyunsaturated fatty acid in which first double bond, starting from the methyl (CH_3^-) end, lies between the sixth and seventh carbon atom, e.g. linoleic acid and its longer chain polyunsaturated fatty acids. They are also referred to as n-6 PUFA.

Omega-9 fatty acid: Any polyunsaturated fatty acid in which the first double bond starting from the methyl (CH_3)-end lies between the ninth and tenth carbon atoms.

Osteoblasts: Bone cells that promote bone deposition and bone growth. They synthesize and excrete the extracellular matrix, which forms the bone structure.

Osteoclasts: Bone cells that promote bone resorption and calcium mobilization. They breakdown bone structure and release calcium and phosphate into the blood.

Osteomalacia: Osteomalacia refers to a disease in adults that results from vitamin D deficiency. It is marked by softening of bones leading to bending of the spine, bowing of legs and increased risk of fractures.

Osteoporosis: A condition of abnormal porousness or thinning of bones.

Over-nutrition: Over-nutrition means long term consumption of excess of nutrients. The most common type of over-nutrition is due to the regular consumption of excess kilocalories, fats, particularly saturated fats and cholesterol.

Pasteurization: Pasteurization is a process for destroying pathogenic bacteria by heating liquid food to a prescribed temperature for a specified time.

Pernicious anemia: It is due to the inability of the body to absorb vitamin B_{12}. Its hallmarks are excess megaloblasts and nerve degeneration that can result in paralysis and death.

Phytochemicals: Phytochemicals are substances present in plants that may possess health positive effects, even though they are not essential for life.

Phytosterols: Phytosterols are sterols found in plants. These are poorly absorbed by humans and reduce intestinal absorption of cholesterol.

Polyunsaturated fatty acids (PUFA): Unsaturated fatty acids with two or more double bonds.

Positive energy balance: Periods of time in which energy intake exceeds energy expenditure, resulting in an increase in body energy stores.

Positive nitrogen balance: Nitrogen intake exceeds the sum of all sources of nitrogen excretion.

Processed foods: Foods that are produced by converting raw food materials into the form suitable for eating.

Pre-eclampsia: A toxemic condition of late pregnancy characterized by increased blood pressure, swelling of feet and excretion of protein in the urine.

Protein energy malnutrition (PEM): A marked dietary deficiency of both energy and protein resulting in undernutrition.

Recommended Dietary Allowance: Recommended Dietary Allowance **(RDA) refers to the daily dietary nutrient intake level** that is sufficient **to meet the nutrient requirements of nearly all (97–98%) the healthy individuals, in a particular life stage and gender group.**

This is derived from ANR/EAR as the mean plus 2SD of the distribution of requirements.

Recommended Nutrient Intake (RNI) or Recommended Dietary Allowance (RDA)

Refined foods: Foods which have been processed to improve their appearance, color, taste, odor or keeping quality.

Saturated fatty acids: Fatty acids containing maximum number of hydrogen atoms that each carbon atom can carry. They do not have double bonds.

Satiety: Feeling of satisfaction after food intake.

Semiessential amino acid: Semiessential amino acid is the one that is normally synthesized in the body but becomes essential under certain circumstances such as during critical illness.

Skin-fold measurement: A method to estimate body fatness by measuring, with calipers, the thickness of a fold of skin.

Soluble fibre: Soluble fiber refers dietary fiber components that dissolve in or absorb water, including pectins, gums, mucilages and some hemicelluloses.

Staple food: A staple food is the one that forms the basis of a diet in terms of both quantity and frequency of consumption and provides the highest proportion of energy. Staple foods vary with geographic region but in general, most important staple foods include cereals and millets.

Steatorrhea: Steatorrhea means production of stool with an abnormally high amount of fat.

Stomatitis: Stomatitis means inflammation of the mouth, a symptom of riboflavin deficiency.

Stroke: Popular term for cerebrovascular disease, a sudden condition that arises from blocking or bleeding of blood vessels in the brain, resulting in paralysis.

Syndrome X: A cluster of risk factors for heart disease associated with insulin resistance. These risk factors include hypertriglyceridemia, low HDL-cholesterol, hyperinsulinemia, often hyperglycemia and hypertension.

Thermic effect of food: The energy used to digest, absorb and metabolize energy-yielding foodstuffs. It constitutes about 10% of total energy expenditure but is influenced by various factors. It is also called dietary-induced thermogenesis or meal-induced thermogenesis.

Thrombosis: The condition in which the blood changes from a liquid to a semi-solid state and produces a blood clot (thrombus) which blocks blood flow.

Total energy expenditure: Total energy expenditure includes resting energy expenditure, energy used in physical activity, energy used in processing food and adaptive thermogenesis. It is expressed in kilocalories per day.

Total parental nutrition: Total parental nutrition means feeding a person by giving all essential nutrients, intravenously.

Trans-fatty acids: These are mainly produced during hydrogenation of oils; a few also occur naturally in very small quantities.

Transferrin: A protein synthesized in the liver that transports iron in the blood to the erythroblasts for use in heme synthesis. It is a globulin that binds and transports iron from the gut wall to tissue cells.

Transferrin saturation: The extent to which transferrin has vacant iron-binding sites.

Transitional milk: Milk that is whiter and thinner than colostrums and is produced in the beginning, may be about 5 to 7 days after delivery. This transitional milk signals the gradual development of mature milk.

Triglycerides (neutral fat): The major type of dietary fat and the principal form in which energy is stored in the body. A complex of fatty acids and glycerol.

Unsaturated fatty acids: Fatty acids in which there is a shortage of hydrogen atoms. The carbon atoms then become linked by double bonds. Unsaturated fatty acids are less stable than saturated fatty acids.

Upper Nutrient level (UNL) or Tolerable Upper Level (TUL) refers to the highest average daily nutrient intake level that is likely to pose no risk of adverse health effects to almost all individuals in the general population.

Visible fats: Fats and oils that can be used directly or in cooking.

Waist circumference: It is the waist measurement, as a marker of abdominal fat content. It can be used to indicate health risks.

Weaning foods: Foods which are used during gradual transition of the infant from breastfeeding to a normal diet.

Wilson disease: It is a genetic disorder of increased copper absorption, which leads to its toxic levels in the liver and heart.

Xerophthalmia: A condition caused by vitamin A deficiency that dries the cornea and mucous membrane of the eye.

Index